MEDICAL CONSEQUENCES OF RADIOLOGICAL AND NUCLEAR WEAPONS

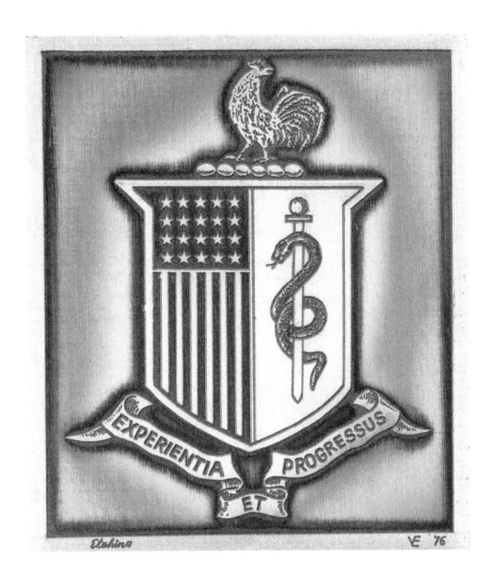

The Coat of Arms
1818
Medical Department of the Army

A 1976 etching by Vassil Ekimov of an
original color print that appeared in
The Military Surgeon, Vol XLI, No 2, 1917

Textbooks of Military Medicine

Published by the

Office of The Surgeon General
Department of the Army, United States of America

and

US Army Medical Department Center and School
Fort Sam Houston, Texas

Editor in Chief
Martha K. Lenhart, MD, PhD
Colonel, MC, US Army
Director, Borden Institute
Assistant Professor of Surgery
F. Edward Hébert School of Medicine
Uniformed Services University of the Health Sciences

The *TMM* Series

Published Textbooks

Medical Consequences of Nuclear Warfare (1989)

Conventional Warfare: Ballistic, Blast, and Burn Injuries (1991)

Occupational Health: The Soldier and the Industrial Base (1993)

Military Dermatology (1994)

Military Psychiatry: Preparing in Peace for War (1994)

Anesthesia and Perioperative Care of the Combat Casualty (1995)

War Psychiatry (1995)

Medical Aspects of Chemical and Biological Warfare (1997)

Rehabilitation of the Injured Soldier, Volume 1 (1998)

Rehabilitation of the Injured Soldier, Volume 2 (1999)

Medical Aspects of Harsh Environments, Volume 1 (2002)

Medical Aspects of Harsh Environments, Volume 2 (2002)

Ophthalmic Care of the Combat Casualty (2003)

Military Medical Ethics, Volume 1 (2003)

Military Medical Ethics, Volume 2 (2003)

Military Preventive Medicine, Volume 1 (2003)

Military Preventive Medicine, Volume 2 (2005)

Recruit Medicine (2006)

Medical Aspects of Biological Warfare (2007)

Medical Aspects of Chemical Warfare (2008)

Care of the Combat Amputee (2009)

Combat and Operational Behavioral Health (2011)

Military Quantitative Physiology: Problems and Concepts in Military Operational Medicine (2012)

Medical Consequences of Radiological and Nuclear Weapons (2012)

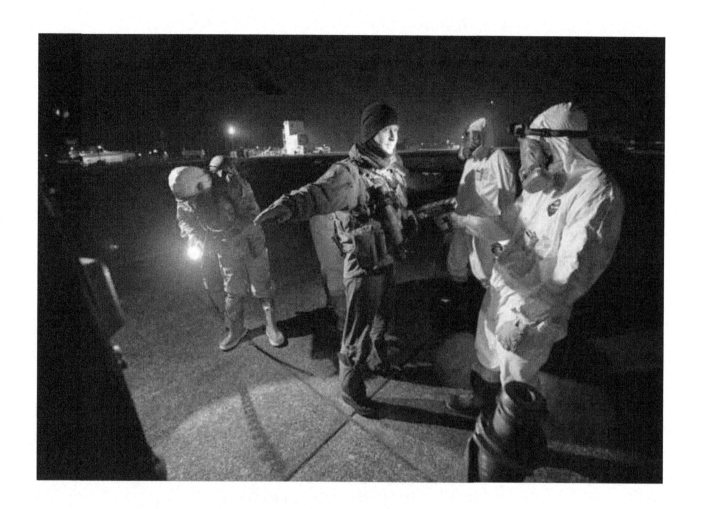

A US Air Force air rescue squadron crew member is checked for radiation by bioenvironmental engineers at Yokota Air Base, Japan, after a flight to northern Japan during relief efforts in response to the Great East Japan Earthquake in March 2011.

Photograph: Courtesy of the US Air Force. Photographer: TSgt Samuel Morse, NCOIC, Photography, 374th Airlift Wing Public Affairs

MEDICAL CONSEQUENCES OF RADIOLOGICAL AND NUCLEAR WEAPONS

Senior Editor

ANTHONY B. MICKELSON, MD
Colonel, Medical Corps, US Army
Director of Military Medical Operations, Armed Forces Radiobiology Research Institute
Uniformed Services University of the Health Sciences

Office of The Surgeon General
United States Army
Falls Church, Virginia

Borden Institute
Fort Detrick, Maryland

2012

Editorial Staff: Ronda Lindsay
                       Volume Editor

                       Douglas Wise
                       Senior Layout Editor

Joan Redding
Senior Production Editor

Bruce G. Maston
Illustrator

This volume was prepared for military medical educational use. The focus of the information is to foster discussion that may form the basis of doctrine and policy. The opinions or assertions contained herein are the private views of the authors and are not to be construed as official or as reflecting the views of the Department of the Army or the Department of Defense.

Dosage Selection:

The authors and publisher have made every effort to ensure the accuracy of dosages cited herein. However, it is the responsibility of every practitioner to consult appropriate information sources to ascertain correct dosages for each clinical situation, especially for new or unfamiliar drugs and procedures. The authors, editors, publisher, and the Department of Defense cannot be held responsible for any errors found in this book.

Use of Trade or Brand Names:

Use of trade or brand names in this publication is for illustrative purposes only and does not imply endorsement by the Department of Defense.

Neutral Language:

Unless this publication states otherwise, masculine nouns and pronouns do not refer exclusively to men.

Published by the Office of The Surgeon General
Borden Institute
Fort Detrick, MD 21702-5000

Library of Congress Cataloging-in-Publication Data

Medical consequences of radiological and nuclear weapons / senior editor, Anthony B. Mickelson, MD.
     p. ; cm. -- (TMM series)
  Includes bibliographical references and index.
  I. Mickelson, Anthony B., editor. II. Borden Institute (U.S.), issuing body. III. Series: Textbooks of military medicine.
  [DNLM: 1. Nuclear Weapons. 2. Radioactive Fallout--adverse effects. 3.Disaster Planning--methods. 4. Environmental Exposure--adverse effects. 5. Nuclear Warfare. 6. Radiation Injuries--therapy. WN 610]

  363.73'5--dc23

                              2012047982

PRINTED IN THE UNITED STATES OF AMERICA

19, 18, 17, 16, 15, 14, 13, 12   5 4 3 2 1

Contents

Contributors

LEONARD A. ALT, MS
Major, US Army; Program Manager, Radiation Sources Department, Armed Forces Radiobiology Research Institute, Bethesda, Maryland 20814

STEVEN M. BECKER, PhD
Professor of Community and Environmental Health, College of Health Sciences, Old Dominion University, Norfolk, Virginia 23529

WILLIAM F. BLAKELY, PhD
Senior Scientist and Biodosimetry Research Program Advisor, Biological Dosimetry Research Group, Scientific Research Department, Armed Forces Radiobiology Research Institute, Uniformed Services University of the Health Sciences, Bethesda, Maryland 20889; Adjunct Assistant Professor, Preventive Medicine and Biometrics Department, Uniformed Services University of the Health Sciences, Bethesda, Maryland

VICTOR BOGO, MA
Armed Forces Radiobiology Research Institute, Bethesda, Maryland 20814

C. NORMAN COLEMAN, MD, FACP, FACR, FASTRO
Senior Medical Advisor and Team Leader, Office of the Assistant Secretary for Preparedness and Response, US Department of Health and Human Services, 200 Independence Avenue, Room 638G, Washington, DC 20201; and Associate Director, Radiation Research Program, Division of Cancer Therapeutics and Diagnosis, National Cancer Institute, National Institutes of Health, Executive Plaza North, Room 6014, 6130 Executive Boulevard, MSC 7440, Bethesda, Maryland 20892; formerly, Professor and Chairman, Harvard Joint Center for Radiation Therapy, Boston, Massachusetts

THOMAS B. ELLIOTT, PhD
Research Microbiologist, Scientific Research Department, Radiation and Combined Injury Infection Group, Uniformed Services University of the Health Sciences, 8901 Wisconsin Avenue, Building 42, National Naval Medical Center, Bethesda, Maryland 20889

DANIEL F. FLYNN, MS, MD
Colonel, US Army Medical Corps (Retired); Visiting Faculty, Radiation Emergency Assistance Center/Training Site, Oak Ridge, Tennessee 37831; New England Radiation Therapy Associates, Radiation Oncology Department, Holy Family Hospital, Methuen, Massachusetts 01884

C. DOUGLAS FORCINO, PhD
Lieutenant, United States Navy; Department of Military Medicine, Uniformed Services University of the Health Sciences, Bethesda, Maryland 20814

RONALD E. GOANS, PhD, MD
Senior Medical Advisor, MJW Corp, Amherst, New York, 14228; Senior Research Advisor/Physician, Radiation Emergency Assistance Center/Training Site, Oak Ridge, Tennessee 37831; Associate Professor, Tulane School of Public Health and Tropical Medicine, New Orleans, Louisiana 70112

MARTIN HAUER-JENSEN, MD, PhD, FACS
Professor of Pharmaceutical Sciences, Surgery, and Pathology; Associate Dean for Research, College of Pharmacy; Director, Division of Radiation Health, University of Arkansas for Medical Sciences, 4301 West Markham, Slot 522-10, Little Rock, Arkansas 72205

JOHN F. KALINICH, PhD
Program Advisor, Internal Contamination and Metal Toxicity Program, Armed Forces Radiobiology Research Institute, Uniformed Services University of the Health Sciences, 8901 Wisconsin Avenue, Building 42, Bethesda, Maryland 20889

JULIANN G. KIANG, PhD
Program Advisor, Combined Injury Program, Scientific Research Department, Armed Forces Radiobiology Research Institute, Professor of Radiation Biology and Medicine, Uniformed Services University of the Health Sciences, 8901 Wisconsin Avenue, Bethesda, Maryland 20889

SHILPA KULKARNI, PhD
Staff Investigator, Scientific Research Department, Armed Forces Radiobiology Research Institute, 8901 Wisconsin Avenue, Building 42, Room 3122, Bethesda, Maryland 20889

K. SREE KUMAR, PhD
Senior Research Scientist, Radiation Countermeasures Program, Scientific Research Department, Armed Forces Radiobiology Research Institute, Uniformed Services University of the Health Sciences, 8901 Wisconsin Avenue, Bethesda, Maryland 20889

G. DAVID LEDNEY, PhD
Research Biologist, Scientific Research Department, Radiation and Combined Injury Infection Group, Uniformed Services University of the Health Sciences, 8901 Wisconsin Avenue, Building 42, National Naval Medical Center, Bethesda, Maryland 20889

JOHN P. MADRID, MS
Captain, United States Army; Health Physicist, Military Medical Operations, Armed Forces Radiobiology Research Institute, 8901 Wisconsin Avenue, Building 42, Bethesda, Maryland 20889

G. ANDREW MICKLEY, PhD
Lieutenant Colonel, United States Air Force; Armed Forces Radiobiology Research Institute, Bethesda, Maryland 20814

ALEXANDRA C. MILLER, PhD
Senior Scientist, Scientific Research Department, Armed Forces Radiobiology Research Institute, 8901 Wisconsin Avenue, Building 42, Room 3122, Bethesda, Maryland 20889

ANDRE OBENAUS, PhD
Departments of Pediatrics, Radiation Medicine, Radiology, and Biophysics and Bioengineering, Loma Linda University, 11175 Campus Street, CSP A-1120, Loma Linda, California 92354

PATAJE G.S. PRASANNA, PhD
Program Director, Radiation Research Program, National Cancer Institute, National Institutes of Health, Executive Plaza North, 6015A, Room 6020, 6130 Executive Boulevard, MSC 7440, Bethesda, Maryland 20889; formerly, Principal Investigator, Armed Forces Radiobiology Research Institute, Bethesda, Maryland

JACOB RABER, PhD
Departments of Behavioral Neuroscience and Neurology, Division of Neuroscience, Oregon National Primate Research Center, Oregon Health & Science University, Department of Behavioral Neuroscience, Oregon Health & Science University, 3181 Southwest Sam Jackson Park Road, L470, Portland, Oregon 97239

MERRILINE SATYAMITRA, PhD
Staff Scientist, Scientific Research Department, Armed Forces Radiobiology Research Institute, 8901 Wisconsin Avenue, Building 42, Room 3122, Bethesda, Maryland 20889

THOMAS WALDEN, PhD, MD
Radiation Oncologist, Gibson Cancer Center, 1200 Pine Run Drive, Lumberton, North Carolina 28358

RICHARD I. WALKER, PhD
Captain, United States Navy; Director, Enteric Diseases Program, Naval Medical Research Institute, Bethesda, MD 20814 and Armed Forces Radiobiology Research Institute, Bethesda, Maryland 20814

BRUCE R. WEST, MS
Major, United States Army; Human Response Officer, Radiation Policy Division, Defense Nuclear Agency, 6801 Telegraph Road, Alexandria, Virginia 22310

MARK H. WHITNALL, PhD
Program Advisor, Radiation Countermeasures Program, Scientific Research Department, Armed Forces Radiobiology Research Institute, Uniformed Services University of the Health Sciences, 8901 Wisconsin Avenue, Bethesda, Maryland 20889

CHARLES R. WOODRUFF JR, BS
Head, Medical Radiobiology Advisory Team, Military Medical Operations Directorate, Armed Forces Radiobiology Research Institute, 8901 Wisconsin Avenue, Building 42, Bethesda, Maryland 20889

Foreword

The events of September 11, 2001, catalyzed a long-recognized terror threat around the world and heightened global concern regarding the management and creation of weapons of mass destruction in the post-Cold War era. The US Army Medical Department, in conjunction with other US military commands and military health services, government agencies, and our allies, has undertaken ambitious programs to meet the unique nuclear and radiation challenges and threats that have grown increasingly complex in today's world. Other long-standing nuclear realities include industrial radiation leaks and associated potential catastrophic events caused by human error and natural disasters, such as the earthquake and tsunami that resulted in the disaster at the Japanese Fukushima Daiichi Nuclear Power Plant. Continual global conversation and collaboration among principal entities is needed to improve medical doctrine and policies that not only address combat operations, but how military medicine influences and works with other agencies—international, federal, state, and local—in large-scale, multi-agency responses.

Military medicine sustains the health of the force regardless of the environment. Weapons of mass destruction and natural disasters pose potential threats to our military forces and their families. Military medicine must be prepared to sustain the force in any environment and ensure they meet the challenges presented by the chemical, biological, radiological, nuclear, and explosive (CBRNE) threat. Military medical providers must also have contingencies that address the environment post-incident and through humanitarian relief efforts. When working internationally with NATO and other military forces in combat operations or in support of humanitarian relief efforts, Army Medicine has the opportunity to strengthen medical response around the world. Frequent technological advances make it imperative to constantly seek improvements in medical procedures, research, equipment, and logistics to sustain the force. The CBRNE threat adds a complex layer to planning for and executing the military medical response if an event was to occur.

Meeting the medical imperatives in the nuclear and radiological CBRNE threat requires a large, comprehensive healthcare system effort. In cooperation with other US and foreign government agencies, civilian academic institutions, and private industry, we know our capabilities progressively improve and create better outcomes for populations affected by natural or manmade disasters. Ongoing research in the realms of protectants, medications, colony-stimulating factors, and decorporation agents that will increase the survival of radiological casualties while decreasing late-term health effects is improved by biodosimetry, in conjunction with radioinformatics, and offers the medical provider a more precise and rapid way to triage radiological casualties during a mass casualty radiological incident. Preventive measures, including the use of robotics, improved personal protective equipment, and detection equipment can minimize the radiation exposure of first responders and medical personnel as well. The Army is currently developing better methods for recording the dose assessment in a permanent database for individuals exposed to radiation, and making the database accessible to the Veterans Administration for long-term monitoring and treatment of our veterans. These are just a few of the efforts military medicine is involved in that will sustain the health of our military forces and their fighting strength well into the future.

I hope you find this *Textbook of Military Medicine* to be an invaluable guide that stimulates your interest in this subject and sharpens your focus on how to best sustain the health of the force as it relates to CBRNE threats. It is our collective responsibility to be prepared and plan for these medical challenges because the threats, both human and natural, are real. It is my hope that this textbook will serve as a definitive reference to influence your current operations and training programs regarding the response to contingent nuclear and radiological medical threats. As past is often prologue, then preparedness is essential.

Patricia D. Horoho
Lieutenant General, US Army
The Surgeon General and
Commanding General, US Army Medical Command

Washington, DC
October 2012

Preface

The initial Medical Consequences of Nuclear Warfare component of the *Textbooks of Military Medicine* series was published in 1989. In the years since that publication, many changes have occurred in areas of research, technology, doctrine, and medical practice. An update for the radiological portion of the textbook in particular was long overdue to address the challenges of a post–September 11, 2001, world.

The radiological and nuclear threat has expanded from Cold War nuclear warfare to radiological terrorism and domestic accidents. Radiological incidents, such as Chernobyl, Goiânia, and the Fukushima Daiichi Nuclear Power Plant disaster demonstrate the importance of continued vigilance and preparedness, as these types of disasters affect the physical and mental health of surrounding populations and result in negative effects on the environment and economy.

To minimize the consequences of radiation exposure, it is important to harness technological and scientific advances of medical radiobiology. Since establishment in 1961, the Armed Forces Radiobiology Research Institute (AFRRI) has been the leader in Department of Defense medical radiobiology research, working alongside other US government agencies, the private sector, and our allies. AFRRI continues work aimed at maximizing use of available technologies that have potential to expand medical radiobiology capabilities. Other initiatives include the development of protectants to minimize the harmful effects of ionizing radiation, the creation of biologically friendly metal alloy alternatives for depleted uranium, and quantifying the radiation required to eradicate various microorganisms.

Along with its research mission, educating the force is an equally important facet of AFRRI. As a subordinate organization to the Uniformed Services University for the Health Sciences, AFRRI continues to educate military and civilian medical providers, including first responders, through activities such as the Medical Effects of Ionizing Radiation course, the Military Radiobiology Advisory Team, and numerous publications to assist in improving our nation's emergency response.

It is by the contributions of many that this book is now a reality. Among individuals who merit specific recognition are Colonel Patricia Lillis-Hearne, MC, US Army (Ret); Colonel Donald Hall, MSC, US Army (Ret); and Captain Christopher Lissner, MSC, US Navy (Ret). They initiated this project and provided expert guidance in developing its content and format. Colonel Lester "Andy" Huff, MC, US Air Force, and Colonel Mark Melanson, MSC, US Army, unflaggingly oversaw this publication project to its completion. And special recognition and sincere appreciation is due to each author who willingly contributed his or her expertise to this valuable resource. Their input will immensely benefit both military and civilian communities by enhancing knowledge of the consequences and management of radiation injuries.

Colonel Anthony B. Mickelson, MC, US Army
Director, Military Medical Operations,
Armed Forces Radiobiology Research Institute

Bethesda, Maryland
August 2012

Chapter 1

RADIOLOGICAL EVENTS AND THEIR CONSEQUENCES

CHARLES R. WOODRUFF JR, BS*; LEONARD A. ALT, MS†; C. DOUGLAS FORCINO, PhD‡; AND RICHARD I. WALKER, PhD§

*Head, Medical Radiobiology Advisory Team, Military Medical Operations Directorate, Armed Forces Radiobiology Research Institute, 8901 Wisconsin Avenue, Building 42, Bethesda, Maryland 20889
†Major, United States Army; Program Manager, Radiation Sources Department, Armed Forces Radiobiology Research Institute, Bethesda, Maryland 20814
‡Lieutenant, United States Navy; Department of Military Medicine, Uniformed Services University of the Health Sciences, Bethesda, Maryland 20814
§Captain, United States Navy; Director, Enteric Diseases Program, Naval Medical Research Institute, Bethesda, Maryland 20814 and Armed Forces Radiobiology Research Institute, Bethesda, Maryland 20814

INTRODUCTION

Understanding the basic concepts of radiation physics, radiobiology, and the mechanisms by which radiation causes damage to the body is important to allow a coherent approach to radiation injury treatment. Wilhelm Conrad Roentgen reported the discovery of X-rays in 1895. Radiation damage to human cells was first recognized just 4 months later in 1896, when Dr John Daniel at Vanderbilt University found the irradiation of his colleague's skull resulted in hair loss, and English physician LG Stevens reported in the *British Medical Journal* that "those who work with X-rays suffer from changes to the skin which are similar in effect from the sun burn." Since then, many other biomedical effects of radiation have been described. Much of our basic understanding of mechanisms of injury has come from animal research and epidemiological studies of populations exposed during accidents and occupationally, and from the survivors of the atomic bombings of Hiroshima and Nagasaki, Japan. More recently, it has been possible to experiment on human cells maintained in tissue cultures.

The understanding of atomic physics increased rapidly in the early 20th century and culminated in the Manhattan Project, which harnessed the power of the atom in a bomb. Thus began the nuclear era in international relations and warfare, bringing new challenges to the military physician. When this volume was first published in 1989, the Cold War was in its final stages. Vast stockpiles of weapons were maintained and mutually targeted by the United States and the Soviet Union. Since the fall of the Soviet Union in December 1991, we have been forced to rethink what constitutes the most likely radiation threat to our country and our forces. Where the previous version of this chapter dealt strictly with nuclear warfare, a section has now been included that discusses radiological weapons; that is, the use of radioactive material to cause harm in a form other than a nuclear weapon.

In the 21st century, although more countries are developing or seeking to develop nuclear weapons (with a few notable exceptions), none is in a position to target them at the United States or our allies. We have, therefore shifted our focus away from all-out nuclear apocalypse and toward the possibility of one or more small tactical detonations carried out by terrorists or agents of a rogue nation, and to a threat not thought of in 1989: the radiation dispersion device (RDD), or "dirty bomb." The most likely situations requiring a military medical response are a terrorist act, an accident or incident involving a nuclear weapon, the use of a weapon against a deployed military force, or a developing-world conflict with collateral US casualties.

However, military medical preparedness must focus beyond nuclear weapon events. Today, nuclear material is used in medicine, industry, and power generation, bringing increased risk of occupational and accidental exposures. Radiation hazards during military operations in countries with limited oversight of radiological sources, or with sources abandoned by former occupiers, is now a cause of concern. Military physicians trained to respond to weapons-related injuries can bring expertise to these situations.

NUCLEAR AND PHYSICAL PROCESSES IN WEAPONS

Weapons-related injuries can be best understood after examining the destructive forces—blast, thermal, and radiation—that produce them. Generally, an explosion results from the very rapid release of a large amount of energy within a limited space. In comparison with a conventional explosive weapon, a nuclear weapon's effectiveness is due to its unequalled capacity to liberate many thousands (up to millions) of times more energy from a much smaller mass of material. This section presents a simple description of the physical processes taking place within the first few thousandths of a second after a nuclear weapon detonation.

Nuclear Energy

Energy may be broadly classified as potential or kinetic. Potential energy is energy of configuration, position, or the capacity to perform work. For example, the relatively unstable chemical bonds among the atoms that comprise trinitrotoluene (TNT) possess chemical potential energy. Potential energy can, under suitable conditions, be transformed into kinetic energy, which is energy of motion. When a conventional explosive such as TNT is detonated, the relatively unstable chemical bonds are converted into bonds that are more stable, producing kinetic energy in the form of blast and thermal energies. This process of transforming a chemical system's bonds from lesser to greater stability is exothermic (there is a net production of energy). Likewise, a nuclear detonation derives its energy from transformations of the powerful nuclear bonds that hold the neutrons and protons together within the nucleus. The conversion of relatively less stable nuclear bonds into bonds with greater stability leads not only to the liberation of vast quantities of kinetic energy in blast and thermal forms, but also to the generation of ionizing radiation.

To discover where these energies come from, consider the nucleus of the helium atom, which is composed of two neutrons and two protons bound tightly together by the strong (or specifically nuclear) force, also referred to as "nuclear binding energy." If we compare the bound neutrons and protons to those in the unbound state, we find that the total mass of the separate neutrons and protons is greater than their mass when they bind together to form the helium nucleus. The mass that has been lost in the process of forming the nuclear bonds is called the mass defect. Einstein's famous equation, $E = mc^2$ (energy equals mass multiplied by the speed of light squared), quantifies the conversion of this missing mass into the binding energy that holds together the helium nucleus. This is the potential energy stored in the bonds of the strong force. A small amount of mass, when multiplied by the speed of light squared (an extremely large number), has a large amount of binding energy. If the total binding energy for each element is calculated and divided by its total number of nucleons (that is, neutrons plus protons; for helium, two neutrons plus two protons equals four nucleons), a measure is obtained of how tightly the average nucleon is bound for that particular atom. Elements from hydrogen to sodium generally exhibit increasing binding energy per nucleon as atomic mass increases. This increase is generated by increasing forces per nucleon in the nucleus, as each additional nucleon is attracted by all of the other nucleons, and thus more tightly bound to the whole. The next region is the saturation region, which is quite stable and includes elements through xenon. In this region the nucleus is large enough that the nuclear forces do not extend all the way across its width. Above xenon, the binding energy per nucleon begins to decrease as the atomic number increases. At this point, electromagnetic repulsive forces start to gain and dominate against the strong nuclear force. A plot of this "average binding energy per nucleon" for each element gives the curve in Figure 1-1.

It is significant that this curve has a broad maximum. At the peak of the binding energy curve is iron-56, with the highest total binding energy (although the three highest binding energies per nucleon, in order

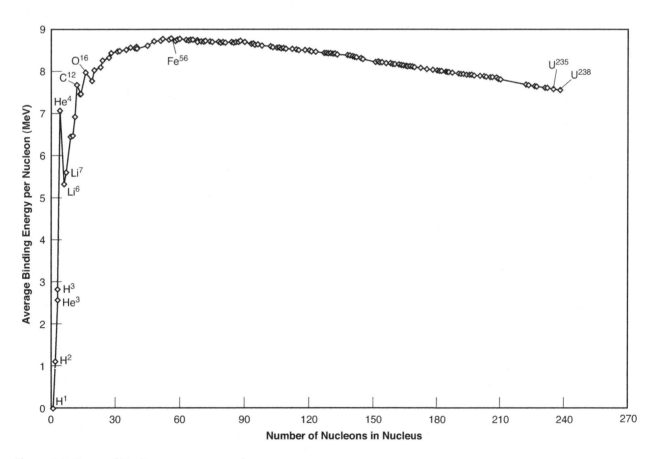

Figure 1-1. Curve of binding energy per nucleon.

highest to lowest, is as follows: nickel-62, iron-58, iron-56). These three isotopes are produced in large amounts as end products in the burn-up of stars. This is generally why iron and nickel are found in large quantities in planetary cores. Since there is a range of elements for which the neutrons and protons are most tightly bound and, thus, have the most stable nuclear bonds, nuclei having less stable nuclear bonds can be converted into ones with more stable bonds, allowing the system to pass from a state of lesser to greater stability and releasing energy. This serves as the energy source of nuclear weapons. The process can occur in two ways: via fission or fusion. Fission is the process of breaking less stable larger elements (such as uranium and plutonium) into two of the more stable midrange elements. Fusion is the process of combining lighter nuclei (such as those of deuterium and tritium, which are isotopes of hydrogen) into heavier elements lying further up the curve of binding energy per nucleon.

Energy Release in Nuclear Weapons

A fission nuclear device is practical for only three elements: uranium-233, uranium-235, and plutonium-239. In order to construct an efficient weapon, instability is induced in one of these nuclei by striking it with a neutron. The unstable nuclear bonds are broken, the nucleus splits apart, and relatively more stable nuclear bonds are reformed by each of the two midrange fission fragments. This is accompanied by the release of a large quantity of energy and the prompt emission of gamma rays and neutrons (initial nuclear radiation). It is important to note that approximately 82% of the fission energy is released as kinetic energy of the two large fission fragments. These fragments, which are massive, highly charged particles, interact readily with matter. They transfer their energy quickly to the surrounding weapon materials, which rapidly become heated. The fission fragments consist of over 300 different isotopes of 38 separate chemical elements. Most of the fragments are highly unstable radioactively and will later contribute to the radiologically and chemically complex fallout field.

One fission event alone does not make a weapon; a weapon requires a self- perpetuating, exponentially escalating chain reaction of fissions. This is achieved by the suitable physical arrangement of certain nuclear materials. Also, since the weapon must not reach the proper, or "critical," configuration until the desired time of detonation, some way must be found to make the transition on demand from a safe, or subcritical, condition to the critical state. In a functioning fission device, this is done by altering the mass, shape, or density of the nuclear materials.

The two basic classes of fission weapons are the gun-assembled device and the implosion device. The gun-assembled weapon is a mechanically simple design that uses a "gun tube" arrangement to blow together two small masses of uranium-235 to form a supercritical mass. The 15-kt yield weapon used at Hiroshima was a gun-assembled device (1 kt equals the energy released by detonation of 1,000 short tons of TNT, and 1 megaton equals 1,000,000 short tons of TNT). The implosion weapon uses an extremely complex system of precisely formed, conventional, chemical-explosive lenses to crush a mass of plutonium-239 to supercritical density. The first tested nuclear weapon (the Trinity device) and the 21-kt-yield weapon used at Nagasaki were implosion devices. From the viewpoint of a weapon's accessibility, it is fortunate that the much more easily constructed gun-assembled weapon cannot effectively use the more readily producible plutonium-239, which can be obtained by using naturally occurring uranium in a breeder reactor. Instead, it must be fueled with uranium-235, which is more difficult to obtain.

The limit on a fission weapon's yield, from an engineering viewpoint, is several hundred kilotons. Therefore, the multimegaton weapons in nuclear inventories are fusion weapons (often referred to as "hydrogen" or "thermonuclear") that derive much of their power from the combination of light isotopes of hydrogen (deuterium and tritium) and heavier nuclei lying farther up the curve of binding energy per nucleon. Because of the powerful forces of electrostatic repulsion, initiating fusion of deuterium and tritium requires extremely high temperatures, about 50,000,000°C. The only practical way to achieve those temperatures in a weapon on earth is to detonate a fission device inside the fusion materials. The deuterium and tritium then fuse and release energy, partly in the form of highly energetic and penetrating fusion neutrons, which have energies about ten times the typical energies of fission-generated neutrons. The fusion weapon then uses these high-energy fusion neutrons to cause secondary fissions. Thus, a fusion weapon actually generates power from both the fission and fusion processes, usually in roughly equal proportions. Only five or six countries have conducted thermonuclear tests (India claims to have tested a thermonuclear device, but many experts are skeptical).[1]

There is one other type of nuclear weapon that bears mention. While technically a small modified thermonuclear device, an enhanced radiation weapon (ERW; neutron bomb) produces a very different damage profile. The goal of this type of weapon is to reduce blast damage and fallout while increasing the radius of the lethal radiation dose. The neutron production of an ERW is around one order of magnitude greater than that of a standard fission weapon of the same yield. The neutrons born from fusion are around 14 mega electron volts (MEV), whereas fission neutrons are only about 2 MEV. The higher yield and energy of neutrons from the weapon increases the radius for a given radiation dose by about 50% and also increases the radiation from activation products. However, since the half-life of the activation products is generally shorter than those of fission fragments, the duration of radiations from induced radiation and fallout materials is lower. Since the radiation dose is distributed over a greater range than a similar or slightly larger-yield fission warhead with less blast and thermal damage, these weapons are considered "surgical strike" weapons. A 1-kt ERW will produce approximately two times the casualties, with one fifth the area of blast damage, compared to a 10-kt fission weapon. Published reports state that five countries, including the United States, have produced these weapons.[2]

Production of Blast and Thermal Effects

The blast and thermal effects of detonation produce by far the greatest number of immediate human casualties in nuclear warfare. One of the important differences between a nuclear and a conventional explosion is the large proportion of thermal energy released by a nuclear weapon. The temperatures reached in a nuclear explosion reach tens of millions of degrees, as opposed to a few thousands in a conventional explo-sive. The nuclear reactions within the weapon have died out after the first one-millionth of a second, and the fission and fusion events have produced a vast quantity of energy that has been rapidly and locally transferred to the bomb materials in the form of heat. The weapon's materials (bomb casing, electronics, chemical explosive residues, and a large percentage of the original nuclear fuels), which, even in a relatively efficient (about 40% maximum efficiency) device re-main unreacted, now exist as a highly energetic plasma of positive ions and free electrons at high temperature and high pressure. Through a process of electron-ion interaction known as "bremsstrahlung," the plasma becomes an intense source of X-rays. These X-rays leave the vicinity of the bomb materials at the speed of light, heat the first several meters of air surround-ing the weapon, and generate a fireball with an initial temperature up to several tens of millions of degrees. The intensely hot fireball reradiates thermal energy of a longer wavelength at infrared, visible, and ultraviolet frequencies. The first pulse delivers approximately 1% of the thermal radiation due to its very short duration (about a tenth of a second). Most of this energy is in the ultraviolet region and is readily attenuated in air. The second pulse may last for several seconds and is of a lower temperature than the first pulse. This means that most of the rays reaching the earth are in the vis-ible and infrared regions. This radiation is the main cause of skin burns and eye injuries suffered by those exposed to a nuclear detonation.

At about the same time, the weapon's materials have started to expand supersonically outward, dra-matically compressing and heating the surrounding air. This high-pressure wave moves outward from the fireball and is the cause of much destruction in the form of the blast wave and further thermal radiations. The high-temperature blast wave travels out from the point

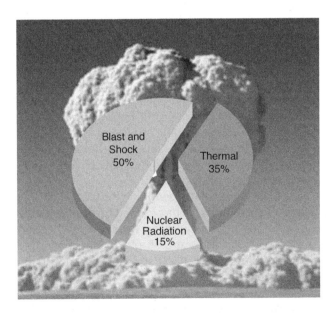

Figure 1-2. Energy distribution of a nuclear weapon.

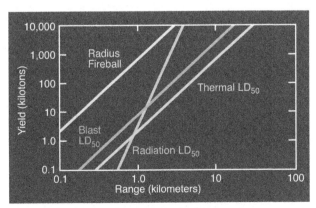

Figure 1-3. Range of nuclear weapon effects.

of detonation, gradually decreasing in velocity and overpressure based on the yield of the weapon. Added to these blast and thermal effects is the initial nuclear radiation (primarily neutrons and gamma rays) that is produced promptly by the fission and fusion processes, and the residual radiation (primarily gamma rays and high-energy electrons), which are produced later by decay of the radioactive fission fragments composing the fallout field (Figure 1-2).

The range of the blast, thermal, and radiation effects produced by the detonation of a nuclear weapon depends on many factors, perhaps the most significant of which, for the battlefield soldier, is total weapon yield (Figure 1-3). Initial radiation is the dominant threat for only very small tactical devices, and thermal effects are dominant for large-yield strategic weapons.

BLAST, THERMAL, AND RADIATION EFFECTS

The destructive blast, thermal, and radiation effects of a fission or fusion weapon all stem from the device's capacity to transform the very strong nuclear bonds of uranium, plutonium, deuterium, and tritium from a relatively unstable state to a more stable one. The quantitative difference between the effects of a nuclear weapon and the effects of a conventional explosive is the result of the dramatically greater strength of the nuclear bonds compared to the chemical bonds of a conventional explosive. A qualitative difference arises from the production of initial nuclear radiations from the fission and fusion processes themselves and from delayed radioactivity resulting from decay of the unstable fission fragment by-products.

Blast Effects

During the detonation of a standard fission or fusion nuclear device, the sudden liberation of a tremendous amount of potential energy causes a huge increase in temperature and pressure, converting everything into hot compressed gases and plasma. This rapidly expanding plasma gives rise to a shock or blast wave that is responsible for dissipating about 50% of the total energy of the weapon into the surrounding air, water, or earth. This represents a tremendous amount of energy, even in small, tactical-sized weapons of a few kilotons. Most of the material damage to structures, vehicles, and other objects caused by a surface or low air burst is due to this blast wave. As the blast wave travels outward from the site of the explosion, it is composed of static and dynamic components that are capable of producing medical injuries and structural damage. The static component of the shock or blast wave is a wall of compressed air that causes an overpressure (an excess over atmospheric pressure) that exerts a crushing effect on objects in its path. The dynamic component is the movement of air caused by and proportional to the difference between the static overpressure and the ambient pressure. In this discussion, the static and dynamic components will be called the blast wave and blast wind, respectively.

In discussing the structural damage to buildings after a nuclear detonation, it is difficult to separate the effects of the static component from those of the dynamic component. For example, the 5-psi blast wave and 160-mph blast winds associated with the blast wave's passage would destroy a two-story brick house. However, the medical problems resulting from exposure to the shock wave can be divided into those that result from the static component and those that result from the dynamic component. Injuries resulting from the blast waves will be caused by exposure to high pressures with very short rise times, and will consist primarily of internal injuries. For example, the threshold level for rupture of the eardrum is about 5 psi. Although this injury is very painful, it would not limit the accomplishment of a critical military mission. The 160-mph winds that accompany the passage of a 5-psi blast wave would be sufficiently strong to cause displacement and possible injuries. At the other end of the spectrum, a pressure level of 15 psi will produce serious intrathoracic injuries, including alveolar and pulmonary vascular rupture, interstitial hemorrhage, edema, and air emboli. If the air emboli make their way into the arterial circulation, cerebral and myocardial infarctions may ensue. The initial outward signs of such pulmonary damage are frothy bleeding through the nostrils, dyspnea, and coughing. Victims may be in shock and lack visible wounds. In addition, serious abdominal injuries, including hepatic and splenic rupture, may result from a rapid and violent compression of the abdomen. The LD_{50} (lethal dose, or fatal injury, for 50% of cases) for static effects occurs at around 50 psi of overpressure.

The blast winds that accompany the blast wave can also produce injuries. Debris carried by the wind may cause missile injuries ranging from lacerations and contusions to fractures and blunt trauma, depending on the projectile's size, shape, and mass. Wind velocity of 100 mph will displace a person, resulting in lacerations, contusions, and fractures from tumbling across the terrain or from being thrown against stationary structures. Winds capable of causing displacement injuries or missile injuries would be produced by a blast wave with an overpressure of less than 5 psi. At this pressure level, the blast winds are more significant in producing injury than is the static component of the blast wave. At high pressure levels, both the static and dynamic components are capable of producing serious injuries.

The LD_{50} from impact occurs when a body strikes a solid surface at about 37 to 38 mph. For a small tactical weapon or terrorist device with a yield of 1 kt, the range for this level of overpressure would extend to slightly over a tenth of a mile. For larger tactical or strategic weapons with yields of 100 and 1,000 kt, the range for the LD_{50} would expand to just under 1 mile and just under 2 ¼ miles, respectively.

Protection from the effects of the blast wave is difficult to achieve because the wave is an engulfing phenomenon. The best protection can be found in a blast-resistant shelter. However, protection from the effects of the blast winds can be achieved in any location offering shielding from the wind. If adequate shelter is not found, the best defense against blast effects is to lie face down on the ground, covering the head, and with head pointed toward ground zero. This reduces the body's surface area that is exposed to wind-borne debris and offers less resistance to the force of the blast wind.

Thermal Effects

One important difference between conventional high-explosive and nuclear detonations is the large proportion of energy released as thermal (heat) radiation during a nuclear explosion. Following the detonation of a standard fission or fusion device, approximately 35% of the weapon's energy is dissipated as thermal energy. The general types of injuries resulting from this energy are burns, including flash burns and flame burns, and certain eye injuries, including flash blindness and retinal burns.

The thermal output after a nuclear detonation occurs in two distinct pulses as a result of the interaction of the shock wave with the leading edge of the fireball. The first pulse contains only about 1% of the total thermal energy output and is composed primarily of energy in the ultraviolet range. Because the first pulse is of very short duration and the ultraviolet energy is rapidly absorbed by the surrounding atmosphere, it does not contribute significantly to producing casualties. The second pulse, which may last for several seconds depending on the weapon yield and is of lower temperature than the first, is composed primarily of energy in the infrared and visible portions of the electromagnetic spectrum. This pulse contains about 99% of the thermal energy liberated by the nuclear detonation and is responsible for subsequent burns and vision problems.

Burn injury. The two types of burn injury—flash burn and flame burn—are caused by different events and have different prognoses. Flash burn results from the skin's exposure to the second pulse of thermal energy. This absorption of a large quantity of thermal energy in a very brief time often leaves the affected area of the skin with a charred appearance. However, since the heat pulse occurs rapidly and the thermal conductivity of the skin is low, the burn is often superficial, killing only the outer dermal layers and leaving the germinal layer essentially undamaged. Often clothing, especially white or light colors, provides enough shielding to prevent flash burns on covered areas of the body. After the bombings of Hiroshima and Nagasaki, the majority of burns were first and second degree and healed fairly quickly. In contrast, flame burn results from contact with a conventional fire, such as clothing or the remains of a building ignited by the fireball's thermal pulse. In most cases, flame burns heal abnormally because the skin's germinal layer has been damaged. Of the Hiroshima casualties who survived to the 20-day point post-irradiation, fewer than 5% had flame burns; the results for the survivors of the Nagasaki bombing are similar. A much larger percentage of the 20-day survivors in both cities had flash burns.[3]

Fires due to nuclear weapons are caused either directly by the heat of the blast or indirectly due to the blast damage. Blast damage to stoves, water heaters, furnaces, electrical circuits, and gas lines would ignite fires where kindling fuel is plentiful. In Hiroshima, individual fires turned into a firestorm that burned a 4.4-square-mile area of the city and caused further burn casualties.

Because the heat pulse travels at the speed of light, protection from burns is not possible unless warning is given in time to find cover. The electromagnetic energy of the thermal pulse travels in a straight line, so any barrier placed in its path will offer some protection. As shown in Hiroshima and Nagasaki, even clothing will provide some protection from the deposition of thermal energy onto the skin. Because light colors tend to reflect rather than absorb thermal energy, light-colored clothing will offer more protection than dark.

For weapons of very low yield, the range for burn injury LD_{50} is about equal to the range for the LD_{50} from blast and radiation (see Figure 1-3). As the weapon yield increases, the range for burn injury increases much more rapidly than does the range for blast or radiation injury. This means that burns will always result after the detonation of a nuclear device, and, for weapons with a yield above 10 kt, burns will be the predominant injury. Because of the large number of burn casualties and the time and labor-intensive treatment that they require, burn injury is the most difficult problem to be faced by the military medical community in a nuclear conflict. Additionally, mortality of thermal burns markedly increases with exposure to radiation. Burns with a 50% normal mortality may increase to 90% or greater mortality after just 1.5 Gy of radiation exposure.

Eye injury. Thermal energy may also cause eye injury. Flash blindness is a temporary condition that results from a depletion of photopigment from the retinal receptors. This happens when a person indirectly (peripherally) observes the brilliant flash of intense light energy from a fireball. The duration of flash blindness can be as short as several seconds during the day, followed by a darkened afterimage for several minutes. At night, flash blindness can last three times longer, with a loss of dark adaptation for up to 30 minutes. This could seriously compromise military operations.

Another type of eye injury is retinal burn, which results from looking directly at the fireball and focusing its image on the retina. This intense light energy is strong enough to kill the retinal receptors and create a permanent blind spot. A retinal burn is no more or less detrimental to mission accomplishment than flash blindness, and neither of these injuries should create a burden on medical facilities.

To protect against injury, individuals can close and shield their eyes after being warned of a detonation. Using lead-lanthanum-zirconium-titanium goggles may provide further protection.

Effects of Initial and Residual Radiations

A detonating fission or fusion weapon produces a variety of nuclear radiations. Initial radiation occurs at the time of the nuclear reactions and residual radiation occurs long after the immediate blast and thermal effects have ended. The nuclear radiations include neutrons, gamma rays, alpha particles, and beta particles, which are biologically damaging and may significantly affect human health and performance. Alpha and beta particles have relatively short ranges and cannot reach the surface of the earth after an airburst. Even when the fireball touches the ground, they are not of great importance. Therefore, initial radiation is considered to consist of neutrons and gamma rays produced within the first minute after detonation. Both gammas and neutrons can travel long distances in air and are highly injurious to the cells in the human body. It is this combination of range and injury that makes these nuclear radiations a significant aspect of a nuclear weapons detonation.

In addition to the gamma rays produced during the actual fission/fusion process, other sources of gamma rays contribute to initial radiation. The mechanisms for producing these are inelastic scatter reactions with elements in the atmosphere surrounding the weapon and other weapons materials, and isomeric-decay and neutron-capture gamma rays. Inelastic scattering gammas are produced when neutrons with a high kinetic energy ("fast" neutrons) collide with certain other atomic nuclei and transfer a portion of their energy, leaving the nuclei in an excited state. The nucleus will then emit its excess energy as gamma rays in order to stabilize itself back to its normal ground energy state. Capture gammas are produced when neutrons are absorbed or captured by nitrogen in the atmosphere and by the nuclei of various weapons materials. These capture reactions are accompanied by the release of secondary gammas. Residual radiation primarily includes gamma rays, beta particles, and alpha particles generated beyond the first minute after detonation. Most of these radiations are produced by the decay of the fission fragments generated by weapon fission processes, but some are activated bomb components and surface materials that are made radioactive by exposure to the intense neutron flux generated by fission and fusion events.

The broad classes of initial radiation and residual radiation come from an analysis of a 20-kt ground burst. The hot fireball produced by this weapon, laden with highly radioactive fission fragments, rises upward through the atmosphere so quickly that, after about 60 seconds, it reaches a height from which the initial radiation can no longer strike the ground. A person on the ground would therefore be safe from the initial radiation after 1 minute. As the yield of the weapon is increased, the fireball rises more quickly, but the 60-second point remains approximately the same. The main hazard from initial radiation is acute, external, whole-body irradiation by neutrons and gamma rays. It is only for very small tactical weapons that the initial radiation is potentially fatal at distances where the blast and thermal effects are survivable (see Figure 1-3). Therefore, significant initial radiation hazards are restricted to the first minute after detonation and to several hundred meters surrounding a small-yield tactical weapon. Conversely, residual, or fallout radiation, covers a wide geographic area and remains a significant biological hazard long after detonation.

Fallout

Residual nuclear radiation from a detonation is defined as radiation that is emitted more than 1 minute after the detonation of the weapon. At this 1-minute point, the fireball for a 20-kiloton-yield weapon will have cooled to the point that it no longer glows and will have risen up to 7 miles into the atmosphere. The convective forces caused by the fireball result in an enormous amount of air and debris being sucked upward. In an airburst, the residual radiation results mostly from the fission products and, to a lesser extent, unused fuel that was not fissioned due to the disassembly (blowing apart) of the core during the detonation. Additionally, there will be activation products formed by the interaction of neutrons with bomb materials such as the case, the shielding, and the neutron reflector. If the fireball touches or is close enough to the earth that materials on the ground are sucked into it, the materials are vaporized and mix with the other materials in the fireball. The debris from a predominately fusion weapon (the ERW mentioned earlier) will not contain the amounts of fission products that a comparable-yield fission weapon will. If the fission yield of the ERW is sufficiently low, most of the residual radiation will be due to neutron interactions in the weapon and the surrounding environment.

The primary hazard of residual radiation is from the creation of fallout particles. Sources of fallout include all those listed in the previous paragraph: fission fragments, unused fuel (uranium, plutonium, and tritium), and activation products. As may be suspected from the previous discussion, an airburst of sufficient height to prevent the introduction of ground-based materials into the fireball will result in far less fallout than a ground or near-ground burst. In Hiroshima and Nagasaki, the bombs were detonated at a height to maximize blast damage and minimize fallout to allow earlier entry into the cities for inspection of the damage. Fallout is categorized as early fallout or late fallout.

Early fallout is radioactive material deposited within the first day after detonation. This fallout is the most significant for the military because it is highly radioactive, geographically concentrated, and local. It tends to consist of larger particles (approximately 0.01–1.0 cm in diameter) usually deposited within a few hundred miles of ground zero. The two largest sources of this early fallout are fission products and activation products formed by neutron interactions. Because the material has had little time to decay, it is initially very radioactive when it falls; however, it tends to decay quite rapidly. An approximation of the decrease in dose rate can be made by using what is referred to as the "seven-ten rule," where for every sevenfold increase in time, the dose rate will decrease by a factor of ten. Using this rule, if you have a dose

rate at 1 hour post-detonation of 30 Gy/h, for example, in 7 hours the dose rate will be 3 Gy/h, and in 49 hours (7 × 7) it will be 0.3 Gy/h. This approximation is accurate within about 25% through about 2 weeks post-detonation. There are around 300 isotopes of 36 elements formed from the fission process in a weapon. Most of these are radioactive, decay by beta radiation, and are often accompanied by gamma emissions (Figure 1-4).[4] The biological hazards from early fallout are primarily external, whole-body, gamma-ray irradiation; secondarily external beta-particle irradiation from beta emitters deposited on the skin; and lastly internal irradiation from isotopes that are ingested, injected, or inhaled.

Delayed fallout generally consists of the smaller particles deposited after the first 24 hours. This material is less significant as an immediate hazard to the military because it has a longer time to decay and it is deposited over a wider area. Delayed fallout is almost exclusively an internal hazard due to ingestion of iodine, strontium, and cesium in food and milk. Under certain circumstances, delayed fallout may be distributed worldwide, presenting a widespread long-term health hazard through internalized exposure.

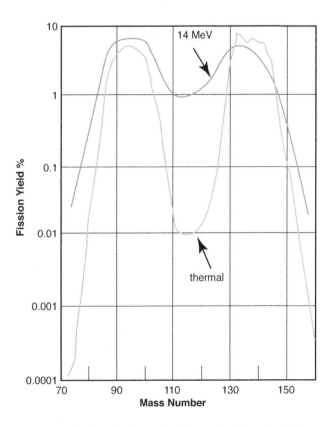

Figure 1-4. Probability curve for the production of radioisotopes due to U-235 fission.

The ultimate deposition of nuclear fallout on the ground is influenced by the physical interactions of the rising fireball with the atmosphere. For a ground, water, or near-surface burst, the interaction of the fireball with ground debris greatly affects the fallout deposition. As the hot gas bubble quickly rises through the atmosphere, it creates and is followed by a strong vacuum directly from below. This generates winds that rush radially inward toward ground zero and upward toward the ascending fireball. These winds can pick up large quantities of dirt and debris from the ground and inject them into the fireball (a process called stem formation). This material, along with any other ground material directly vaporized by a surface burst, then provides condensation centers within the fireball. The gaseous fission fragments condense more quickly on these relatively larger debris particles than they would have otherwise, greatly increasing early local fallout. This fallout is deposited quickly in a concentrated area relatively near ground zero. The activation of surface materials through irradiation of ground elements by the direct neutron flux of a near-surface burst may also increase the local fallout hazard to troops traveling through that area soon after detonation.

In the case of a pure airburst detonation with no secondary ground materials injected into the fireball, the cloud rises and cools and the fission fragment vapors begin to cool and condense at certain temperatures (characteristic of their particular elements). Therefore, because the time for airburst fission-product condensation is delayed and because fission products do not condense on large particles of ground debris, the proportion of fallout activity expressed as early local fallout is greatly reduced.

Characteristics of Fallout and the Prediction of Hazards

The factors that determine the extent of anticipated fallout hazard are as follows:

- The total fission yield (fission fragments are the largest contributor to fallout activity)
- The ratio of energy produced by the fission process versus the fusion process (the higher the fission fraction, the more fission products and consequently the greater the radiological hazard)
- The specific design of the weapon (for example, an ERW will produce proportionately less fallout than an equivalent-yield standard nuclear weapon)
- The altitude of burst (a ground, water, or near-surface detonation produces the greatest early local hazard)
- The composition of surface elements near ground zero in a near-surface burst (accounting for the neutron flux-induced activation potential of surface materials)
- The meteorological conditions (winds and precipitation introduce by far the greatest uncertainties in predicting where and when the fallout will be deposited)
- The time after detonation (the more time allowed for radiological decay, the less the activity of the fallout field)

In terms of absolute quantity of energy from fallout, approximately 10% of the quoted energy yield of a typical fission weapon will be residual radiation; for fusion weapons, it will be approximately 5%.

RADIOLOGICAL WEAPONS

The use of a radiological weapon as a weapon of terrorism is a distinct possibility. This would likely take the form of either a radiation exposure device or an RDD. There are at least three potential difficulties with using radiation sources as weapons. First, a large enough dose must be absorbed by an individual to cause radiation sickness. This would take a relatively large and energetic source and most likely a fairly long contact time. A source placed in a container that people merely walk by is not likely to produce a sufficient dose to be medically detectable, let alone to cause radiation-induced symptoms. Secondly, because the potential dose received by the person who puts the device together or transports it may be extremely high, the viable options of sources that could be used are limited. Thirdly, dispersed radioactive material from even a very large dirty bomb is unlikely to be concentrated enough (other than right at the scene of the explosion) to cause a high enough dose rate to cause radiation sickness.

Radiological Exposure Device

A radiological exposure device is simply a radioactive source placed in an area where it would irradiate unsuspecting persons. It would be difficult to handle a large enough source to cause injury unless the source was placed where people stay in the same location for some length of time. This also tends to limit the number of potential victims and therefore is not a likely choice for those trying to irradiate vast numbers. This type of source is only an external irradiation hazard.

Radiation Dispersal Device

The classic definition of an RDD is a radiation source wrapped with explosives and detonated to cause a spread of radioactive material. However, this is not the only way to disperse radioactive material. Any device that aerosolizes a liquid or powdered radioactive source may also be used to spread contamination. This can be something as simple as a spray bottle used to spray the material on surfaces where it will be touched or otherwise picked up and spread by unsuspecting individuals, or as commonplace as a truck with a sprayer or a crop-dusting aircraft with hundreds of pounds of material.

Potential Radioactive Sources

Legal acquisition of most highly radioactive sources is regulated by federal and state laws requiring licensing of the user and some level of oversight, which depends on the source type and strength. Several common radionuclides are possible sources for use as RDDs (Figure 1-5). Cesium-137, usually in the form of cesium chloride, is commonly used in industry and medicine. It is often sealed in a steel pellet or button and found in teletherapy units, brachytherapy sources, and industrial sources, and sources of over 1,000,000 curies are not uncommon. Cesium emits high-energy gamma radiation and has a half-life of 30 years. Cesium chloride is a salt that can be easily dispersed or dissolved in liquid. In the United States, the Nuclear Regulatory Commission has taken steps to minimize the amount and increase the security of cesium chloride held by licensees because of the potential for it to be used in a terrorist weapon.

Cobalt-60 is used in medical teletherapy units and industrial irradiators. It is commonly found as metallic rods, ribbons, or pellets and emits two high-energy

Radionuclide	Half-life	Typical Activity	Use
Cobalt-60	5 years	15,000 Ci	Cancer therapy
Cesium-137	30 years	1.5×10^6 Ci 10 mCi	Food irradiation Medical source
Iridium-192	74 days	150 Ci 1 mCi	Industrial radiography Medical source
Plutonium-238	88 years	Varies	Satellite power source
Strontium-90	29 years	40,000 Ci	Radio-thermal generator
Iodine-131	8 days	0.15 Ci	Cancer therapy
Americium-241	432 years	5×10^{-6} Ci	Smoke detectors

Figure 1-5. Possible sources of radiological material for terrorist use.

gamma rays. It has a half-life of 5.27 years and is found in sources ranging in strength up to several thousands of curies. Iridium-192 is an industrial radiography and brachytherapy source that is usually in metallic form. It emits high-energy beta particles and several mid- to high-energy gammas. Due to its relatively short half-life (74 days) and the fact that iridium sources are usually fairly small (150 curies or less), it is more likely to be used for a radiological exposure device than a dispersal type of device.

Strontium-90 is a pure beta emitter that releases a very high-energy beta particle. It is used in radiothermal generators, particularly in eastern Europe and Russia. These devices are used to provide power, often in remote areas without electric lines. Strontium is in the form of a ceramic matrix in quantities of tens of thousands of curies. These devices have been responsible for several deaths when unknowing individuals find them and use them to keep warm.

MEDICAL CONSEQUENCES OF NUCLEAR WEAPONS

When preparing for the consequences of nuclear weapons during the Cold War, planners worried about "hardening" (protecting from the detrimental effects of radiation) the electronics and mechanical systems of equipment needed to pursue a conflict. During this same time, the Armed Forces Radiobiology Research Institute and others spent an enormous amount of time, energy, and resources on determining how "hard" the operators of these systems were and how to protect them and allow them to not only survive, but also to function effectively when subjected to doses of radiation that would ordinarily be incapacitating. This also provided data useful to planners and commanders

who need to know what the performance decrement to their personnel will be at various doses. The $LD_{50/60}$ (lethal dose to 50% of the population within 60 days) for ionizing radiation at greater than 0.10 Gy/h is around 4.10 Gy with minimal treatment.

When the United States dropped atomic weapons on Hiroshima and Nagasaki, no one had much experience treating radiation injuries, and certainly not in the setting of a mass casualty situation where tens of thousands of individuals were exposed. As was discussed previously, radiation injury is not the only effect from a nuclear weapon, or even an explosive RDD. Many individuals will also suffer burns and trauma, which is termed "combined injury." These combined injuries have a synergistic effect where a less-than-lethal dose of radiation, when combined with a normally nonlethal injury, becomes a potentially fatal combination. In Hiroshima and Nagasaki, when the magnitude of the numbers of people with radiation exposure and injuries, including burns, was combined with the nearly complete destruction of the medical infrastructure, not to mention the preexisting lack of medical equipment due to the war effort, survival became problematic at even relatively low doses. Even in the 21st century, if medical centers are damaged or destroyed and local medical providers are dead or injured, the situation could initially be much like Japan in August of 1945 (Figure 1-6). With somewhere between 4,000 and 9,000 individuals exposed to a survivable dose but also suffering burns and trauma, the medical system would be immediately overwhelmed and victims would need to be transported out of the area of the blast and fallout to have a chance at survival. As the size of the weapon increases—or if a weapon is used on a major city with a high population density—the number of casualties increases, as does the distance from ground zero in which there will be survivors who will require medical treatment.

Some additional confounders are that doses to individuals will not be uniform, nor is there likely to be good dosimetry information immediately available. An individual on one side of a wall in a building is likely to receive a very different dose than a person on the other side of the wall standing in the street. A partial-body irradiation can have drastically different effects than a whole-body irradiation of the same total dose. A personal dosimeter does not cover the entire body and may be exposed to more or less than the majority of a person's body, resulting in unreliable measurements. Unless an electronic dosimeter is worn, no information about dose rate will be recorded. Dose rate has a dramatic influence on what constitutes a lethal dose of radiation.

The Chernobyl Accident

In 1986 when the reactor in Chernobyl, Union of Soviet Socialist Republics (now independent Ukraine) exploded and burned, many individuals were exposed to a combined field of neutron, gamma, and strong beta radiations. Measuring this type of radiation dose is difficult because the different types of radiation have a wide range of quality factors. Quality factors refer to a radiation's effectiveness at causing biological damage. They range from 1 to 20, depending on the energy and type of radiation. What this means is that an absorbed dose of 1 rad (0.01 Gy) can be an effective dose to the body of anywhere from 1 to 20 rem (0.01–0.2 Sv), depending on the radiation involved. Biological dosimetry is a useful tool to help estimate dose, but at the time of Chernobyl, it was very time consuming and often gave conflicting results. Since that time, many advances have been made using automated assays to look at dicentric chromosome aberrations and translocations to estimate dose.

Bone-marrow transplants were generally unsuccessful in Chernobyl victims, partially because of the survival of some host stem cells in the bone marrow; as surviving marrow was regenerated, it rejected the transplanted marrow cells. Since 1986, we have learned to determine if there are any surviving cells

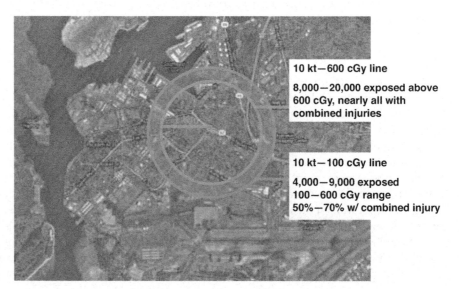

Figure 1-6. Initial radiation effects for a 10-kt yield nuclear weapon. Map: copyright Google, CyberCity 3D, Inc/3D Travel Inc, Digital Globe, GeoEye, US Geological Survey; 2011.

10 kt—600 cGy line

8,000—20,000 exposed above 600 cGy, nearly all with combined injuries

10 kt—100 cGy line

4,000—9,000 exposed 100—600 cGy range 50%—70% w/ combined injury

prior to transplant. If so, we can use newer, much more accurate immune compatibility testing and new antirejection drugs to minimize the incidence of rejection. Also, in 1986 granulocyte colony-stimulating factor was approved for use and there have been other new treatments developed since that help the body produce new granulocytes and stem cells. If there is a surviving fraction of stem cells, these treatments can they stimulate them to produce more cells, making a marrow transplant unnecessary.

A number of the personnel injured at Chernobyl sustained burns as well as radiation exposure. Of the 237 individuals hospitalized in the first 72 hours of the accident, 134 of whom suffered from acute radiation syndrome (ARS), 28 died within 4 months from radiation and thermal burns. Over 2,000 medical personnel were on scene to treat those who were hospitalized (around a 10-to-1 ratio). This ratio would be implausible in the event of a modern nuclear weapons incident. Only about 10%–15% of the victims at Chernobyl suffered combined injury. In a nuclear attack, it is estimated that up to 70% of victims would have combined injury (Table 1-1).[5] The nature of these injuries, as well as their numbers, will require that a mass casualty approach be taken.

Nature of Radiation Injuries

Ionizing radiation deposits energy in the materials within which it interacts. In the case of the human body, this energy deposition occurs within the cells. The body is made up mostly of water and radiation interacts with water molecules, dissociating them into free radicals such as free hydrogen atoms and hydroxyls, which can then go on to form other reactive species, like hydrogen peroxide. Both the free radicals and radiation directly attack targets in the cells. Deoxyribonucleic acid (DNA) is the primary target of lethality, although recent research shows that damage to proteins within the cells can be a major contributor to biological damage. Several single-strand DNA breaks occur every day in our bodies. Almost all of these are recognized and corrected by the body's repair mechanisms. When we are exposed to large amounts of radiation at high dose rates, these repair mechanisms are overwhelmed and the damage cannot be repaired. This leads to cell death, which affects tissues that make up organ systems, which in turn make up major portions of the body. The amount of damage sustained is a direct function of the radiation's quality, dose, and dose rate, and of the individual cell's sensitivity. In general, the more quickly a dose of radiation is delivered to the body, the more severe the consequences. The most sensitive cells are those that tend to divide rapidly, such as the bone-marrow stem cells and the cells lining the crypts of the gastrointestinal tract. Less sensitivity is exhibited by cells that divide more slowly or not at all, such as cells in the central nervous system and muscle cells.

The irradiation of cells has both acute and delayed effects. Acute effects involve cell death, cell injury, and the release of disruptive mediators within the cell, which can lead to performance decrements. Other acute effects are infection and uncontrolled bleeding due to bone marrow destruction, dehydration and electrolyte imbalance due to denuding of the epithelial lining of the intestine, and slow wound healing. Delayed effects include cancer and hereditary effects.

Military attention is focused primarily on acute effects because they are of the most immediate concern to the tactical military commander. Performance decrement occurs within minutes or hours after relatively low exposures to radiation. It includes a phenomenon called early transient incapacitation, a temporary inability to perform physically or cognitively demanding tasks. This inability can be accompanied by hypotension, emesis, or diarrhea. A pilot or a soldier in a nuclear/biological/chemical protective suit could be critically affected by a symptom like emesis, since the suits are only designed to protect the wearer from inhalation or contamination and do not protect against penetrating radiation.

TABLE 1-1

PREDICTED DISTRIBUTION OF INJURIES SUSTAINED FROM A NUCLEAR DETONATION

Injury Types	Percentage of Total Injuries
Radiation only	15
Burn only	15
Wound only	3
Irradiation, burns, and wounds	17
Irradiation and burns	40
Irradiation and wounds	5
Wounds and burns	5
Combined injury total	67

Adapted from US Department of the Army. *Treatment of Nuclear and Radiological Casualties*. Washington, DC: DA; 2001. Field Manual 4-02.283. Table 3-1.

Acute Radiation Syndrome and Associated Subsyndromes

At whole-body or significant partial-body doses around 1 Gy (100 rem) and above, a combination of clinical signs and symptoms occur, which are referred to as ARS. The key mechanisms in the pathophysiology of ARS are depletion of cell lines and microvascular injury.

ARS has four distinct phases or stages, starting with the prodromal phase. During this phase, histamines and other disruptive mediators from free radical effects are released due to cell damage and causing nausea, vomiting, diarrhea, malaise, and, in severe cases, loss of consciousness. Prodromal symptoms can start within minutes, hours, or days after exposure. The time of onset as well as the severity and duration of these symptoms depends on the dose received. Following the prodromal phase is the latent period. During this period, which may last up to 3 to 4 weeks, the patient feels better and appears to recover as symptoms wane. The respite is only temporary; however, and is followed by the manifest illness phase in which the patient is immunocompromised and must be aggressively managed (see Chapter 2). If the patient survives the manifest illness phase, the individual enters the fourth and final phase: recovery.

There are three subsyndromes associated with ARS that are dependent on the total dose received. At the lower end of the spectrum is hematopoietic syndrome, which is seen with doses of around 1 to 5 Gy. The onset of the prodromal symptoms is 3 to 16 hours and they last for less than 48 hours. The prodromal symptoms of the hematological syndrome are characterized by nausea, vomiting, malaise, anorexia, and possibly diarrhea. As the patient enters the latent period, mild weakness becomes the only symptom and will remain for 3 to 4 weeks. If the dose is greater than 3 Gy, there will be epilation or hair loss at around 2 weeks. Manifest illness with bone marrow suppression, infection, and hemorrhage will develop at around 3 to 5 weeks.

The middle subsyndrome is referred to as gastrointestinal subsyndrome and occurs after exposure to around 6 Gy or more. In an unsupported patient with a dose of 6 to 9 Gy, death will occur in 2 to 3 weeks; at greater than 9 Gy, it will occur as early as 1 week after exposure. The prodromal phase for gastrointestinal subsyndrome occurs within 1 to 4 hours and will feature severe nausea and vomiting, possibly watery diarrhea, weakness, and fever. Combat effectiveness will be seriously degraded in the service member with gastrointestinal subsyndrome. A latent period featuring weakness and malaise will last from 5 to 7 days, followed by manifest illness with a return to the prodromal symptoms plus bloody diarrhea, sepsis due to loss of the blood barrier in the intestines, fluid and electrolyte imbalance, shock, and death. At these doses, the intestinal crypt cells are destroyed. As the mature cell layer sloughs off as part of its normal life cycle, there will be no replacement cells to take its place and thus no barrier to keep the intestinal bacteria where they are supposed to be.[6]

Cerebrovascular subsyndrome occurs at around 20 Gy and is always fatal. The prodromal symptoms are erythema, a burning sensation (blush from the endothelial injury and cell breakdown products), vomiting and diarrhea in 30 minutes or less, loss of balance, confusion, and loss of consciousness. The latent period only lasts a few hours and often features euphoria, which is quickly followed by manifest illness. This stage will have severe central nervous system signs due to endothelial cell injury in the brain, unstable blood pressure, respiratory distress, coma, and death.

Combined Injury

ARS and its medical effects are significantly complicated when radiation injury is combined with conventional blast trauma or thermal burn injuries. As has been previously discussed, this combined injury can significantly lower the dose at which fatality occurs. This will lead to significant complications in the treatment strategies employed, and means that there cannot be a "one-treatment-fits-all" mentality for radiation victims. Different doses and confounders will require a very personalized and labor-intensive strategy of treatment.

SUMMARY

Although the Cold War ended many years ago, vast arsenals of nuclear weapons, as well as huge stockpiles of weapons-grade nuclear material, still exist. The number of nations that possess nuclear weapons is at an all-time high, while still more appear to be attempting to join their ranks. In addition to nuclear weapons, the United States is now very concerned with the potential use of radiological weapons such as RDDs. US troops now operate in areas where they may come into contact with abandoned or hidden radiation sources, or may be deliberately targeted with these materials. Our ability to successfully treat radiological casualties has been enhanced by continued research and the availability of new drugs; however, to be successful, treatment must be started soon after exposure by medical personnel who understand the specialized treatment required. US military medical personnel must understand how to treat radiological and nuclear injuries. The country should never underestimate an enemy and assume that they will not use every option available to them against it, including nuclear or radiological weapons.

REFERENCES

1. Federation of American Scientists. Nuclear Weapons—India Nuclear Forces. http://www.fas.org/nuke/guide/india/nuke/. Updated November 8, 2002. Accessed August 11, 2011.

2. Nell PA. *NATO and the "Neutron Bomb"—Necessity or Extravagance.* Fort Leavenworth, KS: Department of the Army; 1987. Technical Report, Army 1987.

3. US Department of the Army. *The Effects of Nuclear Weapons.* Washington, DC: DA; 1977. DA PAM 50-3.

4. US Department of Energy. *DOE Fundamentals Handbook: Nuclear Physics and Reactor Theory.* Washington, DC: DOE; 1993. Department of Energy Handbook 1019/1-93, p 57, Fig 21.

5. US Department of the Army. *Treatment of Nuclear and Radiological Casualties.* Washington, DC: DA; 2001. Field Manual 4-02.283. Table 3-1.

6. US Department of the Army. *The Effects of Nuclear Weapons.* Washington, DC: DA; 1977. DA PAM 50-3.

Chapter 2

ACUTE RADIATION SYNDROME IN HUMANS

RONALD E. GOANS, PhD, MD[*]; DANIEL F. FLYNN, MS, MD[†]

[*]Senior Medical Advisor, MJW Corp, Amherst, New York, 14228; Senior Research Advisor/Physician, Radiation Emergency Assistance Center/Training Site, Oak Ridge, Tennessee 37831; Associate Professor, Tulane School of Public Health and Tropical Medicine, New Orleans, Louisiana 70112
[†]Colonel, US Army Medical Corps (Retired); Visiting Faculty, Radiation Emergency Assistance Center/Training Site, Oak Ridge, Tennessee 37831; New England Radiation Therapy Associates, Radiation Oncology Department, Holy Family Hospital, Methuen, Massachusetts 01884

INTRODUCTION

Victims of acute radiation events in radiological and nuclear incidents require prompt diagnosis and treatment of medical and surgical conditions as well as of conditions related to possible radiation exposure. Emergency personnel should triage victims using traditional military medical and trauma criteria. Radiation dose can be estimated early following the event using rapid-sort, automated biodosimetry and clinical parameters, such as the clinical history and timing of symptom complexes, the time to emesis (TE), lymphocyte depletion kinetics,[1,2] and various multiparameter biochemical tests.[3–17] Acute high-level radiation exposure should generally be treated as a case involving multiorgan failure (MOF).[18] Various radiation severity grading schemes are currently used by the medical community.[7,14,19]

Radiation-induced multiorgan dysfunction (MOD) and MOF refer to progressive dysfunction of two or more organ systems, the etiological agent being radiation damage to cells and tissues over time. Radiation-associated MOD appears to develop in part as a consequence of the systemic inflammatory response syndrome and in part as a consequence of radiation-induced loss of vital organs' functional cell mass. A worldwide consensus conference considering many different historical radiation accidents has recently addressed radiation-related MOD and MOF.[11,20–25] Besides providing modern guidance to medically managing radiation-induced MOF, the conference proceedings are also a comprehensive educational resource for the physician likely to be involved in managing patients in a radiation incident.

As a resource to physicians, the Strategic National Stockpile Radiation Working Group and other working groups have recently issued recommendations on medically managing acute radiation syndrome (ARS).[12,26–28] ARS has been an important part of radiation medicine for many years and the basic pathophysiology and treatment protocols are summarized in various textbooks.[29–34] In addition, the Radiation Emergency Assistance Center/Training Site, a medical asset of the US Department of Energy, sponsors periodic symposia and short courses on the medical management of radiation accidents.[35–38] Likewise, the Armed Forces Radiobiology Research Institute (AFRRI) provides the Medical Effects of Ionizing Radiation course for military and ancillary personnel and has long been a guiding influence in developing improved treatment methods for ARS.

Radiation sensitivity data on humans and animals has made it possible to describe the symptoms associated with ARS. ARS results from high-level external exposure to ionizing radiation, either of the whole body or a significant portion (> 60%) of it. For this purpose, "high-level" means a dose greater than 1 Gy delivered at a relatively high dose rate. From a physiological standpoint, ARS is a combination of syndromes. These syndromes appear in stages and are directly related to the level of radiation received. They begin to occur within hours after exposure and may last for several weeks. ARS includes a subclinical phase (< 1 Gy) and three syndromes resulting from either whole-body irradiation or irradiation to a significant fraction of the body: hematopoietic syndrome (approximately 1–8 Gy), gastrointestinal syndrome (approximately 6–20+ Gy), and neurovascular syndrome (20–50+ Gy).

Radiation accidents have historically fallen into certain major categories, including low-dose incidents in which the patient shows essentially no signs or symptoms; higher dose, acute whole- or partial-body incidents with significant systemic signs and symptoms associated with ARS and often MOF; local radiation injury arising primarily from lost radiation sources and involving a regional portion of the body, often the hands; and inhalation or ingestion of radioactive material, often without systemic signs and symptoms. In a tactical event, it is possible to have ARS from exposure to a lost or stolen source, from an improvised nuclear weapon, or from inhalation or ingestion of radioactive material. However, the latter is expected to be rare. This chapter will focus on evaluation and management of ARS, regardless of the etiology of the event, although high-level external radiation dose will most likely be the etiology. From a medical viewpoint, patient mortality from radiation exposure is generally associated with a high-level gamma or neutron dose delivered over a short period of time.

Goans has provided an analysis of the recent history of radiation medicine that shows many cases of delayed diagnosis, even with the presentation of classical symptoms. In a review of four recent major gamma radiation incidents involving lost high-level gamma sources (Goiânia, Brazil [September 1987]; Tammiku, Estonia [October 1994]; Bangkok, Thailand [February 2000]; and Meet Halfa, Egypt [May 2000]), the average time from beginning of the accident until definitive diagnosis averaged 22 days.[38] However, in the severe criticality event in Tokaimura, Japan (September 1999), awareness of the accident was immediate because it occurred in an industrial environment.[39]

Radiation incidents will be seen by physicians in a dichotomous fashion: either soon after the event or 2 to 4 weeks or more later (as in the case of lost sources found in the public domain or stolen covertly), when the patient becomes ill secondary to radiation-induced neutropenia or pancytopenia. The clinical presentation of the externally irradiated patient will be much different in these two scenarios.[40]

PATHOPHYSIOLOGY

The etiology of organ damage from high-level radiation exposure results from the radiosensitivity of certain cell lines.[41] Cell radiosensitivity in various tissue systems is the basis for the distinction among the three acute radiation syndromes, as described below. Specifically, cells are radiosensitive if they replicate rapidly, are immature (eg, blast cells), and have a long mitotic future (law of Bergonie and Tribondeau). For example, spermatogonia, lymphocytes, blast cells (various types), other hematopoietic cells, and cells of the small intestine, stomach, colon, epithelium, and skin are radiosensitive, while cells of the central nervous system, muscle, bone, and collagen are much less sensitive. In addition, more highly differentiated cells are less radiosensitive. Lymphocytes are an exception to the law of Bergonie and Tribondeau[41] because they have a long life span, but they do have a very large nucleus, encompassing almost all of the cytoplasm, thereby producing an excellent target for radiation damage.

In radiation medicine, ARS is classically divided into hematopoietic, gastrointestinal, and neurovascular syndromes, each with increasing dose, although there is some overlap, particularly within the first two. Each of these syndromes has been further divided into four clinical stages: prodromal, latent, manifest illness, and recovery or death. Prodromal symptoms begin a few hours after exposure and the time of onset is generally related to the severity of dose and dose rate. During the latent period, the patient may appear relatively clinically normal and generally symptom free. In the hematopoietic syndrome, during the period of manifest illness, significant issues to address are neutropenia and possibly pancytopenia. Therefore, medical treatment during the first 6 weeks after exposure to approximately 2 to 6 Gy is focused toward managing pancytopenia, controlling infection, and managing possible MOF in places other than the hematological system.

Hematopoietic Syndrome

Hematopoietic syndrome occurs after whole-body or significant partial-body irradiation of greater than 1 Gy delivered to the bone marrow. The radiosensitive cells of the hematopoietic tissue are the various lineages of stem cells.[42–46] Their anatomical location in the bone marrow distributes them throughout the body. A dose-dependent suppression of bone marrow at doses greater than 2 to 3 Gy leads to eventual neutropenia and possibly pancytopenia. Prompt radiation dose (within minutes to an hour) of approximately 3 to 8 Gy will cause significant damage to the bone marrow. A dose of approximately 3 to 4 Gy may result in death to 50% of exposed individuals without significant medical support.[47–49] Radiation exposure causes the exponential biological death of bone-marrow stem and progenitor cells. If it is possible in tactical situations, shielding is the best method to protect bone marrow.[50,51]

Prodromal symptoms after high-level radiation exposure often last for 1 to 3 days and include nausea, emesis, anorexia, and diarrhea. Generally, the earlier the onset of nausea and emesis, the higher the dose, if one excludes the possibility of psychogenic emesis. An approximate dose dependence for nausea and emesis was compiled from prior, unpublished research at Oak Ridge Associated Universities in the 1970s in conjunction with the US space program. From this research, the ED_{50} (effective dose; the amount of drug that produces a therapeutic response in 50% of the subjects taking it) was found to be approximately 1.6 Gy and 2.4 Gy for nausea and emesis, respectively (Figure 2-1).

The prodromal symptoms are followed by 2 to 3

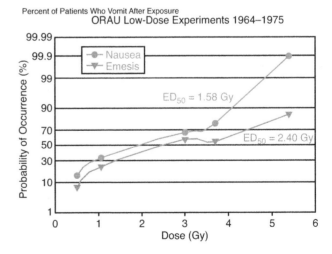

Figure 2-1. Incidence of nausea and emesis as a function of dose. Research performed at Oak Ridge Associated Universities for the National Aeronautics and Space Administration. Adapted with permission from Taylor and Francis and Oak Ridge Associated Universities.

weeks of latency, during which the patient will suffer from significant fatigue and weakness. The clinical symptoms of manifest illness appear approximately 21 to 30 days after exposure and may last up to 2 weeks. Sepsis associated with pancytopenia from bone-marrow suppression and severe hemorrhage from platelet loss are often the lethal factors in hematopoietic subsyndrome.[46,49] Platelet counts of fewer than 20,000/mm[3], moderately decreased erythrocyte counts, and severely suppressed neutrophil counts (fewer than 500/mm[3]) may also be seen. The treating physician will consequently be required to use current medical therapy for severe neutropenia in the setting of MOF.

Clinical hematological profiles over the period of manifest illness generally follow a course similar to that shown in Figure 2-2. There is a progressive decrease in lymphocytes, neutrophils, and platelets with increasing radiation dose. From traditional medical guidance, a 30% to 50% decrease of absolute lymphocytes within the first 24 hours is suggestive of serious and potentially lethal injury.[52] More recently developed guidelines have been presented for early determination of the severity of radiation injury using both hematological kinetics and the appearance and severity of various clinical symptoms.[15,28,40,53–58] Subpopulations of selectively radioresistant stem cells or accessory cells often exist[49,59–62] and play an important role in hematologic reconstitution. Moreover, the radiation exposure is often inhomogeneous. The patient's physical environment and distance from the source may afford

partial shielding, accounting for dose variability, and this may result in areas of viable hematopoietic stem cells. Such a reservoir of stem cells may contribute to the future reestablishment of hematopoiesis.

The onset of radiation-induced cytopenia is variable and dose dependent. Granulocytes may experience a transient rise prior to decrease in patients exposed to less than 5 Gy. The transient increase prior to decline is termed an "abortive" rise, a finding that may be clinically helpful because it may indicate a more survivable exposure. The time to onset and duration of the nadir are variable.[43,63] Indeed, the nadir may not occur for 3 to 4 weeks, particularly at lower doses. The duration of neutropenia is often extensive, requiring prolonged administration of hematopoietic growth factors, blood product support, and antibiotics. Patients with burns or wounds also experience poor wound healing, bleeding, and infection because of hematopoietic suppression. Impaired wound healing may be due in part to radiation-induced endothelial damage, which significantly depresses the revascularization of injured tissue.[52,64,65]

Gastrointestinal Syndrome

Gastrointestinal syndrome and hematopoietic syndrome occur simultaneously at high radiation doses, beginning at 6 to 8 Gy. Consequences of gastrointestinal syndrome are more immediate and less amenable to treatment. The prodromal stage includes severe nausea, vomiting, watery diarrhea, and cramps occurring within hours after irradiation. At higher doses, bloody diarrhea, hypovolemia, shock, and death may ensue.[52,66–70] At radiation doses above 10 to 12 Gy, patients will die sooner than if they just had hematopoietic syndrome. In a mass casualty event, these patients will likely be triaged expectant.

From a pathology viewpoint, the intestinal mucosa experiences severe radiation-induced damage following high-dose exposure.[43,52] A shorter latent period is observed clinically because of the observed turnover time of 3 to 5 days for intestinal mucosal epithelial cells. Damaged crypt stem cells do not divide and therefore the damaged mucosal lining is shed and not replaced.[52] The ability to absorb food is greatly reduced because of the disrupted mucosal lining and because of vascular coalescence. The damage to the mucosal lining also provides a portal for intestinal flora to enter the systemic circulation and serve as a nidus for sepsis.[52] In addition, severe mucosal hemorrhage has been seen in experimental animal models. The overall intestinal pathology includes disturbance of absorption and secretion, glycocalyx disruption, mucosal ulceration, alteration of enteric flora, depletion of gut lymphoid

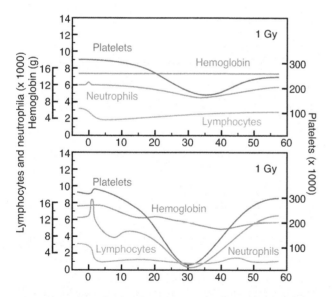

Figure 2-2. Cellular kinetics for the hematopoietic syndrome as a function of days following irradiation.
Graphic courtesy of the US Armed Forces Radiobiology Research Institute.

tissue, and motility disturbances.[34,71,72]

Medical issues associated with the gastrointestinal syndrome include malnutrition resulting from malabsorption, emesis, ileus, dehydration, possible acute renal failure, and cardiovascular collapse resulting from shifts in fluids and electrolytes. It is also possible to observe anemia from prolonged gastrointestinal bleeding and sepsis resulting from entry of bacteria into the systemic system via the damaged endothelial lining.[34,52,69,73–75]

Neurovascular Syndrome

Neurovascular syndrome is less well defined than the others.[76,77] Generally, patients with this syndrome have experienced a lethal dose over 30 Gy, but there is relatively little clinical experience at these doses for human exposure and the mechanism of death is unclear. Cardiovascular shock accompanies such high doses, resulting in a massive loss of serum and electrolytes through leakage into extravascular tissues. The ensuing circulatory problems of edema, increased intracranial pressure, and cerebral anoxia can bring death within 2 days.[23,34,52,77,78]

The prodromal stages of the neurovascular syndrome are compressed. The patient may experience a burning sensation occurring within minutes; nausea and vomiting within 1 hour; and confusion, prostration, and loss of balance (ataxia). During the latent period, apparent improvement for a few hours is likely to be followed by severe manifest illness. Within 5 to 6 hours, the overt clinical picture proceeds with the return of severe watery diarrhea, respiratory distress, and gross central nervous system signs.[34,52] MOF is the final common pathway in the neurovascular syndrome.[11,23,79]

The histopathology of the neurovascular syndrome appears to be due to massive endothelial damage in the microcirculation.[34,52,65] This has been postulated as a causative mechanism in the damage of some organs. Preliminary experimental evidence indicates that the cause of initial hypotension may be an early, overwhelming surge of histamine released from degranulated mast cells.[34] The radiation threshold for the neurovascular symptom complex is not well defined. Experimental evidence in animals and in a few human radiation accidents indicates that 30 to 50 Gy will elicit the neurovascular syndrome and all doses in this range will eventually cause a lethal outcome.[52]

The natural history of ARS shows that the time to death in an untreated patient is approximately 20 to 30 days in a severe hematopoietic case, 8 to 14 days in a patient with gastrointestinal syndrome, and 1 to 3 days with neurovascular syndrome.

DETERMINANTS OF RADIATION EFFECTS ON HUMANS

Radiation Lethality Curve

The slope of a radiation lethality curve is weighted heavily by data at each extreme of its distribution.[34,52] This fact underscores the importance of reliable dosimetry, not only in the experimental situation but also in accurately determining the human exposure after a nuclear incident. In spite of the heterogeneity surrounding LD_{50} values, it is possible to conclude that the doses giving between 90% and 95% mortality in most animal experiments are about twice those giving 5% to 10% mortality.[47,51,80] In a recent review of animal data, a uniform dose (D) normalized to the LD_{50} (D/LD_{50}) revealed that no deaths occurred when D/LD_{50} was less than 0.54. When D/LD_{50} was greater than 1.3, mortality was 100%.[47,48,52,81,82] Therefore, total survival in a population can apparently be changed to total mortality by increasing the radiation dose by a factor of approximately 2.4.[34] Relationships between dose and lethality, drawn from a large number of animal studies, emphasize two important points on extrapolation to the human radiation response: reliable dosimetry is extremely valuable, and either therapy or trauma can significantly shift the dose–response relationship. An error in dosimetry of 0.5 to 1 Gy can result in large shifts along the dose–response curve, and effective therapy can increase the LD_{50} by 1 Gy or more. Radiation lethality appears to be a consequence of changes in the cellular kinetics of renewal systems critical for survival.

Factors such as trauma, stress, and poor nutritional status that compromise or damage the hematopoietic system or the immune system negatively affect the dose–response curve.[34]

The goal of modern medical management of ARS is to shift the mortality curve to the right, which will result in saving more lives.[83–86] This can be accomplished by good medical and nursing care, intravenous (IV) hydration, antibiotic coverage (as indicated), early use of cytokine growth factors, and possibly the use of stem cell transplants in the higher dose ranges (> 6–8 Gy).

Influence of Trauma on LD_{50}

A recent consensus committee has examined modern scientific aspects of combined injury (radiation plus burns or trauma).[86] The combination of radiation exposure and trauma produces a clinical dilemma not encountered by most military and civilian physicians.

In combined injury, two (or more) injuries that are sublethal or minimally lethal when occurring alone will act synergistically with radiation injury, resulting in much greater mortality than the simple sum of what all injuries would have produced.[9,34,52,85–89]

Human radiation exposure events, such as the Hiroshima and Nagasaki bombings[90–94] or the Chernobyl accident,[63,95,96] were often coupled with other forms of injury, such as wounds, burns, blunt trauma, and infection. Radiation-combined injury would also be expected after a radiological or nuclear attack. Few animal models of radiation-combined injury exist, and mechanisms underlying the high mortality associated with complex radiation injuries are poorly understood. Medical countermeasures are currently available for managing the nonradiation components of radiation-combined injury, but it is not known whether treatments for other insults will be effective when the injury is combined with radiation exposure. Further research is needed to elucidate mechanisms behind the synergistic lethality of radiation-combined injury and to identify targets for medical countermeasures.[86]

The mechanisms responsible for combined injury sequelae are unknown, but they can significantly increase the consequences of radiation exposure across the entire dose–response curve.[52] It must be emphasized that the survival of a patient following exposure in the hematopoietic dose range requires the following: (*a*) a minimum critical number of surviving stem cells to regenerate a competent host defense system, (*b*) the functional competence of surviving cells composing the specific and nonspecific immune system, or (*c*) effective replacement or substitution therapy during the critical postexposure cytopenic phase.[52] Trauma alone, depending on its intensity, may also effectively depress host resistance to infection.[97–99]

When trauma is imposed on a physiological system with even mild radiation injury, the outcome can be lethal. In most instances, trauma symptoms will either mask or exacerbate the first reliable signs of radiation injury. This will cloud the situation if one is relying on prodromal symptoms to estimate dose. In addition, the choice of treatment in these cases should include consideration of not only the patient's initial status, but also the condition that will exist 7 to 21 days later, when the radiation effects are seen. An open skin wound (combined injury) markedly increases the chances of infection. Therefore, immediate wound closure has been recommended. Injuries to the abdomen may also present significant problems to the irradiated subject. Blast overpressure, blunt trauma, and penetrating trauma are all significant causes of abdominal injury in a tactical situation.[52]

Effect of Clinical Support on the LD_{50} Dose Effect Curve

Modification of survival throughout the LD_{50} dose range is achievable using a simple regimen of clinical support to replace or substitute the depleted functional cells after stem cell destruction.[34,52–70] Experimental work over the last 20 years showed the efficacy of supportive care centered on systemic antibiotics and transfusions of fresh platelets.[49,100] Several canine studies indicated that antibiotics, individually or in combination, were successful in reducing mortality in the LD_{50} range. Combination antibiotics, in conjunction with fresh whole-blood transfusions and parenteral fluids, have been effective in controlling dehydration and thereby reducing mortality.[34,52] These studies have been extended over a dose range that can determine the significant shift in LD_{50} that results from treatment. It must be emphasized that the practical application of these concepts requires that the damage to the stem cell system be reversible; that is, the surviving fraction of hematopoietic stem cells must be capable of spontaneous regeneration. Carefully controlled experiments clearly indicate that supportive treatment will elevate the estimate of the LD_{50} by as much as 30%. Based on the range of values discussed, the recommended value for the LD_{50} is approximately 3.6 to 3.9 Gy, but a mild dose-rate dependence has been demonstrated.[34]

CLINICAL ASPECTS OF THE US CRITICALITY EXPERIENCE

Only a small number of radiation accidents in the United States have been severe enough to result in ARS-related MOF. Since 1945, four deaths have resulted from criticality accidents. The four criticality cases are particularly relevant for analysis of MOF because medical treatment was supportive and did not appreciably perturb the clinical evolution of radiation injury. In addition, these cases illustrate the clinical and pathological expression of the various ARS syndromes.[101,102]

Two criticality events occurred with the same 6.2-kg, delta-phase plutonium sphere at Los Alamos National Laboratory in New Mexico. The first incident occurred on August 21, 1945, when a worker was preparing a critical assembly by stacking tungsten carbide bricks around the plutonium core as a reflector. He moved the final block over the assembly but, noting that this block would make the assembly supercritical, he withdrew it. The brick fell onto the center of the assembly, resulting in a super-prompt critical state. The worker sustained

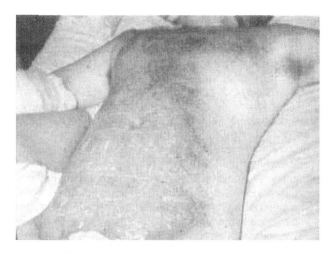

Figure 2-3. Los Alamos criticality victim (LA-1) on day 24, prior to death.
Reproduced with permission from Hempelmann LH, Lisco H, Hoffman JG. The acute radiation syndrome: a study of nine cases and a review of the problem. *Ann Intern Med.* 1952;36:279–510 (Plate XVIII).

an average whole-body dose of approximately 5.1 Gy neutrons and gammas and a dose to the right hand of approximately 100 to 400 Gy. The patient died of sepsis 24 days later (Figure 2-3).[35,103,104]

The second criticality accident occurred in 1946 during an approach-to-criticality demonstration at which several observers were present. The operator used a screwdriver as a lever to lower a hemispherical beryllium shell reflector into place. While holding the top shell with his left thumb in an opening at the spherical pole, the screwdriver slipped and caused a critical configuration. The operator received an estimated acute whole-body dose of approximately 21 Gy, with a dose to the left hand of 150 Gy and somewhat less to the right hand. Seven observers were exposed in the range of 0.27 to 3.6 Gy. The operator died 9 days later.[35,103]

A third Los Alamos event was a liquid criticality event. On December 30, 1958, during purification and concentration of plutonium, unexpected plutonium-rich solids were washed from two vessels into a single large vessel that contained layered, dilute aqueous and organic solutions. The tank contained approximately 295 liters of a caustic stabilized organic emulsion. The added nitric acid wash is believed to have separated the liquid phases. Accident analysis shows that the aqueous layer was initially slightly below delayed critical (approximately 203-mm thick, with critical thickness being 210 mm). When the stirrer was started, the central portion of the liquid system was thickened, changing system reactivity to super-prompt critical. Bubble generation was the negative feedback mechanism for terminating the

first neutron spike. The system was driven permanently subcritical by mixing the two layers. This accident resulted in the death of the operator 36 hours after the accident. The dose to the upper extremity is estimated to have been 120 Gy, plus or minus 50%. Two other persons received acute doses of 1.34 Gy and 0.53 Gy.[105]

The last fatal US criticality case occurred at Wood River Junction, Rhode Island. This liquid process accident occurred on July 24, 1964, at the United Nuclear Fuels Recovery Plant. A chemical processing plant was designed to recover highly enriched uranium from scrap material left over from the production of fuel rods. Uranyl nitrate solution U(93) was poured into a carbonate reagent vessel. The critical excursion occurred when nearly all of the uranium had been transferred. It is probable that the system oscillated, resulting in a series of neutron excursions. The acute dose to the operator was estimated to be 100 Gy. Two supervisory personnel received approximately 1 and 0.6 Gy. The operator died 49 hours later (Figure 2-4).[106,107]

Clinical Course of the Criticality Cases

Radiation histopathology is an important adjunct to the clinical aspects of radiation medicine and has been examined by various authors.[108–114]

Case Study 2-1: Los Alamos Plutonium Sphere (hematopoietic syndrome; cutaneous radiation injury syndrome; whole-body dose approximately 5.1 Gy; dose to right hand 100–400 Gy). The patient was a 26-year-old male whose past

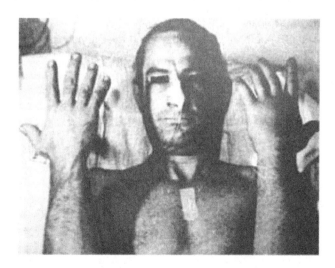

Figure 2-4. Wood River Junction, Rhode Island, patient postaccident.
Reproduced with permission from Karas JS, Stanbury JB. Fatal radiation syndrome from an accidental nuclear excursion. *N Engl J Med.* 1965;272:755–761. Article DOI:10.1056/NEJM196504152721501.

medical history was significant only for Wolff-Parkinson-White syndrome diagnosed 3 years prior to the incident. On admission to the hospital, his vital signs were within normal limits and his only initial complaint was numbness and tingling of both hands. The initial physical examination was also within normal limits.

Within 30 minutes after the accident, the patient's right hand had become diffusely swollen. Emesis began approximately 1.5 hours after the event, and nausea continued intermittently for the next 24 hours. The patient experienced subjective improvement but had a mild temperature, mild gastric distress, and weakness during days 3 to 6. By day 5, the patient experienced a distinct rise in temperature with tachycardia and began to appear increasingly toxic. On day 10, he developed severe stomatitis, a paralytic ileus, and diarrhea. Clinical signs of pericarditis were noted on day 17, and the patient's mental status became irrational. The clinical course is notable for progressive pancytopenia.

Within 36 hours after the accident, blisters were noted on the volar aspect of the right third finger, and within 24 hours thereafter, extensive blistering was noted on both palmar and volar surfaces of the hand. A decision was made on day 3 to surgically drain the blisters, but by the third week the right hand had progressed to a dry gangrene. Desquamation of the epidermis involved almost all of the skin of the dorsum of the forearm and hand. In addition, epilation was almost complete at the time of death.

On day 24, the patient's temperature had risen to 41.1°C. He had lost a great deal of weight, developed thoracic-abdominal erythema, and had signs of sepsis. On day 24, the patient became comatose and died. During the patient's clinical admission, treatment consisted of fluid support, penicillin antibiotic therapy, thiamine, and two blood transfusions.

On autopsy, severe skin necrosis was observed as well as overt dry gangrene. The cardiorespiratory system was significant for pericarditis, cardiac hypertrophy, pulmonary edema, and alveolar hemorrhage. The spleen was noted to have no germinal centers and the mucosa of the large bowel was ulcerated, as well as that in the buccal mucosa. The bone marrow was noted to be hypoplastic with foci of bac-

teria (Figure 2-5) and lymph nodes also showed significant lymphocyte depletion. The testes demonstrated significant atrophy with aspermia. A solitary ulcer was noted in the large colon, as was a right renal infarct.

Case Study 2-2: Los Alamos Plutonium Sphere (gastrointestinal syndrome; cutaneous radiation injury syndrome; acute dose approximately 21 Gy; dose to the left hand 150 Gy). The patient was a 32-year-old male, admitted to the hospital within 1 hour after the accident. His medical history is generally unremarkable. His occupational history is significant only for several prior, generally chronic occupational exposures, none exceeding 0.005 Gy in a week. The patient complained of nausea in the hour prior to admission and vomited once in that time.

The general condition of the patient was quite good in the first 5 days following the accident. On the fifth day, there was a precipitous drop in his leukocyte count, and his condition began to decline rapidly. The patient rapidly lost weight, became mentally confused on day 7, became comatose, and died in cardiovascular shock on the ninth day.

Medical therapy during the 9-day course was largely symptomatic. Penicillin was given (50,000 U every 3 hours intramuscularly) beginning on day 5 because of granulocytopenia. Blood transfusions were also given daily after the fifth day. On day 6, fever and tachycardia developed, and on the seventh day, the patient developed a severe paralytic ileus. At the time of death, both hands showed extensive radiation damage.

On autopsy, examination of the skin was remarkable for early vesicle formation in the abdominal skin and marked epidermal damage. The cardiorespiratory system was remarkable for cardiac hemorrhage and myocardial edema, and the terminal bronchi showed features of aspiration pneumonia. The spleen exhibited no germinal centers and mucosa of most of the gastrointestinal tract showed atrophy and sloughing, most pronounced in the jejunum and ileum (Figure 2-6). Widespread degenerative changes were noted in the adrenal cortex as well as hyaline degeneration in the

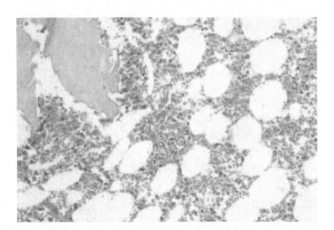

Figure 2-5. Hypocellular marrow with bacteria present centrally (hematopoietic syndrome).
Slide courtesy of the US Department of Energy.

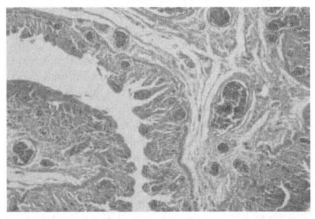

Figure 2-6. Intestinal specimen illustrating villous atrophy, congestion, and hemorrhage (gastrointestinal syndrome).
Slide courtesy of the US Department of Energy.

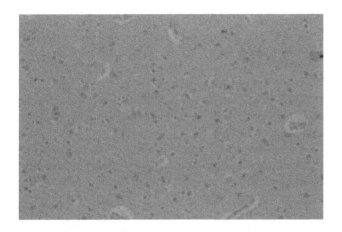

Figure 2-7. Neurovascular syndrome with brain perivascular edema (Virchow-Robins space).
Slide courtesy of the US Department of Energy.

renal tubular epithelium. Examination of the red bone marrow showed it to be of liquid consistency.

Case Study 2-3: Los Alamos Liquid Criticality Event (central nervous system syndrome; dose to the upper extremity 120 Gy ± 50%). The patient was a 50-year-old male with no significant past medical history. The clinical course has been divided into four separate phases. Phase 1 (20–30 min after the event) included immediate physical collapse and mental incapacitation, progressing eventually into semiconsciousness. Phase 2 (90 min after the event) consisted of signs and symptoms of cardiovascular shock accompanied by severe abdominal pain. Phase 3 (4 h after the event) included subjective minimal clinical improvement. Phase 4 (28 h after the event) was characterized by rapidly appearing irritability and mania, progressing to coma and death. The clinical course was remarkable for continuing, profound hypotension; tachycardia; and intense dermal and conjunctival hyperemia. The patient died 35 hours after exposure.

On autopsy, examination of the bone marrow was most significant for absence of mitotic activity. The lungs showed pyknotic, degenerating cells in the pleura, degenerating

lymphocytes and neutrophils in the subpleural connective tissue, and many areas of focal atelectasis interspersed with foci of emphysema. All lymph nodes were markedly atrophic and lymphoid follicles in the spleen were greatly depleted.

Examination of the heart showed acute myocarditis, myocardial edema, cardiac hypertrophy, and a fibrinous pericarditis. Examination of the brain demonstrated cerebral edema, diffuse vasculitis, and cerebral hemorrhage. The gastrointestinal system showed necrosis of the anterior gastric wall parietal cells, acute upper jejunal distention, mitotic suppression throughout the entire gastrointestinal tract, and acute jejunal and ileal enteritis.

Case Study 2-4: Wood River Junction (neurovascular syndrome; approximately 100 Gy). The patient was a 38-year-old male with a negative medical history. Following the initial criticality excursion, the patient appeared stunned, ran from the building, and immediately vomited. He also experienced immediate diarrhea and complained of severe abdominal cramping, headache, thirst, and profuse perspiration. His initial vital signs showed borderline blood-pressure elevation and tachycardia. Approximately 4 hours after the accident, the patient experienced transient difficulty in speaking, hypotension, and tachycardia. A portable chest radiograph 16 hours after admission showed hilar congestion. The physical examination also showed the left hand and forearm to be edematous, as well as left-sided conjunctivitis and periorbital edema. On day 2, the patient became disoriented, hypotensive, and anuric. The patient died 49 hours after the accident in cardiovascular shock.

At autopsy, interstitial edema of the left hand, arm, and abdominal wall was noted. Examination of the heart, lungs, and abdominal cavity revealed acute pulmonary edema, bilateral hydrothorax, hydropericardium, abdominal ascites, acute pericarditis, interstitial myocarditis, and inflammation of the ascending aorta. Examination of the gastrointestinal tract showed severe subserosal edema of the stomach and of the transverse and descending colon. The bone marrow was noted to be aplastic, and lymph nodes, spleen, and thymus were depleted of lymphocytes. The brain showed minimal change, with rare foci of microglial change and perivascular edema (Figure 2-7). The testes also showed interstitial edema and overt necrosis of the spermatogonia.

CURRENT TREATMENT OF ACUTE RADIATION SYNDROME

Radiation damage results from the inherent sensitivity of certain cell types to radiation, with the most undifferentiated and mitotically active cells being the most sensitive to acute effects. The inherent sensitivity of these cells results in a constellation of clinical syndromes that occur with radiation exposure. The clinical components of ARS include hematopoietic, gastrointestinal, and neurovascular syndromes and are reviewed above. The medical management of patients with acute, moderate to severe radiation exposure (effective whole-body dose > 3 Gy) should emphasize early initiation of colony-stimulating factor (CSF),

transfusion support as needed, antibiotic prophylaxis, and treatment of febrile neutropenia.[45,49,53,86,115] Additional supportive medications may include antiemetics, antidiarrheals, fluid and electrolyte replacement, and topical burn creams. In the case of coexisting trauma (combined injury), wound closure should be performed within 24 to 36 hours.[86]

The merits of modern supportive care lie in its significant prolongation of survival. The $LD_{50/60}$ (the dose at which 50% of the exposed population will die within 60 days) is approximately 3.5 Gy in persons managed without supportive care. The $LD_{50/60}$ may be increased to 4 to 5 Gy when antibiotics and transfusion support are provided. The lethal dose may also be somewhat higher with early initiation of CSFs.[83,84,116] Casualties whose radiation doses are most amenable to treatment will be those who receive between 2 and 6 Gy. The primary goal of medical therapy is to shift the survival curve to the right by 2 Gy or more. Many casualties whose doses exceed 6 to 8 Gy will also have significant blast and thermal injuries that will preclude survival when combined with the radiation insult. If there is little to no trauma, some authorities would consider stem cell transplant (peripheral or cord blood) for victims in this dose range.[12]

Currently, the only hematopoietic CSFs that have marketing approval from the US Food and Drug Administration (FDA) for managing treatment-associated neutropenia are the recombinant forms of granulocyte-colony stimulating factor (G-CSF), granulocyte-macrophage-colony stimulating factor (GM-CSF), and the pegylated form of G-CSF. All have been explored and have some efficacy in irradiated preclinical models of radiation-induced marrow aplasia. The rationale for using CSFs in irradiated humans is derived from three sources: their enhancement of neutrophil recovery in oncology patients, their perceived benefit in a small number of radiation-accident victims, and several prospective trials in canines and nonhuman primates exposed to radiation.

The most convincing data, which provides the proof of principle, is the demonstration of not only enhanced neutrophil recovery, but more importantly a significant survival advantage in nonhuman primates and canines if the CSF is given less than 24 hours after irradiation (Figures 2-8 and 2-9).[83,84] However, there appears to be less efficacy with a delay in treatment, but the interval required before the survival advantage is lost is unknown. The current data strongly suggest that CSFs should be initiated as early as possible in those exposed to a survivable whole-body dose of radiation and who are at risk of the hematopoietic syndrome (> 3 Gy).[83,84]

These data collectively demonstrate that CSFs and extensive medical support may not only ameliorate radiation-induced neutropenia[117] but also offer a survival advantage, especially if employed early. These data justify the treatment recommendations recently published by the Strategic National Stockpile Radiation Working Group.[12] The following cytokines are choices available for patients expected to experience severe neutropenia:

- Filgrastim (G-CSF) 2.5–5 μg/kg/d every day subcutaneously, or the equivalent (100–200 μg/m^2/d)
- Sargramostim (GM-CSF) 5–10 μg/kg/d every day subcutaneously, or the equivalent (200–400 μg/m^2/d)
- Pegfilgrastim (pegG-CSF) 6 mg once subcutaneously

Treatment with CSFs for expected exposures greater than 2 Gy should begin within 2 days.[118] CSFs have been associated with rare splenic rupture and, more commonly, bone pain.[119] Allogeneic stem cell transplantation may have limited use due to severe morbidity and mortality associated with concurrent

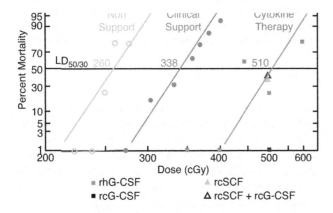

Figure 2-8. Influence of clinical support and cytokine therapy on canine mortality at 3.5 Gy.
Graph courtesy of Dr Thomas MacVittie.

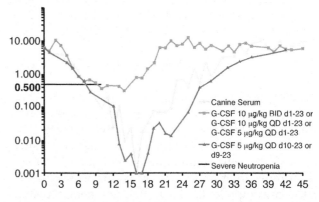

Figure 2-9. Onset of neutropenia and recovery after placebo and colony-stimulating factor given early (day 1) or late (day 10); x-axis is days postirradiation, y-axis is white blood cell count.
Graph courtesy of permission Dr Thomas MacVittie.

nonhematopoietic injuries sustained at marrow-lethal doses of radiation.[18]

Various hospital issues are clinically important when managing patients who have sustained doses greater than 2 to 3 Gy, including:

- antibiotic prophylaxis, as well as antiviral and antifungal agents;
- barrier isolation and gastrointestinal decontamination;
- early cytokine therapy;
- early surgical wound closure and avoidance of unnecessary invasive procedures;
- isolation rooms for ARS patients with whole-body doses greater than 2 to 3 Gy (medical personnel should also be aware of the need for rigorous environmental control, including potential laminar flow isolation, strict hand washing, and surgical scrubs and masks for staff);
- physiological interventions, including maintaining gastric acidity, avoiding antacids and H2 blockers, and using sucralfate for stress-ulcer prophylaxis, when indicated, to reduce gastric colonization and pneumonia (early oral enteral feeding is highly desirable when feasible); and
- povidone-iodine or chlorhexidine for skin disinfection and shampoo, as well as meticulous oral hygiene.

Supportive Care

Transfusion of cellular components, such as packed red blood cells and platelets, is required for patients with severe bone-marrow damage and is an important component of clinical management. Fortunately, this complication does not typically occur for 2 to 4 weeks after the exposure unless losses from concurrent trauma are present. All cellular products must be leukoreduced and irradiated to 25 Gy. The latter prevents transfusion-associated graft-versus-host disease in immunosuppressed patients.

In nonneutropenic patients, antibiotics should be directed toward the foci of infection and the most likely pathogens. For those who experience significant neutropenia (absolute neutrophil count < 500 cells/mm^3), broad-spectrum prophylactic antimicrobials should be given during the potentially long duration of neutropenia.[49] Prophylaxis should include a fluoroquinolone (FQ), an antiviral agent (if indicated, as discussed below), and an antifungal agent. The justification for FQ prophylaxis includes preclinical and clinical studies demonstrating decreased infectious episodes in irradiated animals and neutropenic oncology patients, respectively.[13,120,121] Streptococcal coverage with the addition of penicillin or amoxicillin should also be considered, if not inherently covered by the FQ, given the increased treatment failure observed due to this pathogen and the benefit demonstrated with expanded antistreptococcal coverage in neutropenic animals.[13]

Antimicrobials should be continued until the patient experiences a neutropenic fever and requires alternate coverage or experiences neutrophil recovery (absolute neutrophil count > 500 cells/mm^3). In patients who experience fever first, traditionally the FQ is stopped and therapy is directed at gram-negative bacteria (in particular, *Pseudomonas aeruginosa*), as infections of this type may be rapidly lethal. Antipseudomonal coverage serves as the foundation antibiotic, and additional coverage is then added to address other foci of infection, such as mucosal or integument injury. Empiric therapy of patients with febrile neutropenia with or without a focus of infection should be guided by the current recommendations of the Infectious Diseases Society of America.[122–126] Any focus of infection that develops during the neutropenic period will require a full course of therapy.

MEDICAL ISSUES IN PATIENT MANAGEMENT

ARS is seen to be a sequence of phased symptoms. It is characterized by the relatively rapid onset of nausea, vomiting, malaise, and anorexia. An early onset of prodromal symptoms in the absence of associated trauma suggests a large radiation exposure. The medical management of ARS has two primary goals: hematological support to reduce both the depth and duration of neutropenia, and prevention and management of neutropenic fever.

The onset and depth of neutropenia is directly determined by the severity of the accident. In order to gauge the severity of an incident, radiation dose to a patient can be estimated early after the event using rapid-sort, automated biodosimetry[127–130] and clinical parameters such as the onset of various clinical symptom complexes,[131] TE,[13,54,57,85,132] and lymphocyte depletion kinetics,[13,40,55] and through combinations of various biochemical entities.[3,5,6,127,133] No single technique is satisfactorily sensitive, but multiparameter techniques have been shown to have good predictive value.[5,127,133–135]

For external doses less than 1 Gy, the patient is generally asymptomatic and blood parameters will be within the normal range. Upon admission to emergency care following the incident, it is always appropriate to obtain a complete blood count with differential, either as a baseline level or as a beginning step for lymphocyte kinetic analysis. TE, measured from the irradiating event, generally decreases with increasing dose. For TE between 1 and 2 hours, the effective whole-body dose is likely at least 3 to 4 Gy. If TE is less than 1 hour, the whole-body dose likely exceeds 4 to 6 Gy. In a mass casualty tactical event, patients who experience emesis less than 4 hours after the accident should be triaged to professional medical care, while those with emesis after more than 4 hours can be instructed to receive delayed medical attention. Patients who experience radiation-induced emesis within 1 hour after a radiation incident will require extensive and prolonged medical intervention, and an ultimately fatal outcome will occur in many instances.

Patient radiation dose and expected prognosis in a radiation event may be estimated from the medical history and timing of symptom complexes, serial lymphocyte counts, TE, and confirmatory chromosome-aberration cytogenetics. In addition, close collaboration with health physics experts is critical, since dose reconstruction personnel often have access to an array of sophisticated mathematical analysis techniques to estimate the dose field.

The prodromal symptoms of nausea and emesis will be particularly troublesome to patients. The following dosages of selective 5-HT3 receptor antagonists are recommended for radiation-induced emesis:

- Ondansetron: initially 0.15 mg/kg IV; a continuous IV dose option consists of 8 mg followed by 1 mg/h for the next 24 hours. Oral dose is 8 mg every 8 hours as needed.
- Granisetron (oral dosage form): dose is usually 1 mg initially, then repeated 12 hours after the first dose. Alternatively, 2 mg may be taken as one dose. IV dose is based on body weight; typically 10 µg/kg (4.5 µg/lb) of body weight.

The patient history, physical examination, and early estimate of the severity of the radiation incident may be rapidly analyzed, using multiple clinical and dosimetric parameters, into a clinically meaningful estimate of radiation exposure using the AFRRI Biodosimetry Assessment Tool software package, which is available at no cost (www.afrri.usuhs.mil). Estimation of dose purely from the lymphocyte depletion rate constant is a quantitative enhancement of the classical Andrews model.[1,136,137] Two additional Web resources are useful to the physician charged with treating radiation casualties. The radiation event medical management Web site (http://www.remm.nlm.gov/) developed by the US Department of Health and Human Services, National Cancer Institute, and the National Library of Medicine is an important resource in patient management. In addition, the Centers for Disease Control and Prevention has a useful compendium of radiation medicine information and protocols (http://www.bt.cdc.gov/radiation/). As an additional medical resource, the recommendations of the Strategic National Stockpile Radiation Working Group[12] are considered to be a primary reference document for modern medical management of ARS.

When the irradiated patient is first evaluated, the following laboratory test results are important to acquire, as time permits.

- Required initial laboratory test results (in the field or in the emergency department):
  o complete blood count with differential (repeat every 6 h) to evaluate lymphocyte kinetics and calculate the neutrophil–lymphocyte ratio, and
  o serum amylase (baseline and daily after 24 h). A dose-dependent increase in amylase is expected after 24 hours.
- Other important laboratory test results to obtain:
  o blood FMS-like tyrosine kinase 3 ligand levels (marker for hematopoietic damage),
  o blood citrulline (decreasing citrulline indicates gastrointestinal damage),
  o cytogenetic studies with overdispersion index to evaluate for partial-body exposure,
  o interleukin-6 (blood marker is increased at higher radiation doses),
  o quantitative G-CSF (blood marker is increased at higher radiation doses), and
  o C-reactive protein (increases with dose as an acute-phase reactant; shows promise to discriminate early between minimally and heavily exposed patients).

For a small-volume scenario[12] (< 100 casualties), consider early cytokine therapy, fluid support, and antibiotic prophylaxis in the dose range of 2 to 6 Gy, if there is no significant trauma. At doses greater than 6 Gy without trauma, it is also prudent to consider stem cell transplantation therapy.[12] With doses in the region of 2 to 6 Gy and with burns or trauma, cytokines and antibiotic therapy are warranted. For doses greater than 6 Gy with burns or trauma, the patient is probably expectant. The severely neutropenic patient must be evaluated carefully, using the Infectious Disease Society of America's recommendations and other expert guidelines for the treatment of neutropenic fever.[138–146]

SELECTED ASPECTS OF CURRENT RESEARCH

The field of ARS research is progressing rapidly and any discussion is likely to be just as rapidly dated. However, many promising avenues of treatment have been shown in the preclinical phase or in early clinical evaluations.

AFRRI and a research partner recently achieved FDA clearance for 5-androstenediol (5-AED) to be evaluated in Phase 1 human clinical trials. Cytokines, as discussed above, are useful but costly to transport and store, unstable at room and high environmental temperatures, and must be used under the care of a physician. Those limitations make cytokines impractical for use in a mass casualty radiation scenario, which could leave many victims without access to physicians, hospitals, or roads to access either. Moreover, while G-CSF causes elevations in certain types of white blood cells, it does not stimulate production of platelets. AFRRI's preclinical trials for 5-AED showed an excellent safety and efficacy profile. Therefore it appears to be useful as a single therapy, without need for physician or medical support, in a mass casualty scenario. Research on 5-AED addresses two of the major problems causing mortality after irradiation—loss of infection-fighting white blood cells and loss of platelets—which lead to excessive bleeding. 5-AED also ameliorates the drop in red blood cells seen after high-level external irradiation (Figure 2-10).[147–154] The AFRRI Radiation Countermeasures Branch continues to develop additional pharmacological countermeasures to radiation injury that can be used by military personnel and by emergency responders and to develop a better understanding of the biology of radiation injury and radiation countermeasure drugs. Knowledge of biochemical processes involved in radiation injury and countermeasures can be used to identify and assess novel drug candidates. AFRRI actively collaborates with other research institutions, pharmaceutical firms, and government agencies to develop and obtain approval for radiation countermeasures for use in the field and the clinic.

Possible countermeasures to ionizing radiation can be broadly categorized into three groups: (1) drugs that prevent the initial radiation injury (free-radical antioxidants, hypoxia-generating drugs, and enzymatic detoxification and oncogene targeting agents); (2) drugs that repair the molecular damage caused by radiation either by hydrogen transfer or enzymatic repair; and (3) drugs that stimulate proliferation of surviving stem and progenitor cells, such as immunomodulators and growth factors and cytokines. The availability of medical facilities for radiation casualties after a nuclear detonation near a city will be problem-

atic. In light of the logistical realities of likely nuclear disaster scenarios, much of the current focus is on drug candidates with extremely low toxicity and ease of administration, suitable for use outside the clinic without physician supervision.

Radiation countermeasure candidates tested for efficacy at AFRRI are chosen based on extensive basic research, which increases the probability of eventual clinical success. All four ARS countermeasures currently with FDA investigational new drug status (2010) are AFRRI products. Two (5-AED and BIO 300 [Humanetics, Eden Prairie, MN]) were conceived, initiated, and developed at AFRRI. The two others (Ex-RAD [Onconova, Newtown, PA]; and CBLB502 [Cleveland BioLabs, Inc, Buffalo, NY]) were the subjects of company-initiated research programs that AFRRI joined at early stages. Furthermore and as noted above, the current standard, off-label treatment for ARS, administration of hematopoietic cytokines such as G-CSF, was conceived, initiated, and developed at AFRRI. AFRRI has an ongoing in-vivo efficacy-screening program and is frequently approached by organizations for research collaboration and consultation regarding its promising countermeasure can-

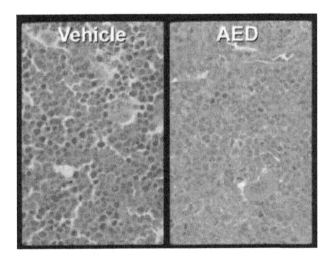

Figure 2-10. Bone marrow from a mouse treated with 5-androstenediol (right), compared with marrow from a mouse treated with placebo (left). The many small, round, dark objects in the control section are nuclei in progenitors of red blood cells. Progenitors of granulocytes (mostly neutrophils) and monocytes possess lighter nuclei, often horseshoe-shaped. Four days after 5-androstenediol treatment, there was a proliferation of granulocyte/monocyte progenitors. Slide courtesy of the US Armed Forces Radiobiology Research Institute.

didates. This screening program is supplemented by a robust research program that provides supporting data for approval of existing drugs and identification of potential drug targets.

Radioprotectants are another class of drugs that are designed to be used before or shortly after exposure. These include antioxidants such as gamma tocotrienol (a vitamin-E moiety),[155,156] or genistein (a soy by-product) to increase survivability. Assessed effects of genistein on hematopoietic progenitor cell recovery in irradiated mice have documented that genistein operates on radiation-responsive gene expression. Genistein also protects against delayed radiation effects in the lungs and induces cytokine production in whole-body gamma-irradiated mice.[157] The use of advanced nutraceuticals as radioprotectants has shown that vitamin E is an effective radioprotectant. This research has also characterized the radioprotectant properties of soy-derived isoflavones and has demonstrated induction of cytokines by vitamin-E–related analogs. In addition, tocopherol succinate has been found to be a promising radiation countermeasure. A tocol antioxidant, gamma-tocotrienol, acts as a potent radioprotector, and alpha-tocopherol succinate has been shown to protect mice from gamma-radiation by induction of G-CSF and by preventing persistent DNA (deoxyribonucleic acid) damage. A recent review

article describes the history and scope of radioprotectants in research and in clinical radiation medicine.[158]

An entity important in the clinical management of ARS is severe mucositis, which often appears in patients with high-dose external irradiation. Keratinocyte growth factor (KGF) has been shown to decrease the incidence and duration of severe oral mucositis in patients with hematologic malignancies who are receiving myelotoxic therapy and require hematopoietic stem cell support. The safety and efficacy of KGF have not been established in patients with nonhematologic malignancies[18]; however, it is likely that KGF would be of use in the treatment of ARS.

Another severe manifestation of high-level dose—gastrointestinal syndrome—has defied effective treatment over the years.[75,159–162] Currently, mixed data is available for treating and mitigating gastrointestinal syndrome. Current treatment modalities include gastrointestinal decontamination with FQs, vancomycin, polymyxin B sulfate, and antifungals (as medically indicated). In addition, L-glutamine has been found to be a helpful adjunct, along with supportive care. Nutrition options include total parenteral nutrition, elemental diets, and fluid and electrolyte repletion. There is also active current research on the use of growth factors to protect intestinal stem cells from radiation-induced apoptosis.[163–165]

SUMMARY

Victims of acute radiation events in radiological and nuclear incidents will require prompt diagnosis and treatment of medical and surgical conditions as well as conditions related to possible radiation exposure. Emergency personnel should triage victims using traditional military medical and trauma criteria. Radiation dose to military personnel can be estimated early after the event using rapid-sort, automated biodosimetry and clinical parameters, such as the clinical history and timing of symptom complexes, TE, lymphocyte depletion kinetics, and various multiparameter biochemical tests. Acute high-level radiation exposure should be clinically treated as a medical case

involving MOF. Radiation-induced MOD and MOF refer to progressive dysfunction of two or more organ systems with the etiological agent as radiation damage to cells and tissues over time. Radiation-associated MOD appears to develop in part as a consequence of the systemic inflammatory response syndrome and in part as a consequence of radiation-induced loss of the functional cell mass of vital organs. Modern guidance to the medical management of radiation-induced MOF is presented in this chapter and it is hoped that this will serve as a comprehensive educational resource for the physician likely to be involved in managing patients in a radiation incident.

REFERENCES

1. Andrews GA. Treatment of radiation injury. *J Miss State Med Assoc*. 1966;7(10):534–538.

2. Andrews GA. Radiation accidents and their management. *Radiat Res Suppl*. 1967;7:390–397.

3. Ossetrova NI, Sandgren DJ, Gallego S, Blakely WF. Combined approach of hematological biomarkers and plasma protein SAA for improvement of radiation dose assessment triage in biodosimetry applications. *Health Phys*. 2010;98(2):204–208.

4. Prasanna PG, Blakely WF, Bertho JM, et al. Synopsis of partial-body radiation diagnostic biomarkers and medical management of radiation injury workshop. *Radiat Res*. 2010;173(2):245–253.

5. Blakely WF, Ossetrova NI, Whitnall MH, et al. Multiple parameter radiation injury assessment using a nonhuman primate radiation model-biodosimetry applications. *Health Phys.* 2010;98(2):153–159.

6. Ossetrova NI, Blakely WF. Multiple blood-proteins approach for early-response exposure assessment using an in vivo murine radiation model. *Int J Radiat Biol.* 2009;85(10):837–850.

7. Wald N, Thoma GE Jr. Radiation accidents: medical aspects of neutron and gamma-ray exposures. *ORNL.* 1961;PtB:1–177.

8. Koenig KL, Goans RE, Hatchett RJ, et al. Medical treatment of radiological casualties: current concepts. *Ann Emerg Med.* 2005;45(6):643–652.

9. Flynn DF, Goans RE. Nuclear terrorism: triage and medical management of radiation and combined-injury casualties. *Surg Clin North Am.* 2006;86(3):601–636.

10. Bader JL, Nemhauser J, Chang F, et al. Radiation event medical management (REMM): website guidance for health care providers. *Prehosp Emerg Care.* 2008;12(1):1–11.

11. Fliedner TM, D Dörr H, Meineke V. Multi-organ involvement as a pathogenetic principle of the radiation syndromes: a study involving 110 case histories documented in SEARCH and classified as the bases of haematopoietic indicators of effect. *BJR Suppl.* 2005;27:1–8.

12. Waselenko JK, MacVittie TJ, Blakely WF, et al. Medical management of the acute radiation syndrome: recommendations of the Strategic National Stockpile Radiation Working Group. *Ann Intern Med.* 2004;140(12):1037–1051.

13. Goans RE, Waselenko JK. Medical management of radiological casualties. *Health Phys.* 2005;89(5):505–512.

14. Kuniak M, Azizova T, Day R, et al. The Radiation Injury Severity Classification system: an early injury assessment tool for the frontline health-care provider. *Br J Radiol.* 2008;81(963):232–243.

15. Azizova TV, Osovets SV, Day RD, et al. Predictability of acute radiation injury severity. *Health Phys.* 2008;94(3):255–263.

16. Berger ME, Christensen DM, Lowry PC, Jones OW, Wiley AL. Medical management of radiation injuries: current approaches. *Occup Med (Lond).* 2006;56(3):162–172.

17. Coleman CN, Hrdina C, Bader JL, et al. Medical response to a radiologic/nuclear event: integrated plan from the Office of the Assistant Secretary for Preparedness and Response, Department of Health and Human Services. *Ann Emerg Med.* 2009;53(2):213–222.

18. Hatchett RJ, Kaminski JM, Goans RE. Nuclear and radiological events. In: Koenig KL, Schultz CH, eds. *Koenig and Schultz's Disaster Medicine: Comprehensive Principles and Practices.* Cambridge, England: Cambridge University Press; 2009: 477–510.

19. Fliedner TM, Powles R, Sirohi B, Niederwieser D. Radiologic and nuclear events: the METREPOL severity of effect grading system. *Blood.* 2008;111(12):5757–5758; author reply 5758–5759.

20. Meineke V, Fliedner TM. Radiation-induced multi-organ involvement and failure: challenges for radiation accident medical management and future research. *BJR Suppl.* 2005;27:196–200.

21. Konchalovsky MV, Baranov AE, Kolganov AV. Multiple organ involvement and failure: selected Russian radiation accident cases re-visited. *BJR Suppl.* 2005;27:26–29.

22. Goans RE, Wald N. Radiation accidents with multi-organ failure in the United States. *BJR Suppl.* 2005;27:41–46.

23. Gourmelon P, Marquette C, Agay D, Mathieu J, Clarencon D. Involvement of the central nervous system in radiation-induced multi-organ dysfunction and/or failure. *BJR Suppl.* 2005;27:62–68.

24. Akashi M. Role of infection and bleeding in multiple organ involvement and failure. *BJR Suppl.* 2005;27:69–74.

25. Boothman DA, Reichrath J. New basic science initiatives for improved understanding of radiation-induced multi-organ dysfunction syndrome (MODS). *BJR Suppl.* 2005;27:157–160.

26. Gorin NC, Fliedner TM, Gourmelon P, et al. Consensus conference on European preparedness for haematological and other medical management of mass radiation accidents. *Ann Hematol.* 2006;85(10):671–679.

27. American Society of Clinical Oncology. Recommendations for the use of hematopoietic colony-stimulating factors: evidence-based, clinical practice guidelines. *J Clin Oncol.* 1994;12(11):2471–2508.

28. Fliedner TM. Nuclear terrorism: the role of hematology in coping with its health consequences. *Curr Opin Hematol.* 2006;13(6):436–444.

29. Mettler FA Jr, Moseley RD Jr. Medical effects of ionizing radiation. Orlando, FL: Grune & Stratton; 1985.

30. Mettler FA Jr, Kelsey CA, Ricks RC. *Medical Management of Radiation Accidents.* Boca Raton, FL: CRC Press; 1990.

31. Mettler FA, Upton AC. *Medical Effects of Ionizing Radiation.* 3rd ed. Philadelphia, PA: Saunders/Elsevier; 2008.

32. Gusev IA, Gus'kova AK, Mettler FA. *Medical Management of Radiation Accidents.* 2nd ed. Boca Raton, FL: CRC Press; 2001.

33. Mettler FA, Johnson JC, Thaul S; Institute of Medicine (US) Committee on Battlefield Radiation Exposure Criteria. *An Evaluation of Radiation Exposure Guidance for Military Operations: Interim Report.* Washington, DC: National Academy Press; 1997.

34. Walker RI, Cerveny TJ, eds. *Medical Consequences of Nuclear Warfare.* In: Zajtchuk R, Bellamy RF, eds. *Textbook of Military Medicine.* Washington, DC: Department of the Army, Office of The Surgeon General, Borden Institute; 1989.

35. Hübner KF, Fry SA, Radiation Emergency Assistance Center/Training Site. *The Medical Basis for Radiation Accident Preparedness: Proceedings of the REAC/TS International Conference: The Medical Basis for Radiation Accident Preparedness, October 18–20, 1979, Oak Ridge, Tennessee, U.S.A.* New York, NY: Elsevier/North-Holland; 1980.

36. Ricks RC, Fry SA, Radiation Emergency Assistance Center/Training Site. *The Medical Basis for Radiation Accident Preparedness II: Clinical Experience and Follow-Up Since 1979: Proceedings of the Second International REAC/TS Conference on the Medical Basis for Radiation Accident Preparedness, Held October 20–22, 1988.* New York, NY: Elsevier; 1990.

37. Ricks RC, Berger ME, O'Hara FM. *The Medical Basis for Radiation-Accident Preparedness III: The Psychological Perspective: Proceedings of the Third International REAC/TS Conference on the Medical Basis for Radiation-Accident Preparedness Held From December 5–7, 1990, in Oak Ridge, Tennessee.* New York, NY: Elsevier; 1991.

38. Ricks RC, Berger ME, O'Hara FM. *The Medical Basis for Radiation-Accident Preparedness: The Clinical Care of Victims: Proceedings of the Fourth International REAC/TS Conference on the Medical Basis for Radiation-Accident Preparedness, Held March 6–8, 2001, in Orlando, Florida.* Boca Raton, FL: Parthenon Publishing Group; 2002.

39. Hirama T, Tanosaki S, Kandatsu S, et al. Initial medical management of patients severely irradiated in the Tokai-mura criticality accident. *Br J Radiol.* 2003;76(904):246–253.

40. Goans RE, Holloway EC, Berger ME, Ricks RC. Early dose assessment following severe radiation accidents. *Health Phys.* 1997;72(4):513–518.

41. Bergonie J, Tribondeau L. De quelques résultats de la radiothérapie et essai de fixation d'une technique rationnelle. *Comptes-Rendus des Séances de l'Académie des Sciences.* 1906;143:983–985.

42. Fliedner TM, Graessle DH. Hematopoietic cell renewal systems: mechanisms of coping and failing after chronic exposure to ionizing radiation. *Radiat Environ Biophys.* 2008;47(1):63–69.

43. Baranov AE, Rozhdestvenskii LM. [The analytical review of the schemes of the acute radiation disease treatment used in experiment and in clinic]. *Radiats Biol Radioecol.* 2008;48(3):287–302.

44. Cronkite EP, Bond VP, Chandra P, Rai KR. *Hematopoietic Cellular Proliferation: An International Conference in Honor of Eugene P. Cronkite.* New York, NY: New York Academy of Sciences; 1985.

45. Dainiak N, Sorba S. Early identification of radiation accident victims for therapy of bone marrow failure. *Stem Cells.* 1997;15(suppl 2):275–285.

46. Doughty HA. Medical management of the haemopoietic syndrome in acute radiation sickness. *J R Army Med Corps.* 2004;150(3 suppl 1):11–16.

47. Jones TD, Morris MD, Young RW. A mathematical model for radiation-induced myelopoiesis. *Radiat Res.* 1991;128(3):258–266.

48. Jones TD, Morris MD, Young RW. Mathematical models of marrow cell kinetics: differential effects of protracted irradiations on stromal and stem cells in mice. *Int J Radiat Oncol Biol Phys.* 1993;26(5):817–830.

49. Dainiak N, Waselenko JK, Armitage JO, MacVittie TJ, Farese AM. The hematologist and radiation casualties. *Hematology Am Soc Hematol Educ Program.* 2003:473–496.

50. Jones TD, Morris MD, Young RW. Dose-rate RBE factors for photons: hematopoietic syndrome in humans vs. stromal cell cytopenia. *Health Phys.* 1994;67(5):495–508.

51. Jones TD, Morris MD, Young RW, Kehlet RA. A cell-kinetics model for radiation-induced myelopoiesis. *Exp Hematol.* 1993;21(6):816-822.

52. Cerveny TJ, MacVittae TJ. Young RW. Acute radiation syndrome in humans. In: Walker RI, Cerveny TJ, eds. *Medical Consequences of Nuclear Warfare.* In: Zajtchuk R, Bellamy RF, eds. *Textbook of Military Medicine.* Washington, DC: Department of the Army, Office of The Surgeon General, Borden Institute; 1989.

53. Fliedner TM, Chao NJ, Bader JL, et al. Stem cells, multiorgan failure in radiation emergency medical preparedness: a U.S./European Consultation Workshop. *Stem Cells.* 2009;27(5):1205–1211.

54. Anno GH, Baum SJ, Withers HR, Young RW. Symptomatology of acute radiation effects in humans after exposure to doses of 0.5–30 Gy. *Health Phys.* 1989;56(6):821–838.

55. Goans RE, Holloway EC, Berger ME, Ricks RC. Early dose assessment in criticality accidents. *Health Phys.* 2001;81(4):446–449.

56. Mettler FA Jr, Gus'kova AK, Gusev I. Health effects in those with acute radiation sickness from the Chernobyl accident. *Health Phys.* 2007;93(5):462–469.

57. Parker DD, Parker JC. Estimating radiation dose from time to emesis and lymphocyte depletion. *Health Phys.* 2007;93(6):701–704.

58. Chaillet MP, Cosset JM, Socie G, et al. Prospective study of the clinical symptoms of therapeutic whole body irradiation. *Health Phys.* 1993;64(4):370–374.

59. Fliedner TM. On the hematology of acute radiation syndrome [in German]. *Strahlentherapie.* 1960;112:543–560.

60. van Bekkum DW. Radiation sensitivity of the hemopoietic stem cell. *Radiat Res.* 1991;128(1 suppl):S4–S8.

61. Vorobiev AI. Acute radiation disease and biological dosimetry in 1993. *Stem Cells.* 1997;15(suppl 2):269–274.

62. Fliedner TM. Physiopathology of radiosensitivity in bone marrow [article in German]. *Strahlenschutz Forsch Prax.* 1973;13:38–48.

63. Gus'kova AK, Baranov AE. The hematological effects in those exposed to radiation in the accident at the Chernobyl Atomic Electric Power Station [article in Russian]. *Med Radiol (Mosk).* 1991;36(8):31–37.

64. Barabanova AV. Significance of beta-radiation skin burns in Chernobyl patients for the theory and practice of radio-pathology. *Vojnosanit Pregl*. 2006;63(5):477–480.

65. Rubin DB. *The Radiation Biology of the Vascular Endothelium*. Boca Raton, FL: CRC Press; 1998.

66. Augustine AD, Gondre-Lewis T, McBride W, Miller L, Pellmar TC, Rockwell S. Animal models for radiation injury, protection and therapy. *Radiat Res*. 2005;164(1):100–109.

67. Bruckner V. Demonstration of gastrointestinal hemorrhages in the acute radiation syndrome [article in German]. *Strahlentherapie*. 1975;149(6):597–601.

68. DuBois A, King GL, Livengood DR. *Radiation and the Gastrointestinal Tract*. Boca Raton, FL: CRC Press; 1995.

69. Igaki H, Nakagawa K, Uozaki H, et al. Pathological changes in the gastrointestinal tract of a heavily radiation-exposed worker at the Tokai-mura criticality accident. *J Radiat Res (Tokyo)*. 2008;49(1):55–62.

70. Potten CS, Hendry JH. *Radiation and Gut*. New York, NY: Elsevier; 1995.

71. Meineke V, van Beuningen D, Sohns T, Fliedner TM. Medical management principles for radiation accidents. *Mil Med*. 2003;168(3):219–222.

72. Maj JG, Paris F, Haimovitz-Friedman A, Venkatraman E, Kolesnick R, Fuks Z. Microvascular function regulates intestinal crypt response to radiation. *Cancer Res*. 2003;63(15):4338–4341.

73. Bories-Azeau A, Dayan L. The radiolesions of the small bowel (author's transl) [article in French]. *Sem Hop*. 1980;56(1–2):65–72.

74. Ende M. Management of the acute radiation syndrome. *Ann Intern Med*. 2004;141(11):891.

75. Freshwater DA. Effects of nuclear weapons on the gastrointestinal system. *J R Army Med Corps*. 2004;150(3 suppl 1):17–21.

76. Hopewell JW. Models of CNS radiation damage during space flight. *Adv Space Res*. 1994;14(10):433–442.

77. Kamarád V. Acute radiation sickness—morphology of CNS syndrome. *Acta Univ Palacki Olomuc Fac Med*. 1989;121:7–144.

78. Slatkin DN, Stoner RD, Rosander KM, Kalef-Ezra JA, Laissue JA. Central nervous system radiation syndrome in mice from preferential 10B(n, alpha)7Li irradiation of brain vasculature. *Proc Natl Acad Sci U S A*. 1988;85(11):4020–4024.

79. Jackson WL Jr, Gallagher C, Myhand RC, Waselenko JK. Medical management of patients with multiple organ dysfunction arising from acute radiation syndrome. *BJR Suppl*. 2005;27:161–168.

80. Baverstock KF, Ash PJ. A review of radiation accidents involving whole body exposure and the relevance to the $LD_{50/60}$ for man. *Br J Radiol*. 1983;56(671):837–844.

81. Jones TD. Hematologic syndrome in man modeled from mammalian lethality. *Health Phys*. 1981;41(1):83–103.

82. Anno GH, Young RW, Bloom RM, Mercier JR. Dose response relationships for acute ionizing-radiation lethality. *Health Phys*. 2003;84(5):565–575.

83. MacVittie TJ. Therapy of radiation injury. *Stem Cells*. 1997;15(suppl 2):263–268.

84. MacVittie TJ, Farese AM. Cytokine-based treatment of radiation injury: potential benefits after low-level radiation exposure. *Mil Med*. 2002;167(2 suppl):68–70.

85. Anno GH, Bloom RM. Combined effects modeling of ionizing radiation and biological agent exposures. *Mil Med*. 2002;167(2 suppl):107–109.

86. DiCarlo AL, Hatchett RJ, Kaminski JM, et al. Medical countermeasures for radiation combined injury: radiation with burn, blast, trauma and/or sepsis. Report of an NIAID Workshop, March 26–27, 2007. *Radiat Res*. 2008;169(6):712–721.

87. Engelhardt M, Kaffenberger W, Abend M, Gerngross H, Willy C. Radiation and burn trauma (combined injury). Considerations in surgical treatment [article in German]. *Unfallchirurg*. 2001;104(4):333–342.

88. Gogin EE. Clinical effects of combined radiation injuries [article in Russian]. *Ter Arkh*. 1987;59(6):8–14.

89. Knudson GB, Elliott TB, Brook I, et al. Nuclear, biological, and chemical combined injuries and countermeasures on the battlefield. *Mil Med*. 2002;167(2 suppl):95–97.

90. Fliedner TM. Hiroshima—then and today [article in German]. *Dtsch Med Wochenschr*. 1977;102(31):1111–1113.

91. Hiroshima Research Group of Atomic Bomb Casualties. *Physical and Medical Effects of the Atomic Bomb in Hiroshima*. Tokyo, Japan: Maruzen Co; 1958.

92. Committee for the Compilation of Materials on Damage Caused by the Atomic Bombs in Hiroshima and Nagasaki. *Hiroshima and Nagasaki, the Physical, Medical, and Social Effects of the Atomic Bombings*. New York, NY: Basic Books; 1981.

93. Oughterson AW, Warren S; Joint Commission for the Investigation of the Effects of the Atomic Bomb in Japan. *Medical Effects of the Atomic Bomb in Japan*. 1st ed. New York, NY: McGraw-Hill; 1956.

94. United States Strategic Bombing Survey. *The Effects of Atomic Bombs on Health and Medical Services in Hiroshima and Nagasaki*. Washington, DC: Medical Division; 1947.

95. Dainiak N; International Consortium for Research on the Health Effects of Radiation. *Radiation Injury and the Chernobyl Catastrophe*. Miamisburg, OH: AlphaMed Press; 1997.

96. Gus'kova AK, Baranov AE, Barabanova AV, Gruzdev GP, Piatkin EK. Acute radiation effects in victims of the accident at the Chernobyl nuclear power station [article in Russian]. *Med Radiol (Mosk)*. 1987;32(12):3–18.

97. Duque RE, Phan SH, Hudson JL, Till GO, Ward PA. Functional defects in phagocytic cells following thermal injury. Application of flow cytometric analysis. *Am J Pathol*. 1985;118(1):116–127.

98. Shires GT, Dineen P. Sepsis following burns, trauma, and intra-abdominal infections. *Arch Intern Med*. 1982;142(11):2012–2022.

99. Munster AM. Post-traumatic immunosuppression is due to activation of suppressor T cells. *Lancet*. 1976;1(7973):1329–1330.

100. Hernadi F, Valyi Nagy T. Role of antibiotics in the treatment of acute radiation syndrome [article in Hungarian]. *Orv Hetil*. 1963;104:913–917.

101. Knief RA. *Nuclear Criticality Safety: Theory and Practice*. La Grange Park, IL: American Nuclear Society; 1991.

102. McLaughlin TPM, Monahan SP, Pruvost NL, Frolov VV, Ryazanov BG, Sviridov VI. *A Review of Criticality Accidents*. Los Alamos, NM: Los Alamos National Laboratory; May 2000. LA-13638.

103. Hempelmann LH, Lisco H, Hoffman JG. The acute radiation syndrome: a study of nine cases and a review of the problem. *Ann Intern Med*. 1952;36(2:1):279–510.

104. Hempelmann LH. Example of the acute radiation syndrome in man. *N Engl J Med*. 1952;246(20):776–782.

105. Shipman TL, Lushbaugh LL, Peterson DF, Langham WH, Harris PS, Lawrence JNP. Acute radiation death resulting from an accidental nuclear critical excursion. *J Occup Med*. 1961;Suppl:145–192.

106. Karas JS, Stanbury JB. Fatal radiation syndrome from an accidental nuclear excursion. *N Engl J Med*. 1965;272:755–761.

107. Fanger H, Lushbaugh CC. Radiation death from cardiovascular shock following a criticality accident. Report of a second death from a newly defined human radiation death syndrome. *Arch Pathol.* 1967;83(5):446–460.

108. Warren S. *The Pathology of Ionizing Radiation.* Springfield, IL: Thomas; 1961.

109. Lapin BA, ed. *Pathogenesis, Clinical Treatment and Therapy of Acute Radiation Sickness Based on Experiments with Monkeys. An All-Union Symposium.* Jerusalem: Israel Program for Scientific Translations; available from the US Department of Commerce, 1967.

110. Berdjis CC. *Pathology of Irradiation.* Baltimore, MD: Williams & Wilkins; 1971.

111. Casarett GW. *Radiation Histopathology.* Boca Raton, FL: CRC Press; 1980.

112. Fajardo LF, Berthrong M, Anderson RE. Radiation pathology. New York, NY: Oxford University Press; 2001.

113. Rubin P, Casarett GW. *Clinical Radiation Pathology.* Philadelphia, PA: Saunders; 1968.

114. White DC. *An Atlas of Radiation Histopathology.* Oak Ridge, TN: Technical Information Center, Office of Public Affairs, US Energy Research and Development Administration; 1975.

115. Fliedner TM, Friesecke I, Beyrer K. *Medical Management of Radiation Accidents: Manual on the Acute Radiation Syndrome.* London, England: British Institute of Radiology; 2001.

116. MacVittie TJ, Farese AM, Jackson W 3rd. Defining the full therapeutic potential of recombinant growth factors in the post radiation-accident environment: the effect of supportive care plus administration of G-CSF. *Health Phys.* 2005;89(5):546–555.

117. Levenga TH, Timmer-Bonte JN. Review of the value of colony stimulating factors for prophylaxis of febrile neutropenic episodes in adult patients treated for haematological malignancies. *Br J Haematol.* 2007;138(2):146–152.

118. Hogan DE, Kellison T. Nuclear terrorism. *Am J Med Sci.* 2002;323(6):341–349.

119. Schneider SB, Nishimura RD, Zimmerman RP, et al. Filgrastim (r-metHuG-CSF) and its potential use in the reduction of radiation-induced oropharyngeal mucositis: an interim look at a randomized, double-blind, placebo-controlled trial. *Cytokines Cell Mol Ther.* 1999;5(3):175–180.

120. Brook I, Elliott TB. Quinolone therapy in the prevention of mortality after irradiation. *Radiat Res.* 1991;128(1):100–103.

121. Brook I, Elliott TB, Ledney GD. Quinolone therapy of *Klebsiella pneumoniae* sepsis following irradiation: comparison of pefloxacin, ciprofloxacin, and ofloxacin. *Radiat Res.* 1990;122(2):215–217.

122. Morrison VA. An overview of the management of infection and febrile neutropenia in patients with cancer. *Support Cancer Ther.* 2005;2(2):88–94.

123. Feld R. Microbial resistance and the Infectious Diseases Society of America (IDSA) guidelines. *Int J Hematol.* 1998;68(suppl 1):S27–S30.

124. Sharma A, Lokeshwar N. Febrile neutropenia in haematological malignancies. *J Postgrad Med.* 2005;51(suppl 1):S42–S48.

125. Groll AH, Ritter J. Diagnosis and management of fungal infections and pneumocystis pneumonitis in pediatric cancer patients [article in German]. *Klin Padiatr.* 2005;217(suppl 1):S37–S66.

126. Zinner SH. Relevant aspects in the Infectious Diseases Society of America (IDSA) guidelines for the use of antimicrobial agents in neutropenic patients with unexplained fever. *Int J Hematol.* 1998;68(suppl 1):S31–S34.

127. Blakely WF. Multiple parameter biodosimetry of exposed workers from the JCO criticality accident in Tokai-mura. *J Radiol Prot.* 2002;22(1):5–6.

128. Prasanna PG, Kolanko CJ, Gerstenberg HM, Blakely WF. Premature chromosome condensation assay for biodosimetry: studies with fission-neutrons. *Health Phys*. 1997;72(4):594–600.

129. Blakely WF, Salter CA, Prasanna PG. Early-response biological dosimetry—recommended countermeasure enhancements for mass-casualty radiological incidents and terrorism. *Health Phys*. 2005;89(5):494–504.

130. Blakely WF, Miller AC, Grace MB, et al. Radiation biodosimetry: applications for spaceflight. *Adv Space Res*. 2003;31(6):1487–1493.

131. Akashi M, Hirama T, Tanosaki S, et al. Initial symptoms of acute radiation syndrome in the JCO criticality accident in Tokai-mura. *J Radiat Res (Tokyo)*. 2001;42(suppl):S157–S166.

132. Demidenko E, Williams BB, Swartz HM. Radiation dose prediction using data on time to emesis in the case of nuclear terrorism. *Radiat Res*. 2009;171(3):310–319.

133. Bertho JM, Roy L. A rapid multiparametric method for victim triage in cases of accidental protracted irradiation or delayed analysis. *Br J Radiol*. 2009;82(981):764–770.

134. Blakely WF, Prasanna PG, Grace MB, Miller AC. Radiation exposure assessment using cytological and molecular biomarkers. *Radiat Prot Dosimetry*. 2001;97(1):17–23.

135. Bertho JM, Roy L, Souidi M, et al. Initial evaluation and follow-up of acute radiation syndrome in two patients from the Dakar accident. *Biomarkers*. 2009;14(2):94–102.

136. Andrews GA, Cloutier RJ. Accidental acute radiation injury. The need for recognition. *Arch Environ Health*. 1965;10:498–507.

137. Andrews GA, Sitterson BW. Hematologic effects of the accidental radiation exposure at Y-12. *ORINS Rep US At Energy Comm*. 1959;252:1–2.

138. Bodey GP. The changing face of febrile neutropenia—from monotherapy to moulds to mucositis. Fever and neutropenia: the early years. *J Antimicrob Chemother*. 2009;63(suppl 1):i3–13.

139. Pascoe J, Steven N. Antibiotics for the prevention of febrile neutropenia. *Curr Opin Hematol*. 2009;16(1):48–52.

140. Ellis M. Febrile neutropenia. *Ann N Y Acad Sci*. 2008;1138:329–350.

141. Jarque I, Salavert M, Sanz MA. Management of febrile neutropenic patients [article in Spanish]. *Enferm Infecc Microbiol Clin*. 2005;23(suppl 5):24–29.

142. Micozzi A, Bucaneve G. Prophylaxis and treatment of bacterial infections: do we need new strategies? *Rev Clin Exp Hematol*. 2005;9(2):E4.

143. Carreras E, Mensa J. Febrile neutropenia: past, present and future [article in Spanish]. *Enferm Infecc Microbiol Clin*. 2005;23(suppl 5):2–6.

144. Bow EJ. Neutropenic fever syndromes in patients undergoing cytotoxic therapy for acute leukemia and myelodysplastic syndromes. *Semin Hematol*. 2009;46(3):259–268.

145. Durakovic N, Nemet D. Therapeutic approach to a patient with febrile neutropenia [article in Croatian]. *Lijec Vjesn*. 2007;129(10–11):344–350.

146. Antoniadou A, Giamarellou H. Fever of unknown origin in febrile leukopenia. *Infect Dis Clin North Am*. 2007;21(4):1055–1090, x.

147. Whitnall MH, Inal CE, Jackson WE 3rd, Miner VL, Villa V, Seed TM. In vivo radioprotection by 5-androstenediol: stimulation of the innate immune system. *Radiat Res*. 2001;156(3):283–293.

148. Whitnall MH, Wilhelmsen CL, McKinney L, Miner V, Seed TM, Jackson WE 3rd. Radioprotective efficacy and acute toxicity of 5-androstenediol after subcutaneous or oral administration in mice. *Immunopharmacol Immunotoxicol.* 2002;24(4):595–626.

149. Singh VK, Grace MB, Jacobsen KO, et al. Administration of 5-androstenediol to mice: pharmacokinetics and cytokine gene expression. *Exp Mol Pathol.* 2008;84(2):178–188.

150. Xiao M, Inal CE, Parekh VI, Chang CM, Whitnall MH. 5-Androstenediol promotes survival of gamma-irradiated human hematopoietic progenitors through induction of nuclear factor-kappaB activation and granulocyte colony-stimulating factor expression. *Mol Pharmacol.* 2007;72(2):370–379.

151. Stickney DR, Dowding C, Garsd A, et al. 5-androstenediol stimulates multilineage hematopoiesis in rhesus monkeys with radiation-induced myelosuppression. *Int Immunopharmacol.* 2006;6(11):1706–1713.

152. Singh VK, Shafran RL, Inal CE, Jackson WE 3rd, Whitnall MH. Effects of whole-body gamma irradiation and 5-androstenediol administration on serum G-CSF. *Immunopharmacol Immunotoxicol.* 2005;27(4):521–534.

153. Whitnall MH, Villa V, Seed TM, et al. Molecular specificity of 5-androstenediol as a systemic radioprotectant in mice. *Immunopharmacol Immunotoxicol.* 2005;27(1):15–32.

154. Whitnall MH, Elliott TB, Landauer MR, et al. Protection against gamma-irradiation with 5-androstenediol. *Mil Med.* 2002;167(2 suppl):64–65.

155. Singh VK, Shafran RL, Jackson WE 3rd, Seed TM, Kumar KS. Induction of cytokines by radioprotective tocopherol analogs. *Exp Mol Pathol.* 2006;81(1):55–61.

156. Kumar KS, Srinivasan V, Toles R, Jobe L, Seed TM. Nutritional approaches to radioprotection: vitamin E. *Mil Med.* 2002;167(2 suppl):57–59.

157. Singh VK, Grace MB, Parekh VI, Whitnall MH, Landauer MR. Effects of genistein administration on cytokine induction in whole-body gamma irradiated mice. *Int Immunopharmacol.* 2009;9(12):1401–1410.

158. Weiss JF, Landauer MR. History and development of radiation-protective agents. *Int J Radiat Biol.* 2009;85(7):539–573.

159. Francois A, Milliat F. Radiation-induced gastrointestinal syndrome: who is the culprit? [article in French]. *Med Sci (Paris).* 2010;26(5):449–452.

160. Jacob A, Shah KG, Wu R, Wang P. Ghrelin as a novel therapy for radiation combined injury. *Mol Med.* 2010;16(3-4):137–143.

161. Rotolo JA, Kolesnick R, Fuks Z. Timing of lethality from gastrointestinal syndrome in mice revisited. *Int J Radiat Oncol Biol Phys.* 2009;73(1):6–8.

162. Brown M. What causes the radiation gastrointestinal syndrome? Overview. *Int J Radiat Oncol Biol Phys.* 2008;70(3):799–800.

163. Zhang L, Sun W, Wang J, et al. Mitigation effect of an FGF-2 peptide on acute gastrointestinal syndrome after high-dose ionizing radiation. *Int J Radiat Oncol Biol Phys.* 2010;77(1):261–268.

164. Qiu W, Leibowitz B, Zhang L, Yu J. Growth factors protect intestinal stem cells from radiation-induced apoptosis by suppressing PUMA through the PI3K/AKT/p53 axis. *Oncogene.* 2010;29(11):1622–1632.

165. Bhanja P, Saha S, Kabarriti R, et al. Protective role of R-spondin1, an intestinal stem cell growth factor, against radiation-induced gastrointestinal syndrome in mice. *PLoS One.* 2009;4(11):e8014.

Chapter 3

TRIAGE AND TREATMENT OF RADIATION AND COMBINED-INJURY MASS CASUALTIES

DANIEL F. FLYNN, MS, MD,* AND RONALD E. GOANS, PhD, MD†

*Colonel, US Army Medical Corps (Retired); Visiting Faculty, Radiation Emergency Assistance Center/Training Site, Oak Ridge, Tennessee 37831; New England Radiation Therapy Associates, Radiation Oncology Department, Holy Family Hospital, Methuen, Massachusetts 01884
†Senior Medical Advisor, MJW Corporation, Amherst, New York 14228; Senior Research Advisor/Physician, Radiation Emergency Assistance Center/Training Site, Oak Ridge, Tennessee 37831; Associate Professor, Tulane School of Public Health and Tropical Medicine, New Orleans, Louisiana 70112

INTRODUCTION

In today's society, nuclear war between the world's major powers is considered by most to be an unlikely scenario; the threat of nuclear terrorism is now the major concern.[1] The current National Planning Scenario for the detonation of a nuclear weapon involves a 10-kiloton tactical weapon exploded at ground level in a major city.[2] This scenario would result in both a civilian and a subsequent military response, and it is a useful template for military medical preparedness for any nuclear detonation. Ten kilotons is a credible weapon yield, and in the worst-case scenario, an attack with such a weapon would involve a ground-level detonation in a densely populated area, resulting in radioactive fallout. Military operations could be impeded. Whether in the lead role or in a supporting role to civilian authority, military medical planning must account for this worst-case scenario, both in the United States and abroad.

The most severe consequence of a nuclear detonation in a densely populated area will be the surge of overwhelming casualties, which will have a tremendous impact on both military and civilian medical systems. Casualties in the immediate area will sustain various combinations of thermal burns, physical trauma, and radiation injuries. In addition, because the ground-level detonation will create a downwind, radioactive fallout plume, radioactive contamination will cause further casualties, primarily due to radiation-alone injury. The death toll, particularly during the first few days, will be high; however, there is the potential to save many thousands of seriously injured people by implementing appropriate triage and treatment strategies. The goal of this chapter is to address the triage and medical management of casualties primarily during the first 24 to 72 hours following a 10-kiloton, ground-level nuclear detonation.

TYPES OF NUCLEAR AND RADIOLOGICAL EXPLOSIVE WEAPONS

Military medical planning and preparation for a 10-kiloton yield detonation is the same as preparation for a wide range of weapon yields: 1 kiloton, 100 kilotons, and 1,000 kilotons (1 megaton). Although the weapon yields are very different, the range (distance from the detonation point) at which a given effect occurs does not differ for explosions of different yields as much as one might expect. For example, the estimated distance for 50% lethality from nuclear radiation is about half a mile for a 1-kiloton explosion, about three

quarters of a mile for a 10-kiloton explosion, a little over a mile for a 100-kiloton explosion, and 1.62 miles for a 1-megaton explosion. The same trend is true for blast and thermal effects (Table 3-1).

An improvised nuclear device can be a modification of an existing nuclear weapon by a nongovernmental entity. It produces a nuclear detonation at full or partial yield, resulting in the identical pattern of damage and medical effects as a conventional nuclear weapon. A nuclear detonation results in an electromagnetic pulse

TABLE 3-1

NUCLEAR DETONATION CASUALTY ESTIMATES VERSUS WEAPON YIELD BY MECHANISM OF INJURY*

Mechanism of Injury	1 kiloton	10 kiloton	100 kiloton	1,000 kiloton (1 megaton)
Indirect blast (winds; 50% lethality, estimated 6 psi)[1]	0.43 km	1.0 km	2.1 km	4.4 km
Direct blast (50% lethality)[2]	0.14 km	0.30 km	0.65 km	1.4 km
Thermal radiation (50% second-degree burns)[2]	0.86 km	2.5 km	6.5 km	14 km
Ionizing radiation (50% lethality in weeks, estimated 450 cGy)[2]	0.77 km	1.2 km	1.7 km	2.6 km

*The estimates of the effects were calculated using a Hotspot (Lawrence Livermore National Laboratory, Lawrence, CA) version 8.0, simulating a surface burst with no intervening shielding or sheltering.
(1) Walker RI, Cerveny TJ, eds. *Medical Consequences of Nuclear Warfare*. In: Zajtchuk R, Jenkins DP, Bellamy RF, Ingram VM, eds. *Textbooks of Military Medicine*. Washington, DC: Office of the Surgeon General, Department of the Army, Borden Institute; 1989. (2) US Department of the Army. *Treatment of Nuclear and Radiological Casualties*. Washington, DC: DA; 2001. Field Manual 4-02.283. Table 2-2.

that has no known medical effects but that damages electronic equipment, including communications and computers. The electromagnetic pulse effect for a surface detonation is not well understood and could extend for at least several miles from the detonation point, thereby affecting some emergency medical response operations. A radiological dispersal device, or "dirty bomb," disseminates radioactive material across an area by means of a conventional explosive without a nuclear detonation (Table 3-2).[3]

MEDICAL EFFECTS OF NUCLEAR WEAPON DETONATION

The medical effects of nuclear weapon detonation include blast, thermal, and radiation effects, all of which cause significant injury.[4–6] Casualties at Hiroshima were generally due to a combination of effects; initial deaths during the first few days were attributed to serious blast and thermal injuries, rather than radiation injuries. However, many casualties had combined injuries.[6]

Blast Injury

Two types of blast forces occur simultaneously in the shock front of a nuclear detonation: direct blast wave peak overpressure, which is measured by the magnitude of the sudden rise in pressure over ambient pressure, and indirect blast wind forces, which are measured by wind velocities. The intensity of both blast forces decreases with increasing distance from the detonation site.

Direct Blast Wave Peak Overpressure

Overpressure refers to sudden pressure changes above the stable ambient pressure, which, at sea level,

is 14.7 pounds per square inch (psi). At a sudden peak overpressure of 1 psi (15.7 psi total), some windows may shatter. With respect to medical effects, rapid compression and decompression with transmission of pressure waves though tissues results in damage at junctions between tissues of different densities.[7,8] This damage is noted particularly at interfaces between air and tissue, such as the eardrums and lungs (Table 3-3). Tympanic membrane rupture may cause tinnitus, pain, and hearing loss, and there may be otoscopic evidence of perforation and blood in the external canal. The threshold overpressure for eardrum rupture is 5 psi. About 50% of eardrums rupture at 18 psi, which is nearly the threshold for lung injury. Thus, ruptured eardrums signal possible lung injury because pressure levels high enough to cause serious injury to the lungs have probably already ruptured the eardrums.

Injury to the lungs is the major cause of morbidity and mortality in direct blast injuries.[7,8] Clinically diffuse pulmonary contusions become apparent as local or diffuse infiltrates on radiographs over the course of hours. Symptoms may include chest tightness, pain, tachypnea, and hemoptysis. At the interface between soft tissue and air in the lung, the direct blast pressure wave results in local tensions that cause micro-

TABLE 3-2

EFFECTS OF DETONATION OF A RADIOLOGICAL DISPERSAL DEVICE AND AN IMPROVISED NUCLEAR DEVICE

Effect	Radiological Dispersal Device ("Dirty Bomb")	Improvised Nuclear Device (Nuclear Weapon)
Major damage to infrastructure	No	Yes
Expected casualty range	10–1,000	50,000–1,000,000
Risk of fatal contamination	Unlikely	Possible in high-fallout zone
Range of significant contamination	A few city blocks	Hundreds of square miles (or more with fallout)

TABLE 3-3

DIRECT BLAST EFFECTS

Effect	Overpressure (psi)
Windows shatter threshold	1
Some vehicles overturn	5
Some houses collapse	5
Eardrum rupture threshold	5
Eardrum rupture (50% risk)	18
Severe lung injury threshold	20
Lethality (lung injury) threshold	40
Lethality (lung injury) 50%	62

Adapted from: Glasstone S, Dolan PJ. *The Effects of Nuclear Weapons.* 3rd edition. Washington, DC: US Department of Defense; 1977.

scopic tears; hemorrhage and edema then develop. An alveolar-pulmonary venous communication can be the source of air emboli, which can be immediately life-threatening. Pneumothorax, hemothorax, and mediastinal extravasation of air are all possible manifestations of very severe direct blast injury.

Indirect Blast Wind Force

A nuclear explosion generates winds much greater than hurricane force that cause flying debris to strike people, or that project people into the air to impact with other objects downwind. Traumatic injuries from blast wind effects, including penetrating trauma (eg, caused by glass or other debris at high velocity) and blunt trauma, are much more common than injuries from direct blast effects. Crush injuries may result from the collapse or fragmentation and displacement of buildings or large, heavy objects due to blast winds. Soldiers in armored vehicles, as well as people in well-constructed buildings, may be protected from most thermal and blast wind effects, but they may still be subject to direct blast effects (overpressures). For eardrum rupture in that scenario, treatment can be delayed.

There is a relationship between the direct blast wave peak overpressure and the maximum wind velocity at the blast wind shock front (Table 3-4). Both the blast wind velocity and the direct blast wave peak overpressure decline with increasing distance from the detonation. For example, for a 20-kiloton nuclear detonation,

TABLE 3-4

INDIRECT BLAST WIND EFFECTS: MAXIMUM WIND VELOCITY OF SHOCK FRONT AND ASSOCIATED DIRECT BLAST PEAK OVERPRESSURE*

Indirect Blast Maximum Wind Velocity (mph)	Direct Blast Peak Overpressure (psi)
2,078	200
1,415	100
934	50
294	10
163	5
70	2

*The actual distance is not listed because it depends on the magnitude of the nuclear detonation yield.
Adapted from: Glasstone S, Dolan PJ. *The Effects of Nuclear Weapons.* 3rd edition. Washington, DC: US Department of Defense; 1977. Chapter 3.

the blast wind velocity is estimated at 180 mph at 0.8 mile. For a 1-megaton detonation, the estimated velocity of the blast wind is 400 mph at 1.1 miles, 180 mph at 3.0 miles, and 40 mph at 9 miles.[4,5]

Thermal Injury

Thermal burns will probably be the most common immediate serious injury following nuclear weapon detonation. The intense heat of the expanding fireball and thermal infrared radiation cause thermal injury consisting of flash burns, flame burns, temporary flash blindness (ranging in duration from seconds to a few minutes as a result of a sudden peripheral observation of intense light), and retinal burns (relatively rare). Thermal effects also decrease with increasing distance from the detonation. In a 10-kiloton detonation, second-degree burns on exposed skin are seen on people located up to 1.4 miles from the site, and first-degree burns (similar in appearance to severe sunburn) are seen on those up to 2 miles from the site. In a 1-megaton detonation, second-degree burns are seen on people at distances up to 10 miles, and first-degree burns are seen on those up to 15 miles away.[4-6]

Flash Burns

Flash burns are caused by thermal infrared radiation that travels in a straight line. Exposed skin absorbs the infrared radiation, and the victim is burned on the side of the body facing the explosion (profile burns). At a sufficient distance from the detonation, objects covering the skin, including clothing, may shield against this injury. A little closer to the detonation, where thermal energy is higher, thermal radiation can cause burns through clothing, even at temperatures below those required to cause ignition of clothing. Light-colored clothing reflects infrared radiation and dark-colored clothing absorbs it, which can result in pattern burns if the clothing is in actual contact with the skin.

Flame Burns

Flame burns are caused by ignition of clothing on those closer to the detonation than those with flash burns. Flame burns also result from secondary effects of fires. Firestorms cause many burn injuries and deaths as damaged buildings burn with people trapped inside. Severe thermal injuries include respiratory injuries from hot gases; respiratory system burns are associated with severe morbidity and high mortality rates. Close to the fireball of the explosion, everything is totally incinerated, with immediate 100% lethality.

Nuclear Radiation Injury

Types of Ionizing Radiation After a Nuclear Detonation

Radioisotopes are characterized by the energy and types of radiation they emit and by their half-lives (the time for radioactive decay to 50% strength). Heavy nuclei, as found in elements such as uranium, plutonium, and americium, emit charged alpha particles, which are not an external hazard because they cannot travel into tissue and are fully stopped by the outer clothing or by the outer (dead) layer of exposed skin. Absorption from wounds or inhalation is sometimes medically significant, but absorption by ingestion is generally not.

Radioisotopes, such as tritium and strontium, found in weapons fallout emit beta particles. Unlike alpha particles, beta particles can travel a short distance in tissue. Large quantities of beta particles deposited on the skin can damage the basal layer and cause radiation burns; large quantities are also important if they are inhaled or ingested.

Neutrons are uncharged particles that are emitted as prompt radiation in a nuclear detonation. They are deeply penetrating, causing a significant whole-body dose, but are not present in fallout radiation. Gamma rays are massless photons with characteristics similar to x-rays. They are produced by the nuclear decay of radioisotopes and account for a significant whole-body dose in both prompt and fallout radiation injuries. In fallout, they are also medically important if inhaled or ingested in significant quantities.[9–13]

Radiation Units and Measurements

The conventional unit of radioactivity used to quantify contamination is the curie, defined as 3.7×10^{10} Bq, where 1 Bq is defined as 1 disintegration per second and is the International System of Units unit of radioactivity (Table 3-5). Published reports and information on the Internet may use different units to express radiation measurements. After a nuclear detonation, gamma and beta radiation levels, but not neutron irradiation, affect decontamination and response decisions.

For dose, 1 R is equal to:

- 1 rem (1,000 millirem),
- 0.01 Gy (1 cGy), or
- 0.01 Sv (10 millisievert).

For dose rate, 1 R/h is equal to:

- 1,000 mR/h,

TABLE 3-5

COMMON UNITS USED IN RADIATION AND THEIR CONVERSIONS IN THE INTERNATIONAL SYSTEM OF UNITS

Conventional Unit	International System of Units (SI)
1 rad	0.01 Gy or 1 cGy
1 rem	0.01 Sv
100 rad	1 Gy
100 rem	1 Sv

- 1 rem/h,
- 0.01 Gy/h, or
- 0.01 Sv/h.

Dosimeters measure the total dose accumulated in rems, millirems, or sieverts. They are used by responders and healthcare providers to determine their own cumulative, total dose at the end of the mission or a defined period of time. Dose-rate instruments, such as radiation detection, indication, and computation (RADIAC) meters, can measure the radiation exposure rate at a certain point in roentgens per hour or milliroentgens per hour. Such instruments are essential in certain circumstances; for example, to assess a casualty's contamination level, potentially guide external decontamination efforts, and assess the effectiveness of decontamination efforts. These instruments are also used by emergency responders as they move through contaminated areas with varying radiation levels.

The AN/VDR-2 military dose-rate meter (or equivalent, commercially available Geiger-Müller counter) can measure and distinguish gamma and beta radiation over an extended range with an adjustable single probe. The military RADIAC meter AN/PDR-77 comes with different probes, including a separate probe to detect alpha particles. However, in the event of a nuclear detonation, it will likely be used for special purposes rather than as a general-purpose instrument like the AN/VDR-2 or the Geiger-Müller counter, which is commonly used by first responders. In a nuclear detonation scenario, it is not necessary for first responders to have an instrument to measure alpha particles. Contamination after the explosion will involve a mixture of many radioisotopes. When gamma (and beta) contamination is localized, all isotopes are localized, including alpha emitters. External decontamination of beta- and gamma-emitting isotopes decontaminates for all isotopes.

Clinical Manifestations of Nuclear Radiation Injury

Acute radiation injury can occur either as the result of instantaneous exposure to radiation at the time of detonation in the impact area or as the result of early deposition of radioactive contamination from the immediate, downwind fallout zone (within minutes or hours following the detonation). The effects of whole-body irradiation increase with increasing radiation dose (Table 3-6), but a low dose of radiation does not produce acute effects (Table 3-7). The most reliable early clinical indicator of whole-body radiation injury is vomiting, which can be seen within minutes to hours after exposure. The most reliable early hematological indicator is reduced lymphocyte count, which is seen in less than 48 hours. Reduced neutrophil and platelet counts are seen at approximately 2 to 6 weeks. For an acute whole-body exposure, the lethal dose that will kill 50% (LD_{50}) of an exposed group in 60 days is expressed as $LD_{50/60}$. For untreated humans, $LD_{50/60}$ is approximately 3.5 to 4.0 Gy (350–400 cGy), which can

be increased to 5.0 to 6.0 Gy when antibiotics and transfusion support are provided.[9] With aggressive treatment in select patients, the $LD_{50/60}$ may rise further to 6 to 8 Gy with the use of hematopoietic growth factors (bone marrow colony-stimulating factors [CSFs]) and the availability of intensive-care-unit management.

Prompt radiation injuries are caused by instantaneous exposure to radiation at the time of the detonation. Most patients with prompt radiation injuries also have injuries from mechanical trauma and thermal burns. As with blast and thermal effects, radiation effects decrease with increasing distance from the detonation. With a 10-kiloton detonation, an absorbed prompt radiation dose of 4.5 Gy would be noted at a distance of about 0.7 mile from the detonation site, whereas this dose would be seen at a distance of 1.6 miles from the site of a 1-megaton detonation.[4,5,13]

Fallout injuries without significant mechanical or thermal trauma (radiation-alone injuries) are seen in the downwind area outside the impact zone within minutes to several hours. There, radiation exposure levels can be so high that a person outdoors can acquire a potentially lethal radiation-alone injury within a relatively short time. People should either take shelter or move from the dangerous fallout area when outside ambient radiation levels are low enough, as determined by command guidance.

Whether they are caused by prompt radiation or by fallout, the acute clinical effects of whole-body or significant (> 60%) partial-body radiation are characterized as acute radiation syndrome.[14,15] In addition

TABLE 3-6

WHOLE-BODY RADIATION DOSE-EFFECT RELATIONSHIP*

Dose	Effect
10 cGy	No observable effects; threshold for minor chromosome changes in circulating blood lymphocytes
50 cGy	Minor lymphocyte depression
1 Gy	Symptom threshold for nausea and vomiting; mild lymphocyte depression at 48 hours; no deaths from acute effects of radiation
2 Gy	Nausea and vomiting within hours are commonly seen; moderate lymphocyte depression at 48 hours; few, if any, deaths, provided no combined injuries are present
3.5–4 Gy	Probable nausea and vomiting within hours; significant lymphocyte depression at 48 hours; 50% lethal within 60 days if untreated; more lethal if combined injuries are present
5–6 Gy	Nearly 100% nausea and vomiting within 2 hours; severe lymphocyte depression at 48 hours; 100% lethal within 60 days if untreated; nearly 100% lethal, even with treatment, if significant combined injuries are present

*1 Gy = 1 Sv
Reproduced with permission from: Flynn DF, Goans RE. Nuclear terrorism: triage and medical management of radiation and combined-injury casualties. *Surg Clin N Am.* 2006;86:601–636.

TABLE 3-7

TYPICAL RADIATION DOSES RECEIVED IN THE UNITED STATES*

Type of Dose	Amount of Radiation
Overseas roundtrip flight or a chest radiograph	10 mrem (0.01 cGy or 0.1 mSv)
Average annual absorbed dose (from natural background radiation to US population)	295 mrem (0.295 cGy or 2.95 mSv)
Diagnostic radiology computed tomography scan (chest and abdomen)	500 mrem (0.5 cGy or 5 mSv)
Maximum annual dose allowed a radiation worker	5,000 mrem (5 cGy or 50 mSv)

*Asymptomatic and not associated with acute injury
Reproduced with permission from: Flynn DF, Goans RE. Nuclear terrorism: triage and medical management of radiation and combined-injury casualties. *Surg Clin N Am.* 2006;86:601–636.

TABLE 3-8

CLASSIC ACUTE RADIATION SYNDROMES*

Dose	Clinical Status	Description
1–8 Gy	Hematopoietic syndrome	Results from the radiation-sensitivity of the rapid cell renewal system of the bone marrow (hematopoietic) stem cells. Clinical effects may include nausea, vomiting, skin erythema, fatigue, fever, mucositis, and diarrhea. The syndrome is not generally clinically significant for doses of 1–2 Gy. Laboratory analysis in cases with acute whole-body exposure greater than 2 Gy can show lymphocytopenia (8–48 h), neutropenia, and thrombocytopenia (20–30 days). Other common effects in the weeks following exposure include impaired wound healing (if there is concomitant trauma), bleeding (frequent gingival bleeding, petechiae, and ecchymoses of skin or mucous membranes), anemia, hair loss (scalp), increased infectious complications, and (if the radiation dose was high enough) death. With a sublethal dose, the bone marrow will recover. Death from hematopoietic syndrome may occur about 3–8 weeks after exposure.
8–20 Gy	Gastrointestinal syndrome	Results from the radiation sensitivity of the rapid-cell renewal system of the gastrointestinal stem cells in the small intestine crypts. Clinical effects include onset of severe nausea and vomiting, from minutes up to 1 hour after exposure, diarrhea (hours later, with or without rectal bleeding), fever, headache, fatigue, and dehydration. Death from gastrointestinal syndrome (added to severe hematopoietic syndrome) usually occurs 1–2 weeks after exposure.
> 20 Gy	Neurovascular/ central nervous system syndrome	Clinical effects within minutes of exposure include early vomiting, early burning sensation, and prostration. Neurological signs include dizziness, ataxia, and confusion. Hypotension, high fever, and explosive diarrhea are seen. Death is inevitable, usually within 24–48 hours.
Varied	Cutaneous syndrome	May occur with any of the above three syndromes because radiation contamination on the skin can cause severe effects (beta burns) without contributing significantly to the whole-body dose. Clinical effects include a possible early but transient skin erythema. The principal effects are not noted until about 2–4 weeks after exposure. They include a brisk erythema, with blistering and wet desquamation at higher doses. At very high doses, ulcerations with necrosis may evolve.

*Approximate dose ranges are a rough guide.
Adapted from: US Department of Homeland Security. *Department of Homeland Security Working Group on Radiological Dispersal Device (RDD) Preparedness.* Washington, DC: DHS; 2003. www.au.af.mil/au/awc/awcgate/va/radiologic_medical_countermeasures.pdf. Accessed March 23, 2012.

to nausea and vomiting, other clinical effects (sometimes delayed) may be noted, including erythema, fever, headache, diarrhea, hair loss, delayed radiation skin burns (as distinguished from prompt thermal burns), and fatigue. The three classic acute-radiation syndromes are hematopoietic, gastrointestinal, and neurovascular (Table 3-8). Persons with whole-body exposures up to 1 Gy are generally asymptomatic. Potentially survivable exposures are generally in the range of those associated with the hematopoietic syndrome (1–8 Gy). Even with aggressive treatment, no

one with a total body dose in excess of approximately 12 Gy will survive for more than about 4 months. Death results not only from the severe hematological and gastrointestinal effects, but also from the lungs' intolerance of a high single dose. For the very few who survive the combined bone marrow and gastrointestinal effects within the first 60 days, death from radiation pneumonitis is likely within 3 to 4 months after exposure. Other organ systems, such as the heart, kidneys, and liver, will sustain severe damage, resulting in organ dysfunction.

URBAN CASUALTY AND DESTRUCTION PATTERNS AFTER THE LOW-ALTITUDE NUCLEAR DETONATION AT HIROSHIMA

In 1945, the two nuclear bombs that exploded in Hiroshima and Nagasaki, Japan, were low-altitude bursts (2,000 ft) in the 15- to 20-kiloton range (equivalent to 30,000–40,000 lb of trinitrotoluene [TNT]). Rivers and concrete bridges throughout Hiroshima served as natural firebreaks. Nevertheless, immediately after the explosion, thousands of independent fires ignited and eventually merged inside a roughly circular area of 4.5 square miles (1.2-mile radius) around ground zero. Firefighting resources were inadequate and made ineffective by wreckage in the streets. There were also broken water pipes in buildings, hydrants buried in debris, and pumping stations disabled by loss of electrical power with resultant low water pressure. Firefighting was limited to the perimeter of the firestorm. Most fires burned themselves out or were extinguished by the second day. Beyond the 1.2-mile-radius fire zone, the destruction or severe damage extended as far as another mile, affecting numerous buildings and other structures.[6]

Rescue, emergency medical care, and first aid in the 1.2-mile radius from ground zero were hampered by communication breakdown, blocking of streets and bridges by rubble, fires, and heavy smoke and dust in the air. Survivors fled to riverbanks and parks or were taken away in boats. An overwhelming number of casualties flooded the few functioning hospitals and first aid stations. It was initially impossible to give even basic medical care to more than a few people. A large part of the care was initially given by patients' relatives. There was a shortage of supplies in first-aid stations, particularly dressings to cover burns and

wounds, even before the surge of casualties was seen. Treatment in the first several days consisted largely of providing places of refuge. Patients were kept warm and administered analgesics. Additional first-aid and alternative care stations were established in schools and other buildings and on an island in the harbor. The mortality rate in first-aid stations was high.[6]

At Hiroshima, about 80% of the area's approximately 200 to 300 physicians and 1,800 nurses were dead or incapacitated. About 60 physicians and a number of nurses were able to give medical care despite their own injuries. However, the shortage of trained personnel was so grave that nursing students, medical students, and many untrained volunteers, especially patients' family members, were pressed into service.[6] Some hospitals and many clinics were located in wooden buildings, and many within a 2-mile radius of the detonation were damaged or destroyed. Only 3 of the city's 45 hospitals and clinics were initially usable: none had functioning blood banks. It is reported that blood transfusions were given to only a few patients during the first 4 days after the detonation. Medical supplies for Hiroshima were stored in adjacent villages but were inadequate. Dressings were scarce, and antibiotics, such as sulfonamides, were in short supply, given the extent of the casualties. There was

TABLE 3-9

ZONAL CASUALTY (KILLED PLUS INJURED) RATES 4 MONTHS AFTER DETONATION IN RELATION TO DISTANCE FROM HYPOCENTER AT HIROSHIMA*

Zone	Distance† from Hypocenter	Population	Casualty Rates (%)		
			Killed	Injured	Uninjured
1A	0–0.3 mi (0–0.5 km)	6,230	96.5	2.7	0.8
1B	0.3–0.6 mi (0.5–1.0 km)	24,950	83.0	11.3	5.7
2	0.6–0.9 mi (1.0–1.5 km)	45,270	51.6	32.9	15.5
3	0.9–1.2 mi (1.5–2.0 km)	67,900	21.9	41.2	36.9
4	1.2–1.6 mi (2.0–2.5 km)	30,600	4.9	34.0	61.1
5	1.6–1.9 mi (2.5–3.0 km)	30,600	2.7	38.4	58.9
6	1.9–2.5 mi (3.0–4.0 km)	29,400	2.5	22.7	74.8
7	2.5–3.1 mi (4.0–5.0 km)	20,310	1.1	8.2	90.7

*The Joint Commission for the Investigation of the Effects of the Atomic Bomb on Japan was established within a few weeks to investigate medical effects of the bombings at Hiroshima and Nagasaki. It was composed of US military and civilian medical doctors, physicists, and other support staff, in addition to Japanese medical doctors and support staff. The US team entered Hiroshima on September 8, 1945, 33 days after the nuclear detonation, formed a joint medical team with the Japanese, and closely coordinated medical investigations. They investigated the effects up to 4 months after the detonation in seven zones at increasing distance from the hypocenter, for an estimated total at-risk population of approximately 255,000 people.
†Approximate miles/kilometers conversion.
Adapted from: Oughterson AW, Warren S. *Medical Effects of the Atomic Bomb in Japan*. National Nuclear Energy Series. Washington, DC: US Atomic Energy Agency; 1956:84.

a shortage of lactated Ringer's and other solutions, as well as blood products. Due to rapidly dwindling supplies, antibiotics and other medications had to be given in such low doses that they may not have been therapeutic.[6]

On the day following the bombing, some help (civil defense and police) was received from adjacent villages. Their principal activities were first aid, evacuation, disposal of the dead, and looting prevention. After the first day, 33 small relief stations were in operation and up to 150 physicians were on duty. However, there was still no substantial organized medical care for several days after the explosion. When some medical teams arrived from larger cities, they were still handicapped by limited supplies and poor conditions. When the public learned that there was radiation associated with the bomb, thousands of uninjured people reportedly crowded into the already overburdened first-aid stations and hospitals believing they might have been injured by radiation.[6] There were a number of military medical facilities in Hiroshima, away from the city center or on the outskirts. Within a few days, the military assumed responsibility for both civilian and military casualties for the subsequent 2 weeks. Surviving casualties were then gradually transferred to civilian hospitals.

The data from Hiroshima demonstrate the striking effect of distance from detonation on the rates of death and injury (Table 3-9). Distance and shielding are the principal factors influencing casualty rates. Both factors should be considered in combination whenever possible. One conclusion, based on the casualty volume and on the life-threatening but potentially survivable injuries, was that the peak of the medical load was located between 0.9 and 1.2 miles from the center.[6] Operationally, this could be expanded to 0.6 to 1.5 miles. Individuals located less than 0.6 mile from the center were unlikely to survive; those more than 1.5 miles away were less likely to have a life-threatening injury, and most injured casualties were ambulatory.

There were special situations at Hiroshima in which both the distance and the shielding factors for casualties were known. During the late wartime years, workers and volunteers in Japan were organized into groups to create firebreaks. The outcome of that effort demonstrates the effects of both distance and partial shielding.[6]

Outcome data were derived from several groups. One group consisted of a large population of students who were well defined in terms of location and shielding, and nearly all could be traced for outcome. Approximately 4,000 students were working outside on the firebreak project at various locations. They were considered unshielded from heat and radiation. Another 13,000 students were in school, most of them in typical wooden buildings. These were considered largely shielded against the thermal pulse, but unshielded against ionizing radiation. Table 3-10 demonstrates the effects of both distance and thermal shielding on casualty rates at Hiroshima. Between 1.5 and 2.0 km (0.9 and 1.2 miles), 14.2% of those who were thermally shielded versus 83.7% of those who were unshielded were dead or missing following the explosion.

TABLE 3-10

ZONAL MORTALITY FOR THERMALLY SHIELDED (WOODEN SCHOOL BUILDINGS) AND THERMALLY UNSHIELDED STUDENTS ACCORDING TO DISTANCE FROM HYPOCENTER AT HIROSHIMA

Thermally Shielded Students		
Distance	Number Shielded	Dead or Missing
0–0.6 mi (0–1.0 km)	969	588 (60.5%)
0.6–0.9 mi (1.0–1.5 km)	3,959	761 (19.2%)
0.9–1.2 mi (1.5–2.0 km)	957	136 (14.2%)
1.2–1.9 mi (2.0–3.0 km)	3,922	99 (2.5%)
1.9–2.5 mi (3.0–4.0 km)	2,077	11 (0.5%)

Thermally Unshielded Students		
Distance	Number Unshielded	Dead or Missing
0–0.6 mi (0–1.0 km)	2,436	2,282 (93.7%)
0.6–0.9 mi (1.0–1.5 km)	484	413 (85.3%)
0.9–1.2 mi (1.5–2.0 km)	135	113 (83.7%)
1.2–1.9 mi (2.0–3.0 km)	76	11 (14.5%)
1.9–2.5 mi (3.0–4.0 km)	No data available	No data available

Reproduced from: Oughterson AW, Warren S. *Medical Effects of the Atomic Bomb in Japan*. National Nuclear Energy Series. Washington, DC: US Atomic Energy Agency; 1956. Table 3.3 (p 35) and Table 5.2 (p 103).

A second group of firebreak workers was divided into two subgroups. The first subgroup consisted of 168 workers at 0.62 mile from the hypocenter. All but three of them were shielded from direct thermal effects, but not from ionizing radiation, by a row of two-story, light, wooden structures. They were standing in formation, awaiting roll call for the beginning of the workday, in the shadow of the thermal pulse of the detonation. Six died of crush injuries from the blast effects, and all three of those who were exposed to the thermal pulse soon died of burns. The 159 immediate survivors later developed some hair loss, and 90% developed cutaneous petechiae (purpura). Ninety-three of the immediate survivors (58.5%) died, primarily of radiation injuries, all between days 20 and 38,[6] consistent with the hematopoietic syndrome timeline following a fatal whole-body exposure.

The second subgroup of 166 workers had just started their workday near the first subgroup, also at 0.62 mile from the hypocenter. All were in the open and completely unshielded from the explosion. Following the detonation, all showed evidence of immediate, severe thermal burns; 101 died on the first day, and 55 died within 2 weeks (most within the first 4 days). The 10 who survived for 2 weeks showed evidence of radiation injury. At 14 weeks, all 10 were still alive but were reported to be too weak to work. No further follow-up was reported.

The death rate, in general, was highest among those who were outdoors; it was lower for those in residential structures, and lowest for those in reinforced concrete buildings. The reinforced buildings provided protection from blast, thermal, and radiation injuries, unless they were very close to ground zero. For 1,600 individuals (combined total from Hiroshima and Nagasaki) in reinforced concrete buildings, between 0.3 and 0.75 mile from ground zero, the following immediate fatality rates were correlated with the severity of the structural damage[5]:

- Severe damage: 88% fatality rate
- Moderate damage: 14% fatality rate
- Light damage: 8% fatality rate

In addition, 11% of those in severely damaged buildings were reported as seriously injured, for a total rate of death or serious injury of 99%.[5]

The high fatality rates in severely damaged buildings compared with less damaged buildings is believed to be due primarily to two effects: first, from severe, often fatal crush injuries resulting when concrete buildings collapse; and second, from inescapable secondary fires after entrapment in a building. Photographic evidence from Hiroshima and Nagasaki showed that a number of reinforced concrete buildings within half a mile of ground zero were still standing, but most of them had severe thermal damage inside, where everything flammable was incinerated with the thermal pulse and ensuing fires.[4-6] In the event of a nuclear detonation today in a major city center, this observation raises concern for tall buildings exposed directly to a thermal pulse and located less than half a mile from ground zero. Buildings that do not collapse may contain large internal fires that prevent people from escaping.

Among the three causes of death in Hiroshima (blast, thermal, and radiation injuries), it has been estimated that perhaps 50% of the deaths were due primarily to thermal burns.[4-6] Flash burns from direct exposure to the thermal pulse were more common than flame burns from secondary fires. First-degree flash (profile) burns occurred at distances of up to 2.8 miles, but second-degree burns with blistering were rarely seen beyond 2 miles. Flash burns of skin directly exposed within 1.2 miles were usually third-degree burns or mixed second- and third-degree burns, and third-degree burns were most common within 0.6 mile. However, many of those within 0.6 mile died quickly, before the severity of the burns could be manifested. It was also difficult to distinguish and classify between a second- and third-degree burn in the early stages.[5]

In addition, people sheltered or trapped in buildings or tunnels close to ground zero may have been killed by the depletion of oxygen or inhalation of hot gases, smoke, and dust as a result of the firestorm. Almost all deaths of those out in the open and unsheltered within 1.1 miles of ground zero are thought to have been caused primarily by thermal burns, although the burns were usually combined with other injuries.[4-6]

There are fewer data on casualties caused by blast winds, since those caught in the open with severe blast wound trauma also had severe burns and injuries that often resulted in death. Direct blast injuries occurred in people who were shielded inside reinforced concrete buildings up to 0.6 mile from ground zero.[6] Most immediate deaths from blast wind injuries near ground zero were due to crush injuries from falling buildings. Outside the ground zero area, there were cases of fractures as a result of blast winds, although fewer were reported than expected. Blunt and penetrating trauma also occurred, usually caused by multiple projectiles causing multiple wounds. Beyond 1 mile, flying debris, such as glass, caused the greatest number of blast wind injuries, most of them nonfatal.[6] The degree of injury was related to the velocity of the glass or other debris, which, in turn, was related to the distance from the explosion. Many casualties who were between 1 and 2.5 miles from ground zero were treated for lacerations from glass fragments and small debris lodged superficially in the skin and subcutaneous tissues; those closer to the explosion had more serious, deeper, more penetrating wounds.[4–6] Complications after treatment were usually associated with infections and slow wound healing.[5]

Among the casualties who survived the first few days following the explosion, a number died weeks later, with symptoms ascribed to nuclear radiation. These fatalities were estimated at 5% to 15% of the total number of deaths. A rough estimate indicated that about 30% of those who died at Hiroshima had received a lethal dose of nuclear radiation, although this was not always the immediate cause of death. A more recent International Atomic Energy Agency review, referring to the inner blast area around ground zero, indicated that the immediate deaths were due to blast and thermal effects, not to radiation exposure, since no one would have been able to survive the lethal blast and thermal effects only to die of radiation effects later.[16]

For injuries due to radiation, the data collected at Hiroshima[6] were based on studies of patients known to be alive 20 days or more after the detonation. A history of vomiting on day 1 and of epilation, purpura, and oropharyngeal lesions later correlated with the radiation dose, as estimated by the distance from the explosion and the degree of shielding. The higher the dose, the earlier the manifestation of radiation injury. The Joint Commission's summary report noted that in the most heavily exposed patients, a severe, dysentery-like diarrhea started early following detonation and persisted until death. This often occurred together with gastrointestinal bleeding. Bleeding sometimes developed from other sites, such as the gums. Vomiting within 3 hours after the explosion was associated with severe cases of radiation injury.[6] Vomiting is not specific for radiation injuries because it may result from other causes, such as physical or psychological trauma, following such an explosion. Some casualties did not vomit, including even some who were within 0.6 mile of the explosion; however, those who were that close would have had a significant degree of ionizing radiation shielding, since they obviously had shielding that protected them from being killed on the first day by the thermal or blast effects. Nevertheless, vomiting, which later correlated with radiation injury, was reported as the most common early symptom at both Hiroshima and Nagasaki. Oropharyngeal lesions (painful oral mucositis) caused by radiation sometimes appeared 3 to 5 weeks after the explosion. These lesions were considered suggestive of radiation injury but not specific. In a study of a large sample of 20-day survivors, the criterion for the diagnosis of significant whole-body radiation injury by the Hiroshima joint medical teams was determined to be the development of epilation and/or purpura. The peak onset of epilation occurred 14 to 21 days after the explosion, and that of purpura 20 to 35 days after the explosion. The occurrence of epilation and purpura together, particularly with an earlier onset for either, was associated with very severe radiation injury. The incidence of such injury according to this criterion was 86% up to 0.62 mile from the explosion, 39% at 0.62 to 0.93 mile, and 10% at 0.93 to 1.24 miles.[6] Partial shielding from ionizing radiation may have prevented the percentage of epilation or purpura from being higher. The degree of radiation injury was not well defined quantitatively in terms of hematological laboratory studies, such as the degree of neutropenia, because data were limited and fragmented, and because no blood tests were done on the vast majority of casualties due to resource limitations. Generally, only one blood specimen was obtained from those who did undergo blood testing; however, a limited number of patients with presumed radiation injuries who survived the first 20 days had variable blood counts done between the third and fifth weeks after detonation. The Joint Commission concluded that "few instances were reported where recovery occurred with white-blood-cell counts of less than 500 [per cubic millimeter]."[6]

The data on delayed epilation, purpura, and oropharyngeal lesions are relevant for current medical planning for a nuclear detonation. Some individuals who have little or no trauma injury may self-evacuate the area, unaware of having sustained significant radiation injury. This would be particularly true for those who were outside the thermal blast zone but were in the dangerous fallout zone for a sufficient period of time. Two weeks after a detonation, public health advisories could target symptoms of epilation, purpura, or oropharyngeal lesions and urge anyone who has or subsequently develops these symptoms to immediately seek medical attention. Unexplained persistent fever and burns 2 or more weeks after the detonation could be warning signs of bone marrow or cutaneous radiation injury. Therefore, the public health advisory should also urge these individuals to immediately seek a medical checkup. A simple physical examination and blood tests 2 or more weeks after the detonation would include, at a minimum, hemoglobin, hematocrit and lymphocyte, neutrophil, and platelet counts to help determine whether there was a clinically significant, whole-body radiation exposure.

In a 1962 updated analysis of the casualty zones after the Hiroshima bombing, the number of zones was reduced from seven to three.[5] Although some information is lost, the three-zone approach is easier in terms of medical planning, particularly for rescue operations. The updated estimates of the number of people at risk and the number of casualties are within 1% of the estimates given in Table 3-9 for 4 months after detonation.

- **Inner zone or severe damage zone (ground zero up to 0.6 mile)**: Population 31,200, with 86% killed and 10% injured. Extensive destruction with a high fatality rate and survivors with very serious injuries. Most concrete buildings collapsed except for a few, most of which had some serious damage. Photographic evidence of large piles of rubble blocking streets; many concrete buildings, which had initially appeared to be relatively sound from the outside, were internally damaged and gutted by fire.
- **Middle zone or moderate damage zone (0.6–1.6 miles)**: Population 144,800, with 27% killed and 37% injured. Many concrete buildings standing but severe destruction of most small masonry and lightweight structures, including residences, as well as overturned vehicles and some secondary fires. Significant fatality rate and many serious life-threatening injuries.
- **Outer zone or light damage zone (1.6–3.1 miles)**: Population 80,300, with 2% killed and 25% injured. Destruction of some lightweight structures. Low fatality rate. Many casualties were ambulatory, with minimal injuries. Others who were in locations nearer to the border of the middle zone had moderately serious injuries. First-degree burns (profile burns) were very common among those who were outdoors.[6]

The differences in early fatality rates between zones are striking: 86% in the inner zone, 27% in the middle zone, and 2% in the outer zone. The injuries among the few survivors in the inner zone were usually severe, whereas there were very few severe injuries in the outer zone. A conclusion for casualties in the middle zone (0.6–1.6 miles) was that "a larger proportion of the population would probably have survived if immediate medical attention had been available."[4,5] This is consistent with the 1956 published report on the seven-zone analysis of casualties.[6] There were 91,000 injured who survived day one who would potentially have benefited from some level of medical care (Table 3-11). Many of the 45,000 who died on day one were killed immediately. Many others who were severely injured also died on day one before receiving medical care. However, today, some of the severely injured might have survived long enough to be triaged and

TABLE 3-11

APPROXIMATE CASUALTY RATE AT HIROSHIMA FROM DAY 1 TO 4 MONTHS AFTER DETONATION

Estimated population at risk	255,000
Uninjured	119,000
Total casualties	136,000
Dead day 1	45,000 (33% of total casualties)
Surviving casualties day 1	91,000
Dead day 2 to month 4	19,000 (86% of those died within 20 days)
Total dead month 4	64,000
Surviving casualties month 4	72,000

Adapted from: Oughterson AW, Warren S. *Medical Effects of the Atomic Bomb in Japan*. National Nuclear Energy Series. Washington, DC: US Atomic Energy Agency; 1956: 86.

provided emergency medical care. Therefore, medical treatment planning for a Hiroshima-like scenario would mean planning for 100,000 or more injuries exclusive of radiation-alone injuries from fallout.

For medical planning, it is necessary to consider not only the number of injured requiring care but also estimates of the numbers of people with each different type of injury. In Hiroshima, the core of the medical load was reported between 0.6 and 1.6 miles (1.0–2.5 km), after which there was a sharp drop in zonal population density, in addition to the lower percentage of dead or severely injured people with increasing distance from ground zero (see Table 3-9). Much effort was put into the post-detonation analysis and quantification of types of single injuries (thermal, blast, or radiation) and the major injury components for combined injuries. An estimated 70% of survivors had blast injuries, 65% had thermal burns, and 30% had radiation injuries. However, there are no precise data available on the relative significance of each injury type.[4-6] Although the predominant type of serious injury was often thermal, it is expected that those who died early with very severe, visually obvious burns also may have had undiagnosed, underlying, fatal, internal traumatic injuries. Therefore, for those fatalities in the inner zone, trauma as the primary cause of death is likely to be underreported. With a ground-level detonation, additional radiation injuries would be expected for those in the heavy fallout zone because of radioactive contamination.

Military medical planning for operations also

involves a review of previous after-action reports for lessons learned from similar past military operations. At Hiroshima, after several months of investigation, it was concluded that "the methods adopted for treating casualties were far below standard because of the shortage of supplies and equipment and the extraordinary demands made on crippled staffs."[6] Members of a Joint Commission of US and Japanese physicians speculated as to what the mortality rate would have been if there had been satisfactory facilities available, with enough medical personnel and adequate supplies to treat the casualties soon after the explosion. In addition to sufficient personnel and basic supplies for burns and wounds, they also recommended having sufficient quantities of resuscitative fluids available, including parenteral fluids (eg, lactated Ringer's), plasma (and plasma volume expanders), and whole blood; equipment for sterile techniques and wound debridement; and an ample supply of antibiotics.[6] However, in this government report, finally published in 1956 after some years of delay, the commission concluded it was doubtful whether more than 5% to 10% of the deaths from all injuries could have been prevented.[6] More resources, such as broad-spectrum antimicrobial agents and cytokines (CSFs), have become available since the Hiroshima bombing. However, the need for adequate basic supplies for overwhelming casualties remains unchanged.

CURRENT PROJECTIONS OF URBAN CASUALTY, DESTRUCTION, AND FALLOUT PATTERNS AFTER A GROUND-LEVEL NUCLEAR DETONATION

The US Department of Homeland Security National Planning Scenario No. 1 involves planning for a ground-level, 10-kiloton nuclear detonation in a major urban environment.[2] The nuclear blast would result in physical destruction of buildings and other structures, with the amount of damage decreasing with increasing distance from ground zero.

For a nuclear detonation at ground level, the three-zone (light damage, moderate damage, and severe damage) approach at Hiroshima will be similar in terms of severity of structural damage and survivability of casualties. However, unlike Hiroshima in 1945, a major city center today is typically surrounded by a great number of tall buildings. There would be significant shadowing (shielding) effects from blast winds, thermal radiation, and prompt nuclear radiation provided by these buildings. Shielding would also be provided by any hills and rolling terrain around ground zero. The zones, therefore, would not be concentric circles, as in Hiroshima. However, in some directions around ground zero, there are likely to be some relatively open sectors between groups of tall buildings where the blast, thermal, and radiation effects would be channeled in full force along corridors. The outer boundary of the light damage zone along these unshielded open corridors is estimated at 3 miles, similar to the outer boundary of the light damage zone at Hiroshima.

Zones are defined by the degree of structural damage as emergency responders move in the direction of ground zero.[2] There are no clear boundaries between the three zones, but the visual evidence of degree of structural damage and measured radiation levels will help responders and their commanding authorities define the operational boundaries. There will also be a dangerous fallout zone that overlaps with and extends beyond the three blast zones[2]:

- **Light damage zone**: At the outer boundary, the incidence of shattered glass windows is roughly 25%. As emergency responders move inward, the damage gradually worsens, with increased litter, rubble, light wooden-structure damage, some downed power lines, and detectable radiation levels. The zone is characterized by minimal injuries to individuals, the most common being very superficial injuries from flying glass and debris carried by blast winds of diminished velocity, and some thermal profile (flash) first-degree burns. More significant injuries will be noted as responders approach the moderate damage zone boundary.

- **Moderate damage zone**: There will be overturned automobiles, downed power lines, some ruptured gas and water lines, significant structural damage, and substantial rubble; many light commercial and residential buildings will be unstable or collapsed (most brick or wood-framed structures will have collapsed); there will be poor visibility as a result of smoke from secondary fires and dust from collapsed buildings. There will be elevated radiation levels, but monitored early entry of emergency responders is possible. Many injuries in the moderate damage zone will be serious or life threatening but potentially survivable. Injuries from high-velocity flying glass and debris will be more severe than in the light damage zone because the higher velocity of the blast winds will cause deeper tissue penetration. Responders should focus their medical attention primarily on this zone and not be distracted by minimally injured individuals when they pass through the light damage zone, which would delay their deployment into the moderate damage zone. Victims in this zone, compared to those in other zones, will benefit the most from priority emergency care. These conclusions are in agreement with the conclusions of the Hiroshima studies conducted more than 60 years ago.

- **Severe damage zone**: This is a no-go zone for responders, best characterized by the complete destruction of most buildings. Very few reinforced buildings will still be standing, but all will be damaged, structurally unstable, and most will probably be gutted by fire. As a consequence, there will be large mounds of rubble. All effects will be more severe than those in the moderate damage zone. There may be more extensive fires, smoke, and dust from collapsed buildings that will limit visibility, and there will be high levels of radiation. Most of the initial survivors will have nonsurvivable injuries. This zone is characterized as a no-go zone for responders until radiation levels are sufficiently reduced through nuclear decay of most isotopes.

- **Dangerous fallout zone**: This zone is not defined by structural damage but by an exposure rate of 10 R/h (10 cGy/h) at the boundary.[2] For example, for a 10-kiloton weapon, if the outer boundary of the blast zones is about 3 miles, the dangerous fallout zone may extend 20 miles away from ground zero in the direction of the prevailing winds.[17,18] The fallout zone overlaps sectors of the severe, moderate, and light damage zones. For example, if the fallout moves northeast from ground zero, the northeast sectors of the moderate and light damage zones will have very high radiation levels during the first day. The severe damage zone will already have very high levels, regardless of the fallout direction.

A massive amount of downwind fallout is produced in a ground-level detonation, unlike in the low-altitude detonations in Japan.[17–20] A nuclear explosion at ground level results in vaporized and irradiated earth and debris being pulled up into the fireball, which rises rapidly into a towering mushroom cloud; as the fireball cools off, the material is carried in the direction of the prevailing winds before falling to the ground. The detonation creates radioactive fission products that attach to particles of debris to form fallout, which becomes the main source of ground contamination.

The larger, heavier particles, which are visible as fine, sand-sized grains, fall to earth in a few minutes. The lighter, fine particles, which are not necessarily visible, travel farther downwind. The fallout will reach the ground in less than a day, with the most intense fallout reaching the ground in the proximal area in less than an hour. The primary medically significant types of radiation will be due to gamma and beta radiation. In the dangerous fallout zone, external exposure to gamma radiation is the predominant risk because of the whole-body effects; however, beta radiation can cause severe cutaneous burns (beta burns) if uncovered skin sustains prolonged contact with fallout.

The fallout will not exactly follow the computerized plume-modeling projections. In the atmosphere, the descending fallout is blown by winds whose speed and direction vary at different elevations, so that the fallout pattern may not be evident from ground-level wind direction alone. Therefore, in addition to the use of computerized fallout-plume models, appropriate ongoing radiation monitoring must be performed to define the dangerous fallout zone, which changes as a function of time. Computerized modeling estimates the maximum dose rate 15 minutes after a ground-level 10-kiloton detonation to be about 1,500 cGy/h (15 Gy/h) at a location on the ground under the middle of the fallout plume 1.6 miles downwind from the explosion.[17,18] This would result in a probable lethal dose in only about 20 minutes. This dose rate decreases to 180 cGy/h at 2 hours, and to about 7 cGy/h at 2 days, due to the rapid decay of many of the short-lived radionuclide fission products. During the first 2 hours, the cumulative dose for a person outdoors and under the center of the plume would be approximately 600 cGy at 2.5 miles downwind of the detonation, 300 cGy at 5 miles, 100 cGy at 9 miles, and only 50 cGy at 12 miles, at which point there would be no symptoms and no acute radiation injury.

Therefore, not only does fallout decrease sharply with distance, it also decays quickly with time. Fallout is most dangerous in the first few hours after an explosion. The rapid decay in fallout radiation dose rate follows a standard 7-to-10 rule for decay: for every sevenfold increase in time after the detonation, the radiation dose rate decreases tenfold.[2] For example, if the radiation dose rate at 2 hours after detonation is known, in 14 hours ($7 \times 2 = 14$) the dose rate will be decreased to one tenth of the dose rate at 2 hours. At 98 hours after detonation ($7 \times 7 \times 2$), the dose rate will be decreased to one hundredth of the dose rate at 2 hours. Therefore, it is prudent for the public to seek shelter immediately after a detonation, such as in the basement of a home, workplace, or school, or in an underground metro station. Military personnel will receive a degree of protection in lightly armored vehicles.

The first public response should generally be to find shelter. Sheltering (particularly at home) is prudent early in a radiological event because families can congregate at home where showers, uncontaminated replacement clothing, food, and water are available. Sheltering also provides authorities time to assess the situation more completely. Evacuation might be indicated later for people in some locations, depending on the specific situation and the extended dose estimates. In other locations, remaining sheltered may result in much lower radiation exposure. This underscores the importance of sheltering immediately following the detonation. Unfortunately, many civilians who choose to self-evacuate immediately after the blast may find themselves stuck in traffic, which would become gridlocked due to mass panic and possibly damaged roads and bridges. Those under the plume area will be exposed to a higher radiation dose if they are outdoors or in a vehicle, where their proximity to the radioactive material on the vehicle's roof will result in a much higher dose than if they were in a basement, far removed from the radioactive material on the roof of the house or building. The policy guidance today should be early, adequate shielding followed by informed, delayed evacuation.

Uncontrolled mass self-evacuation will not only hinder emergency responders and supplies from entering the area, but it will also hinder the evacuation of the critically injured. Contamination from fallout may impede military and civilian response operations. This will delay some actions, such as rescue operations, until sufficient radioactive decay has occurred. Since the fallout is subject to rapid radioactive decay, the radiation exposure rate at a given location will diminish rather quickly with time. The dangerous fallout zone will subsequently shrink dramatically in size each day, which will be taken into account in implementing operations. Continuous monitoring of ground radiation levels is imperative.

PERSONAL PROTECTION AND LONG-TERM HEALTH RISKS FOR EMERGENCY RESPONSE PERSONNEL

Both military and civilian emergency responders have operating guidelines to ensure their safety during rescue operations. They also have protective equipment to help safeguard them against acute and long-term effects of radiation. Both have dosimetry equipment and are under their respective command authorities. In any mission, command authority always weighs the importance of the mission, whether military or civilian, against the possible risks to the responders' health and safety.[2,20–27]

Medics and Military Personnel

Military emergency responders train for chemical, biological, radiological, and nuclear (CBRN) attacks. Under military CBRN policy, decontamination of persons exposed to chemical and biological agents takes place before they are admitted to a medical facility (such as a combat support hospital) because even small amounts of some chemical or biological agents create a potential risk. Persons with radiological contamination, however, pose no significant medical risk to healthcare personnel who use proper decontamination techniques. In addition, unlike biological and chemical contamination, the level of radiation contamination can be monitored easily by hand-held instruments, such as a RADIAC meter.[9,25]

Standard military-issue protective masks plus complete protective overgarments (mission-oriented protective posture level 4 [MOPP 4]) protect against inhalation of most radioactive material and contamination, as well as against chemical and biological agents. Military emergency responders will have personal dosimeters and RADIAC meters. In most radiation environments outside the high-radiation zone, a lower degree of protection is adequate compared to that needed for chemical and biological threats. Because it is difficult to accomplish sustained rescue operations in MOPP 4, the command authority will determine the appropriate MOPP level of protection based on the risks of the specific situation. In some situations where the protective mask and heavy gloves are not required, rescue operations can be accomplished faster and with greater efficiency without undue risk. In other situations, anticontamination suits may be preferred if heat stress in MOPP suits is a concern, and when the contamination threat is only ionizing radiation (not combined with chemical agents, for example). This would require approval from the command authority.

Mission-specific, risk-based dose limits include limits for those engaged in lifesaving activities, as seen in current military doctrine.[2,20] Whereas military commanders set their operational exposure guidance (ie, dose limits to military personnel) at any level in a nuclear war, the risk analysis for extremely high-priority missions, which includes saving lives, yields a maximum operational exposure guidance of 125 cGy (1.25 Sv). If this dose is reached, some soldiers may be symptomatic (with temporary nausea and possible vomiting) but will not be at risk for acute lethal effects.

For operations other than war, and based also on mission priorities and risk analysis, military commanders limit maximum operational exposure guidance levels to 75 cGy (0.75 Sv).

Civilian Personnel

Civilian emergency responders who enter an area after a nuclear detonation may be knowingly exposed to certain levels of radiation to save lives, but they need to stay as safe as possible.[2] Civilian responders need personal protective equipment, such as anticontamination suits and respirators similar to those used by the military, while working under the guidance of the civilian incident commander.[2] Initial emergency responders should have meters, such as Geiger-Müller counters, to measure dose rates and dosimeters to show the total accumulated dose received.[25,26] Incident commanders will make every effort to employ the "as low as reasonably achievable" principle when supervising emergency responders on such a mission.[27] The incident commander will weigh the likelihood and significance of a proposed mission's success against the health and safety risks to emergency response personnel. The risks involve not only high radiation levels but also widespread fires, smoke, dust, chemicals, downed power lines, and unstable structures. For radiation limits, some nonmilitary government agencies have established a maximum-dose guideline of 50 cGy (0.5 Sv, 50 rem) for first responders trying to rescue people who would otherwise die. There are no expected acute symptomatic effects at this dose and no risk of acute lethal effects. The "turn-back" dose for emergency responders can be lower (or higher) than the guideline based on the case-specific circumstances. In higher-radiation areas, where 50 cGy or more could be received, emergency responders should have proper training to understand the risks and be allowed to volunteer for the mission.[2] Any rescuer who

vomits should be removed from the site and medically screened. Vomiting would imply that although the accumulated dose was estimated to be 50 cGy, it might have been higher, since vomiting is not common at a dose of 50 cGy.

Long-Term Health Risks

In addition to considering a high dose of ionizing radiation that may result in acute effects, both military commanders and civilian incident commanders should consider possible long-term effects (primarily lifetime cancer risks) on emergency response personnel under their command.

Data from the National Academy of Sciences report Biological Effects of Ionizing Radiation (BEIR VIII)[28,29] estimate that 43 of every 100 people in the United States will be diagnosed with cancer in their lifetime. It is also estimated that one cancer per 100 people (1%), or about one fatal cancer per 200 people (0.5%), would eventually result from a single exposure of 10 cGy (0.1 Sv) above average natural background radiation levels. A 10-cGy dose is roughly equivalent to that obtained from 20 diagnostic chest and abdominal computed tomography scans and is a dose causing no acute side effects (see Table 3–7). Therefore, a medic or other emergency responder (police officer, firefighter, etc) who received a whole-body gamma dose of 10 cGy (0.1 Gy) from an exposure during a rescue mission would not have acute symptoms, but the additional lifetime risk of developing cancer would be about 1%, for a total risk of 44% instead of the projected 43%. If the dose were 20 cGy (0.2 Gy), the person would be asymptomatic, but the additional risk would be 2%, yielding a 45% chance of cancer in a lifetime versus 43% without such acute exposure. However, the delay in acquiring a radiation-induced cancer may range from 5 to 40-plus years, and about half of all cancers are curable with treatments available today.

TRIAGE: CONVENTIONAL, RADIATION-ALONE, AND COMBINED INJURIES

US Military Triage System

Military triage is a dynamic process and occurs at every level of care, from initial casualty sorting, first-responder care, clinical triage, prioritizing for surgery, and intensive care, to the evacuation system. The conventional military triage system used today to sort and prioritize trauma patients is referred to as "DIME" (delayed, immediate, minimal, expectant; Exhibit 3-1).[8] The DIME system is currently used to train medical and evacuation personnel and is helpful when mass casualties may overwhelm available

medical resources. US Army medical units and hospitals currently drill using this triage system for mass casualties, and it has been applied in operations in Iraq and Afghanistan. The DIME system, sometimes with minor variations, is used by the North Atlantic Treaty Organization (NATO) and also by individual countries, among them Russia, Japan, Finland, Israel, Germany, France, and the United Kingdom.

There are a number of other triage systems available for mass casualty events, such as START (simple triage and rapid treatment), a similar system often used in the civilian sector, and SALT (sort, assess,

---

EXHIBIT 3-1

"DIME" TRIAGE CATEGORIES

Delayed (D): Patients require less urgent treatment than those in the immediate treatment category. This group includes those wounded and in need of surgery but whose general condition permits delay without unduly endangering life. The types of injuries in this category include fractures of major bones, relatively stable intraabdominal or thoracic wounds, and burns on less than 50% of the total body surface area (and not involving the face and without respiratory distress). Preoperative resuscitative treatment will be required (eg, stabilizing intravenous fluids, blood transfusions, antibiotics, and pain relief). Delayed-treatment patients will be monitored in case there is a significant change in condition that warrants a change in triage category.

Immediate (I): Patients require immediate treatment to save life, limb, or sight (highest triage priority). This group includes those requiring immediate life-saving surgery. The surgical procedures should not be time consuming and should involve only those unstable patients with a high chance of survival (eg, surgically correctable respiratory compromise, such as with upper airway obstruction or pneumothorax, or surgically correctable hypovolemic shock due to hemorrhage, etc).

Minimal (M): Patients require outpatient treatment and are often returned to duty. These casualties (the "walking wounded") have relatively minor injuries (eg, minor lacerations, abrasions, contusions, sprains, fractures of small bones, and minor burns) and can effectively care for themselves or can often be helped by nonmedical personnel. They may sometimes be returned after a short time to some form of duty, depending on their condition and on military needs.

Expectant (E): Patients require extensive treatment and resources and usually have a very poor prognosis, even with treatment (lowest triage priority). Casualties in this category have wounds that are so extensive that even if they received the benefit of optimal medical resource application, their chances of survival would be poor. Expectant-treatment casualties are unresponsive patients with penetrating head wounds, mutilating explosive wounds involving multiple anatomical sites and organs, second- and third-degree burns in excess of 60% of total body surface area, profound shock with multiple injuries, open pelvic injuries with uncontrollable bleeding, and agonal respiration.

---

lifesaving interventions, treatment and/or transport), a more recently proposed system.[2] Because there are no established and widely accepted medical triage systems for a nuclear detonation, the existing DIME triage algorithms are used with modification for the impact of radiation injury.

Triage and Emergency Medical Treatment of Mass Casualties

The first responders to casualties, whether military or civilian, will be under protective-action command control that will limit their radiation dose exposure by determining which areas they may enter. Medical treatment facilities (MTFs) will be at a sufficient distance from very high-radiation areas to avoid excessive radiation exposure. Healthcare personnel have never received a significant radiation dose, in the military or civilian setting, while providing care to contaminated radiation casualties.

For overwhelming mass casualties, the speed of assessing and categorizing patients' status is key to effective triage. A patient's location at the time of the detonation is extremely important. Patients who were in the open (unshielded) and relatively close to the detonation site will have serious blast and thermal injuries and significant whole-body radiation exposure

and are presumed to be expectant. Resources will be limited, and transferring obviously expectant patients to the MTF, where they would be clinically triaged, is inappropriate. At the other end of the spectrum, those who were not close to the detonation and were not near the dangerous fallout zone, and who are ambulatory and without significant symptoms, burns, or blast injuries, can be given a brief evaluation and initially presumed to have experienced insignificant trauma and radiation dose. They can be classified in the minimal category and not sent to an MTF.

Emergency rescuers and medics must make decisions as to which trauma patients require priority evacuation to an MTF, particularly to one with surgical assets. Some of these priority patients may require timely lifesaving surgery and must therefore be transferred immediately, regardless of whether there is radioactive contamination on them. Simple, hasty decontamination can be performed as long as it does not delay transfers. Lives will be lost if there are inappropriate delays in transporting critical patients who are contaminated, or if potentially lifesaving surgery is delayed.

Conventional-Injury Triage

Initial primary clinical triage is based on conventional injuries (mechanical trauma and burns), not on radiation dose. In the first days after a nuclear detonation event with overwhelming mass casualties, trauma will be the life-threatening problem to address.[2,3,8–12] Upon the patient's arrival at the MTF, rapid triage will be performed by a triage officer. The surgeon will make the final decision as to whether surgery is needed, the timing of surgery, and the priority of multiple surgical patients. The triage officer and surgeons should identify patients who require early evacuation. Casualties must be moved expeditiously to the next echelon of care when appropriate; otherwise, valuable resources will be consumed in maintaining patients, thereby preventing other casualties from receiving care. After a nuclear detonation, as in wartime, it cannot be assumed that it is possible to rapidly and reliably transport the wounded. In the confusion, casualties with a wide variety of injuries might arrive at the nearest MTF, regardless of its capability. Extra effort will be needed to keep patients moving forward in the system to an appropriate level of care. The greatest number of lives will be saved only by ensuring that time and materials are not allocated to expectant cases or to those whose injuries are such that definitive care can be postponed (minimal trauma or radiation-alone casualties). Knowing how and when to resupply internal resources may prove critical in decision-making for casualty treatment.

All patients receive a triage evaluation, but only some receive priority operative intervention. With an overwhelming number of trauma patients, time on the operating room table is the chokepoint. Trying to include all the factors that influence triage decision-making would be encyclopedic and of little benefit in a mass casualty situation; it is best to rely on the judgment of the trauma surgeons at the various MTFs.

DIME is the first approach in a mass casualty situation. Many patients in the immediate- and delayed-treatment categories require surgical intervention within minutes or hours, respectively. In forward locations where there are no surgical capabilities, patients classified as immediate who require surgery will need rapid transport to facilities capable of performing emergency surgery. It is likely that there will be many more patients in the immediate category than the operating room has the capacity to handle. Given two equally compelling immediate patients requiring emergency surgery, the one estimated to require less operating room table time should be taken first. A patient requiring only one surgical procedure generally has a higher priority than one requiring multiple procedures. Occasionally, with the operating rooms full, emergency lifesaving surgery may be performed outside the operating room; for

example, a patient bleeding uncontrollably from a dysfunctional extremity who requires an emergency amputation.

Surgeons will prioritize operative management. In the initial surge of patients received at an MTF (such as a combat support hospital or a fixed civilian or military medical center), those immediate and delayed patients awaiting surgery will be resuscitated and stabilized as much as possible. For example, at a combat support hospital, if the preoperative area becomes full, the critical presurgery patients can be stabilized in available intensive-care and medical or surgical beds. Thus, while awaiting surgery, immediate- and delayed- treatment patients receive respiratory support, stabilizing intravenous (IV) fluids, efforts to control bleeding, blood transfusions, antibiotics, and pain control, along with any additional external decontamination that may be necessary.

A patient presenting with hypotension must be presumed to be hypovolemic as a result of trauma and not as a result of a massive radiation dose. Therefore, hypotensive patients must be evaluated quickly to determine if their hypotension has a surgically correctable cause (eg, hemorrhage). The medical condition of those awaiting surgery will be monitored, and changes in triage category can be made. For example, given two patients in the immediate category, the patient who fails to respond rapidly to initial fluid resuscitation but who is still considered salvageable can be retriaged (or prioritized) ahead of a patient with a good response to fluid replacement. Alternatively, a nonresponder who is deteriorating rapidly and judged unlikely to be resuscitated and stabilized may be retriaged into the expectant category.

In a mass casualty situation, time itself is a resource that must be carefully managed. Aborting a surgical procedure and retriaging a patient to the expectant category may be necessary if the patient's condition deteriorates during surgery (for example, when extensive injuries are discovered intraoperatively that are not likely to be surgically correctable, with low chances of survival, compared to other patients who are potentially salvageable and urgently awaiting lifesaving surgery).

The decision to delay or withhold care from a wounded patient who, in another less-overwhelming situation, might be salvaged is difficult both for the medic or first responder out in the field and for the surgeon at the MTF. Nonetheless, making the difficult decisions in sorting casualties as quickly as possible is the essence of military triage. The goal is to save as many lives as possible with the available resources. Patients in the expectant category are given comfort care. Once the immediate and delayed patients have been cleared, available treatment resources should be focused on surviving expectant patients, followed by any minimal patients still requiring care

Radiation-Injury Triage

Trauma patients take priority over all radiation-alone patients. Casualties who have no trauma or burns because they were outside the immediate detonation impact area, but who were in the adjacent, downwind, heavy-fallout area, may have been exposed to a high radiation dose if they were unsheltered on the first day. For radiation-alone patients, four basic treatment categories, based on the severity of presumed radiation exposure, can be used to guide triage and treatment. The four categories are:

Mild (< 2 Gy)
- Triage by symptoms, lymphocyte count
- Close observation and complete blood cell count with differential
- Outpatient management is appropriate in the absence of significant mechanical trauma or burns

Moderate (2–5 Gy)
- Possible hospitalization
- Consider early growth factor (cytokine) therapy
- Consider viral prophylaxis
- Consider early antifungal therapy
- Administer antibiotics for febrile neutropenia; consider elective antibiotics for afrebrile neutropenia in certain cases

Severe (5–10 Gy)
- Hospitalization
- Reverse isolation and intensive care, if possible
- Early growth factor (cytokine) therapy
- Early viral prophylaxis
- Early antifungal therapy
- Early antibiotics for anticipated profound neutropenia

Lethal (> 10 Gy)
- Symptomatic and supportive care only; if there are no mass casualties or if resources become adequate, some of these patients can be treated as if in the severe group.[30,31]

The assumption is that these patients do not have significant conventional injuries (trauma or burns). The four groups are roughly parallel to the four groups in the military triage DIME system for conventional injuries.

People who have received a mild radiation dose without other injury can be placed in a minimal treatment category because they are expected to survive with no immediate treatment. Those who have received a lethal radiation dose would be placed in the expectant category and given comfort care. Clinical resources would be prioritized to treat casualties in the moderate and severe groups, parallel to trauma and burn patients in the delayed and immediate trauma triage categories. Patients in these two groups require the assistance of a hematologist knowledgeable in treating severe pancytopenia, and the assistance of an infectious disease expert knowledgeable in treating resistant opportunistic infections with anticipation of profound febrile neutropenia. However, the care of radiation-alone patients can be deferred for a few days, if necessary, until the priority trauma and burn patients are cleared. Patients in the military immediate-treatment category, by strict definition, are those requiring immediate lifesaving intervention. No patients with radiation-alone injuries require immediate intervention in a mass casualty situation. Those exposed to a treatable, life-threatening radiation dose are in the hematopoietic syndrome range and will not die during the first week (but are at risk after several weeks)[32]; however, trauma patients with potentially treatable, life-threatening injuries may die within an hour if untreated. Therefore, patients who have trauma and are triaged to the immediate or delayed categories will take priority over all radiation-alone patients, regardless of their triage category.

Combined-Injury Triage

Combined injury is defined as concurrent trauma (mechanical or thermal) and significant whole-body radiation injury. The prognosis is much worse for victims who have serious combined injuries than it is for those with the same degree of trauma without radiation injury.[3,9–12]

A major difference between conventional and radiation injuries is the time line. Many immediate-treatment patients with only trauma die within hours. Survivable injuries caused by radiation alone do not cause death in the first week. Thermal burns manifest immediately, but radiation burns do not manifest themselves for several weeks. A death caused by radiation alone within the first week indicates a dose so high that it would have been nonsurvivable regardless of treatment (eg, a dose high in the gastrointestinal syndrome or the neurovascular syndrome range; see Table 3-8). For this reason, initial care within the first 24 to 72 hours in a combined-injury scenario focuses on serious mechanical trauma and thermal burns.[33]

A theoretical combined-injury triage guide that

tried to factor in radiation dose would be difficult to implement because of the uncertainty of radiation dose during initial overwhelming mass casualty triage. In the 2004 recommendations of the Strategic National Stockpile Working Group (Table 3-12), delayed-treatment patients with a dose of 1.5 to 4.5 Gy were placed in variable triage categories depending on the nature of the trauma. However, those with a dose of 4.5 Gy have a much worse prognosis than those with a dose of 1.5 Gy. All patients in the minimal-treatment category were kept in that category regardless of how high the radiation dose because treatment for the presumed minor conventional injury plus the significant radiation injury could be postponed without appreciably affecting the chances of survival. However, early group evacuation of significantly radiation-injured individuals would be advantageous. Also in the Strategic National Stockpile Working Group schema, immediate-treatment trauma patients are kept in the immediate category even if they also have serious whole-body radiation injuries. However, suppose two immediate-treatment trauma patients, whose conventional injuries are equally compelling, require lifesaving surgery. If one of them has received an estimated radiation dose of 1.5 to 4.5 Gy, the surgeon will take the other, nonirradiated patient first because the patient with significant combined injuries requires more resources and has a poorer prognosis than the patient with trauma-alone injury. The essence of military triage is to operate first on casualties with life-threatening injuries that require limited resources and have the greatest likelihood of survival. Therefore, an immediate-treatment

trauma patient who was also exposed to an estimated radiation dose of 1.5 to 4.5 Gy would either be kept as a lower-priority immediate patient or retriaged to expectant. What will actually happen depends on the number of immediate casualties without significant radiation injury (< 1.6 Gy), the available resources, and the available evacuation options. It is sometimes difficult to prescribe in advance an appropriate triage category for some combined-injury patients.

Regardless of the triage schema used, it is probable that some combined-injury patients who should have been in the expectant category will have received treatment for immediate trauma injuries. This is because there will be cases where life-threatening injuries will be treated immediately, before a radiation dose estimate is available. In an overwhelming mass casualty situation in which patients need immediate lifesaving treatment, including surgery, there would be limited opportunity to accurately estimate, early on, the absorbed radiation dose. Furthermore, a patient could receive a nonuniform dose due to partial shielding that protected viable hematopoietic bone marrow stem cells from injury. Information on the patient's distance from the detonation and the degree of shielding is important for estimating the radiation dose; however, even if such information is available, unknown shielding factors of the physical environment could partially block the

TABLE 3-12

CONVENTIONAL VERSUS COMBINED-INJURY TRIAGE (2004 RECOMMENDATIONS)

Conventional Triage Categories	Expected Change*		
	< 1.5 Gy	1.5–4.5 Gy	> 4.5– < 10 Gy
Immediate (I)	I	I	E
Delayed (D)	D	Variable†	E
Minimal (M)	M	M	M
Expectant (E)	E	E	E

*Conventional triage categories with added whole-body irradiation
†Triage category depends on the nature and extent of physical injury
Data source: Waselenko JK, MacVittie TJ, Blakely WF, et al. Medical management of the acute radiation syndrome: recommendations of the Strategic National Stockpile Radiation Working Group. *Ann Intern Med.* 2004;140(12):1037–1051.

TABLE 3-13

CONVENTIONAL VERSUS COMBINED-INJURY TRIAGE (2009 RECOMMENDATIONS)

Conventional Triage Categories	Expected Changes*		
	< 2 Gy (Vomit > 4 h)	2–6 Gy (Vomit 1–4 h)	> 6 Gy (Vomit < 1 h)
Immediate (I)	I	Variable (I, E)	E
Delayed (D)	D	Variable (D, I)	E
Minimal (M)	M	D	Variable (D, E)
Expectant (E)	E	E	E

*Changes in triage categories after whole-body irradiation
Data sources: (1) Radiation Event Medical Management Web site. www.remm.nlm.gov. Accessed February 22, 2010. (2) Homeland Security Interagency Policy Coordination Subcommittee for Preparedness and Response to Radiological and Nuclear Threats. *Planning Guidance for Response to a Nuclear Detonation.* Washington, DC: Office of Science and Technology Policy, Executive Office of the President; 2009. www.usuhs.mil/afrri/outreach/pdf/planning-guidance.pdf. Accessed March 23, 2012.

amount of radiation received.

Using clinical symptoms, specifically time to first emesis, is very helpful for a triage officer (Table 3-13). This measure is much more reliable than early erythema for a dose greater than 6 Gy; early erythema is an unreliable indicator of radiation injury because it may be related to thermal or medical treatment effects, rather than ionizing radiation effects, and therefore is subject to misinterpretation. All minimal-treatment trauma patients, primarily the "walking wounded," who are also irradiated can be evacuated by mass transit to centers well outside the impact area that can deal with radiation injury in the hematopoietic syndrome range.

Immediate- and delayed-treatment trauma patients who have received a dose of 2 to 6 Gy or more than 6 Gy can be made lower-priority patients in their same triage categories, since trauma patients without irradi-

ation, or having sustained doses less than 2 Gy, would have priority over patients with greater radiation doses in the same triage category. Alternatively, immediate-treatment trauma patients who have received doses of 2 to 6 Gy or more than 6 Gy could be temporarily designated as expectant until the immediate-treatment patients without irradiation and those exposed to doses less than 2 Gy are cleared. Close and urgent attention must be paid to those patients classified as immediate or delayed upon initial clinical triage who may be potential candidates for priority evacuation. The medical facilities in the area around the impact and fallout zones will be overwhelmed. It is likely there will be many more immediate and delayed patients requiring surgery than the available area resources can handle. This could result in a significant delay in surgery for some immediate-treatment patients unless they can be quickly evacuated.

EVACUATION, RESUPPLY, AND AUSTERE MEDICAL CONDITIONS

Evacuation assets should be mobilized simultaneously with the medical response for triage and treatment. There can be many thousands of individuals inside the dangerous fallout zone who have received a significant whole-body radiation dose. Some may also have minimal conventional injuries. Public transportation assets, such as chartered airplanes, trains, and bus convoys, could be used to evacuate many people in less than 48 hours. They could be organized and escorted in groups of up to 500 individuals or more and sent to distant sites that are able to deal with serious, but potentially survivable, radiation injuries long before such injuries manifest clinically. Individuals with radiation-alone injuries or with minimal trauma do not need medical care during transport in a mass casualty scenario; an early group evacuation policy would take a major burden off local medical resources.

For more serious immediate- and delayed-injury patients, medical evacuation assets can sometimes be expanded under austere conditions. Medical transportation assets, such as air and ground ambulance, with the ability to provide medical care in transit, will be in short supply. The hospitals in the broad area around the detonation site will be overwhelmed with casualties. It is expected that some critical trauma patients who would normally be treated locally may need to be evacuated even when their injuries cannot be completely stabilized prior to transport. In an overwhelming mass casualty scenario, definitive care may be substantially delayed because too many casualties will require immediate care and resources will be taxed. A recent review of the aftermath of a potential 10-kiloton detonation in a major US city concluded

there were not enough burn beds in the United States to handle the expected patients with serious burns, even if all the beds were empty and available.[2,17] Under austere conditions, the "burn bed" should be redefined as any bed or cot set up where at least some basic burn care can be provided, such as IV fluid and electrolyte replacement, pain control, systemic antibiotics, and skin care. Those with minimal or no trauma injuries but with serious yet potentially salvageable radiation injuries can afford to have treatment delayed while they are evacuated to appropriate medical centers throughout the country. Critical trauma patients cannot afford such a delay.

In addition to evacuating casualties, immediate resupply of resources and personnel needs to be addressed. Within a day or two, there will be local shortages of supplies, such as IV fluids and blood, needed for the enormous number of thermal burn and trauma patients awaiting treatment or evacuation. Supplies of drugs, such as narcotics and antibiotics, may be depleted quickly. When first-choice drugs run out, alternative antibiotic regimens can be considered, as recommended by infectious disease clinicians. Oral drugs, including antibiotics, are preferred whenever possible because they can be administered by nonmedical personnel under medical supervision. It is also important that limited medical resources not be used in excess for those with minimal injuries or for hopeless expectant casualties.

Within 24 hours after the start of a mass casualty situation, many healthcare personnel, including surgeons and operating room personnel, will be totally exhausted. Work shifts will be extended throughout the hospital, and extreme fatigue will rapidly set in. Traditionally, two surgeons operate as a team on a complicated trauma case. Insufficient surgical staff levels could be augmented by incorporating the skills of other healthcare personnel. For example, under austere conditions, retired surgeons, surgical resident physicians-in-training, and experienced veterinary surgeons could play a role in assisting surgeons. This would depend on the specific case and the judgment of the primary surgeon in charge; however, using these resources would allow short sleep intervals for some surgeons on the brink of exhaustion after a prolonged surge of trauma cases. The surgical surge period could last up to a week.

Nonmedical volunteers, nursing students, and medical students could also be allowed to work under medical oversight. Each volunteer could be trained to perform a single function (eg, starting IVs, cleaning wounds, decontaminating casualties, acting as litter-bearers, distributing specific oral medication, giving intramuscular pain medication to expectant casualties). Most doctors and nurses at Hiroshima were casualties, and most hospitals were damaged. However, there was an innovative response from available medical and many nonmedical personnel, including those who themselves had minimal injuries.[5,6] The nonmedical personnel provided whatever assistance they could to others, usually under some medical direction.

In a present-day situation, the number of people with radiation contamination, whether minor or significant, will be overwhelming. Initially, there will be severe shortages of trained personnel and instrumentation to address contamination issues. There will be a great need to mobilize health physicists, medical physicists, and associated technical staff, such as health physics technologists or nuclear medicine technologists. All provide critical support in assessing contamination and evaluating decontamination. These individuals may bring their own instrumentation with them to assigned areas requiring health physics support.

ASSESSMENT OF RADIATION DOSE: CLINICAL AND LABORATORY

Clinical Assessment

Once the immediate medical needs of a patient with mechanical or thermal trauma have been met, radiation decontamination should begin and the radiation dose should be estimated. Assessing the radiation dose can be important for modifying patient triage, and it can be estimated by the time to first emesis. The Radiation Emergency Assistance Center/Training Site (REAC/TS) in Oak Ridge, Tenneessee, records and maintains worldwide accident data (Table 3-14) and reports that the time to first emesis decreases with increasing radiation dose in a predictable pattern.[14] The estimated average whole-body dose resulting in emesis in 50% of patients was 2.4 Gy. When a dose is absorbed over a short period of time (ie, at a high dose rate), the dose resulting in emesis in 50% of the patients is expected to be significantly lower, as consistent with clinical experience in radiation oncology treatment where the dose is delivered in a few minutes. Although a relatively small percentage of patients acutely exposed to a dose of 1 Gy vomit, most vomit when the dose is higher than 2 Gy, provided the dose is absorbed over a very short time rather than over many hours or days. As a guide for rapid clinical radiological triage in a mass casualty situation, it has been proposed, based on REAC/TS data, that individuals who vomit within 4 hours after exposure be referred for hospital evaluation and possible admission.[34] Those who do not vomit within 4 hours can be referred for delayed evaluation some days later. If they have no serious concurrent injury, outpatient care is probably appropriate. If no vomiting occurs during the first 4 hours after an acute exposure, one may assume that severe clinical effects are unlikely unless there are significant conventional injuries. If there is insufficient laboratory support in a mass casualty situation, casualty triage according to radiation dose depends on the length of time to initial vomiting. More recently, REAC/TS reported that if the time to emesis is less than 2 hours after exposure, the effective whole-body dose is probably at least 3 Gy.[35] Patients who have radiation-induced emesis within 1 hour have received a whole-body dose that probably exceeds 4 to 6 Gy. The median radiation dose for

TABLE 3-14

ESTIMATES OF TIME TO VOMITING AFTER WHOLE-BODY RADIATION DOSE

Percentile of Dose	Radiation Dose	
	> 4 h to Vomiting	< 4 h to Vomiting
25th	0.5 Gy	2.5 Gy
Median	0.9 Gy	3.6 Gy
75th	1.7 Gy	6.0 Gy

Data source: US Department of Homeland Security. *Department of Homeland Security Working Group on Radiological Dispersal Device (RDD) Preparedness.* Washington, DC: DHS; 2003. www.au.af.mil/au/awc/awcgate/va/radiologic_medical_countermeasures.pdf. Accessed March 23, 2012.

patients vomiting less than 1 hour after exposure is 6.5 Gy, with an interquartile range (25%–75%) of approximately 5 to 11 Gy.[34] Conversely, if the patient has not vomited within 8 to 10 hours after the event, the whole-body dose is probably less than 1 Gy. However, vomiting can occur for reasons other than radiation (eg, as a result of psychological effects).

Laboratory Assessment

Lymphocyte Count Depression

Ideally, a complete blood cell count with differential to evaluate lymphocytes (and neutrophils) should be performed initially, then every 6 hours if resources permit, or at least at 24 and 48 hours. The peripheral blood lymphocyte count (lymphocytes/mm³) is a sensitive indicator of radiation dose and follows a predictable, radiation dose-dependent, exponential decline in the first few days after a significant whole-body dose. For example, at 24 hours after exposure, if the lymphocyte count is less than 10% of normal, the exposure is lethal, even with treatment. If it is 90% or more of normal, survival is likely, even without treatment.[36] If it is about 50% of normal, the corresponding dose is in the mid-hematopoietic syndrome range. In that case, aggressive treatment should ideally be started before the end of the first week to decrease the risk of death in the following weeks.[37,38] REAC/ TS developed a predictive algorithm to estimate the effective whole-body dose soon after an exposure.[34] The method uses the measured lymphocyte depletion rate from serial complete blood cell counts performed within the first 8 to 12 hours after exposure. This algorithm was developed to provide physicians and health physicists with an early approximation of the dose so that cytokine therapy, if indicated, can begin early. A rough estimate of the whole-body dose may be obtained by using the REAC/TS data and taking the absolute lymphocyte count at approximately 8 to 12 hours after exposure (Table 3-15). The dose estimate is independent of the preirradiation lymphocyte count, which is often unknown. This technique is designed to be a radiation triage mechanism applied early after exposure and should be considered along with the time to radiation-induced emesis. Between 12 and 48 hours after exposure, the lymphocyte count continues to drop exponentially. The lymphocyte counts of patients receiving different radiation doses will differ more at 48 hours than at 12 hours because the counts decrease at different dose-dependent depletion rates; therefore, a better estimate of dose and prognosis can be made at the 48-hour point (Table 3-16).[39]

Algorithms from the Armed Forces Radiobiology

TABLE 3-15

WHOLE-BODY, APPROXIMATE DOSE ESTIMATES BASED ON EARLY LYMPHOCYTE COUNT DEPRESSION*

Absolute Lymphocyte Count 8–12 Hours After Exposure*	Estimated Absorbed Dose (Gy)
1,700–2,500/mm³	1–5
1,200–1,700/mm³	5–9
< 1,000/mm³	> 10

*A whole-body dose of 1 Gy or less should not noticeably depress the lymphocyte count below the normal range, taken as 1,500 to 3,500/mm³.
Data source: US Department of Homeland Security. *Department of Homeland Security Working Group on Radiological Dispersal Device (RDD) Preparedness*. Washington, DC: DHS; 2003. www.au.af.mil/au/awc/awcgate/va/radiologic_medical_countermeasures.pdf. Accessed March 23, 2012.

Research Institute biodosimetry assessment tool combine various factors, including time to emesis and lymphocyte depletion rate, to estimate the radiation dose and help guide therapy (see www.afrri.usuhs.mil).[9]

TABLE 3-16

PROGNOSIS AT 48 HOURS BASED ON LYMPHOCYTE COUNT DEPRESSION AFTER ACUTE WHOLE-BODY EXPOSURE

Minimal Lymphocyte Count 48 Hours After Exposure	Aproximate Absorbed Dose (Gy)	Prognosis
1,000–3,000/ mm³ (normal range)	0–0.5	No significant injury
1,000–1,500/ mm³	1–2	Significant but probably nonlethal injury, good prognosis.
500–1,000/ mm³	2–4	Severe injury; fair prognosis
100–500/ mm³	4–8	Very severe injury; poor prognosis
< 100/mm³	> 8	High incidence of lethality even with hemapoeitic stimulation

Reproduced with permission from: Koenig KL, Goans RE, Hatchett RJ, et al. Medical treatment of radiological casualties and current concepts. *Ann Emerg Med.* 2005;45:643–652.

Cytogenetic Studies

The radiation dose may be subsequently confirmed with a chromosome-aberration bioassay in cultured peripheral blood lymphocytes.[40] Chromosome dicentrics are interchanges between two chromosomes that form a distorted chromosome with two centromeres. The frequency of chromosome dicentrics correlates better with the absorbed dose than does lymphocyte count depression, and changes may be detected with a dose as low as 0.2 Gy. The technique is labor intensive, however, and results cannot be obtained rapidly; even in ideal situations, results may not be available until days after exposure. Thus, the method has limited usefulness in a mass casualty situation. However, cytogenetics can guide crucial therapy in selected cases. In the United States, the current laboratories with cytogenetic capability that are dedicated to radiation dose assessment are at the Armed Forces Radiobiology Research Institute in Bethesda, Maryland, and at REAC/TS in Oak Ridge, Tennessee.

EMERGENCY TREATMENT OF COMBINED INJURIES

Basic life-support concerns need to be addressed quickly for casualties in the immediate category; airway, adequate ventilation, and circulatory function should be ensured for patients whose injuries are correctable. Concerns about internal or external contamination from radioactive material should be secondary. During the first 72 hours, the initial phase of treatment will be directed toward trauma and burns, with simultaneous integration of external decontamination, as appropriate. After detonation of a nuclear weapon, most casualties will be combined-injury patients.

Emergency surgical care involves resuscitation, hemorrhage control, and minimizing sepsis with debridement. Traditionally, combat and traumatic wounds are left open. However, there has been concern that in the significantly irradiated patient (hematopoietic syndrome range), wounds left open may serve as a nidus for infection, based in part on animal studies and on observations at Hiroshima. However, in the Hiroshima experience, when wounds were open, antibiotics were in extremely short supply, so they were often diluted and may not have reached therapeutic blood levels.[6] Wounds in the combined-injury patient might be debrided thoroughly and closed early, when possible. However, early closure may not be possible or practical in many circumstances, such as when multiple debridements are needed or in the case of significant devitalized tissue and subsequent morbidity of closed-space contamination. For a patient who has received a whole-body radiation dose over 2 Gy and also has a traumatic wound, therapeutic countermeasures are available today to reduce the risk of radiation-induced neutropenia and subsequent sepsis when a wound must be left open: specifically, cytokines to stimulate the bone-marrow stem cells and more potent antibiotics to prevent or treat infection.

Topical antibiotics and nonadherent dressings are essential to treating wounds and burns, with systemic antibiotics added if appropriate. Major surgical procedures are prioritized for unstable but salvageable patients. Ideally, if surgical correction of major injuries is required, it should be performed as soon as possible. Otherwise, major surgical procedures should be postponed, when possible, until late in the convalescent period following hematopoietic recovery. However, patients requiring critical surgery during the first 2 months should receive it even without full hematopoietic recovery.

For vomiting, treatment includes drugs such as granisetron and ondansetron. Vomiting usually abates within 48 hours, making prolonged antiemetic therapy unnecessary. For diarrhea, treatment includes drugs such as loperamide and diphenoxylate hydrochloride with atropine sulfate.

Casualties who have mild, uncomplicated injuries may be kept in alternative care facilities established in response to the overwhelming mass casualties. Patients who have significant (2–6 Gy) but potentially salvageable whole-body radiation injury should begin to receive aggressive treatment within the first week. They may be transferred to oncology centers equipped to treat potential opportunistic infectious complications of bone marrow failure. One national resource, the Radiation Injury Treatment Network, is partnered with the US Department of Health and Human Services and provides coordinated medical care with a large number of specialty centers.[41,42]

DEFINITIVE TREATMENT OF RADIATION INJURIES

Hematopoietic Injury

During the first 72 hours of the emergency treatment phase, while clinical and laboratory whole-body dose assessments are being made, potentially salvageable patients may be identified who are destined to develop radiation-induced bone marrow aplasia of the hematopoietic syndrome. Early in the definitive treatment phase of casualties, within the first week in an overwhelming mass casualty scenario, the initiation of cytokines (such as granulocyte CSF) and antimicrobials will improve the chances of survival for these patients.[33,35,41–45] Essentially, of the patients treated for significant radiation exposure, those with a chance for survival will be those without serious mechanical or thermal trauma, with a dose limited to the hematopoietic syndrome range (up to 8 Gy). Both in the immediate posttraumatic period and later during the manifestation of hematopoietic radiation injury, blood products should be transfused when indicated.

Hematopoietic growth factors or cytokines (CSFs) are endogenous glycoproteins that induce bone marrow stem cells to proliferate and differentiate into specific mature blood cell types. For those who receive radiation doses above 3 Gy, successful treatment depends on maintaining a surviving fraction of stem cells capable of spontaneous regeneration, assuming that any nonhematopoietic injuries are survivable. For neutropenic patients receiving myelosuppressive chemotherapy, available CSFs include filgrastim, pegfilgrastim, and sargramostim (granulocyte-macrophage CSF). These, along with newer growth factors under development, are potent stimulators of hematopoiesis by the bone marrow. CSFs will usually decrease the duration of radiation-induced neutropenia and stimulate neutrophil recovery. The results of several radiation accidents suggest that prophylactic CSFs should be initiated early, within 3 to 4 days whenever possible, in patients who have been exposed to potentially survivable whole-body doses of radiation and are at risk for hematopoietic syndrome. This may not always be possible in a mass casualty scenario. For patients who were not given early granulocyte-macrophage CSF and who later become profoundly neutropenic (ie, an absolute neutrophil count < 500/mm^3), a CSF should be employed. This can sometimes be effective, as demonstrated in patients who received chemotherapy and subsequently developed febrile neutropenia.

In a nuclear detonation, most casualties exposed to a dose exceeding 6 to 8 Gy may also have significant blast and thermal injuries that preclude survival, regardless of treatment. Bone marrow transplantation and other aggressive treatment cannot salvage anyone who has received a whole-body dose of about 12 Gy because serious radiation injury to the lungs and other vital organs would result in nonsurvivable conditions. For patients who undergo bone marrow transplantation after radiation accidents, outcomes have been poor. Bone marrow transplantation would have no role in a mass casualty situation given the presence of current alternative therapies (such as cytokine therapy), the probability of combined injuries,

uncertainties about radiation dose, and nonuniform exposure of radiation victims.[42,46] The patient's physical environment often affords partial shielding, resulting in variability in the absorbed dose. Because the absorbed radiation dose is nonuniform, there may be unexpected reservoirs of viable hematopoietic stem cells that received a lower dose than the average whole-body dose. Both spared and radiation-resistant stem cells are capable of promoting hematologic reconstitution. This ability appears to be augmented by CSF therapy.

Infectious Complications

Controlling infection during the critical neutropenic phase is a major factor for producing a successful outcome in patients who have absorbed a radiation dose in the hematopoietic syndrome range.[33,43,44] Infections are a major cause of mortality in irradiated casualties because of the immunosuppressive effects that result from declining lymphohematopoietic elements secondary to radiation-induced bone marrow aplasia (reversible or irreversible). Life-threatening, gram-negative bacterial infections are universal among neutropenic patients. Oral fluoroquinolones may be used electively in severely neutropenic patients. Managing established or suspected infection in irradiated patients with fever and neutropenia is similar to managing infection in febrile neutropenic patients undergoing chemotherapy. For those who have significant neutropenia (absolute neutrophil count < 500/mm^3), the use of broad-spectrum prophylactic antimicrobials is indicated because the duration of neutropenia is likely to be prolonged. Treatment might include a fluoroquinolone with streptococcal coverage (with penicillin or amoxicillin, if the streptococci are not inherently covered by the fluoroquinolone); an oral antiviral agent, such as acyclovir; and an oral antifungal agent, such as fluconazole. Acyclovir is effective against herpesvirus, which has a high risk of reactivation during periods of immunosuppression. Fluconazole has been shown to reduce fungal infections and mortality in immunosuppressed patients undergoing allogeneic bone marrow transplantation.[47] Other antifungals, such as voriconazole, could be used for infections that do not respond to fluconazole, such as those from *Aspergillus* or resistant *Candida* species.

Antimicrobial agents should be continued until the treatment fails, the patient has a neutropenic fever, or the patient shows evidence of neutrophil recovery (absolute neutrophil count rising and > 500/mm^3). The fluoroquinolone should be stopped in patients who develop fever while receiving it. Urgent parenteral therapy should be used if fluoroquinolone-resistant, gram-negative bacteria are suspected, in particular *Pseudomonas aeruginosa*, because gram-negative infections may be rapidly fatal. Vancomycin should be added if a resistant gram-positive infection is suspected. The prevalence of life-threatening, gram-positive bacterial infections varies greatly among hospitals, and therefore antimicrobial therapy should be matched against hospital susceptibility patterns.

The specific hematopoietic and antimicrobial treatment described are examples of several approaches to treating victims who have received radiation doses in the hematopoietic syndrome range. Hematologists and infectious disease physicians will determine the actual approaches to treatment. Infectious disease physicians will be the center of the decision-making process regarding opportunistic, drug-resistant infections in patients who have altered immunity or burns. For patients who develop febrile radiation-induced neutropenia, adherence to the new guidelines of the Infectious Disease Society of America[48] is recommended. The society has also endorsed comprehensive new guidelines for preventing infections associated with combat-related injuries,[49] and it periodically updates its treatment guidelines on its website. A truly overwhelming mass casualty situation may, to some degree, preclude the strict application of a formulated approach. For example, oral antimicrobials might be used when there is limited capability for IV therapy,[50] or injections of a specific cytokine might not be given daily because of resource limitations. Because some drug supplies would run short in a mass casualty scenario, available second-choice drugs could be used on the basis of ongoing expert guidance.

Cutaneous Syndrome

In contrast to thermal skin burns appearing immediately following a nuclear detonation and release of thermal radiation, radiation burns occur later, with delayed erythema and desquamation or blistering developing in 2 to 3 weeks. This radiation injury can be caused either by the prompt ionizing radiation released immediately by the detonation or by the radioactive fallout, particularly on the first day. If there is radioactive contamination on the skin, decontamination needs to be done early because reducing the time the radioisotopes remain in contact with the skin reduces the severity of the injury that develops later (Table 3-17).

Skin injury effects, as a function of increasing dose from ionizing radiation after a nuclear detonation, are similar to those seen when normal skin is irradiated as part of cancer treatment. Unlike the erythema that develops in a dose-dependent fashion at 2 weeks, the early transient erythema threshold reported at 6 Gy is not reliably observed, particularly in radiation oncology treatments with 6 Gy given to skin in a single

TABLE 3-17

CUTANEOUS EFFECTS AS A FUNCTION OF A RADIATION DOSE (SINGLE ACUTE EXPOSURE)

Dose	Cutaneous Effects
3 Gy	Epilation of the scalp threshold, typically beginning at 14–21 days after incident
10–15 Gy	Dry desquamation* of the skin usually seen about 3 weeks after incident; desquamation of large, macroscopic flakes of skin
20–50 Gy	Wet desquamation* (partial thickness injury) at least 2–3 weeks after exposure
> 50 Gy	Overt radionecrosis* and ulceration

*Dry desquamation, wet desquamation, and radionecrosis are preceded by erythema, which starts around the second week after exposure.
Data source: Goans RE. Critical care of the radiation-accident patient: patient presentation, assessment and initial diagnosis. In: Ricks RC, Berger ME, O'Hara FM, eds. *The Medical Basis of Radiation-Accident Preparedness: The Clinical Care of Victims*. Boca Raton, FL: Parthenon Publishing Group, CRC Press; 2002.

dose. After a nuclear detonation, early erythema from ionizing radiation may be masked by the immediate effects of thermal radiation.

The two main approaches to managing radiation skin injury are nonoperative and operative treatment. Sometimes both approaches are necessary to manage the cutaneous syndrome. Generally, nonoperative treatment is the initial approach. Treatment consists of gentle flushing and early superficial debridement of potentially septic tissue. Steroid ointment should be used for relatively intact skin, a topical antibiotic with dressings should be used for the blistering phase, and silver sulfadiazine cream and nonadherent dressings (without topical antibiotic treatment) should be used for wet desquamation. Wet desquamation may be complicated by secondary infections. Depending on the specific case, systemic antibiotics may be added. Decisions regarding surgical treatment may be impossible at an early stage because it may be many weeks before the radiation burn fully evolves. Once indications for surgery appear (eg, radiation ulcers, localized necrosis without signs of regeneration, and severe, intractable pain), surgical intervention, such as amputation of a necrotic extremity, should not be delayed. Tissue grafts may be required for some cases; necrotic tissue must be excised and the least irradiated skin harvested or transposed for coverage. Cutaneous injuries in some individuals may be protracted and eventually require the expertise of reconstructive surgeons and other specialists.

DECONTAMINATION: EXTERNAL AND INTERNAL

Initial Management

The initial management of a casualty contaminated by radioactive material involved performing all life- and limb-saving actions without regard to contamination.[2,3,9–12] Decontamination should be integrated with medical care in a way that does not interfere with urgent care.[31,51] Contaminated casualties should never be barred entry to a medical facility if entry is necessary for emergency care. Significant decontamination can be achieved by clothing removal. After a nuclear detonation, it is not possible for a living patient to be contaminated enough to become an immediate threat to healthcare providers; therefore, radiological decontamination should never interfere with medical care priorities.

Radiological decontamination is performed in a manner similar to chemical decontamination. However, whereas chemical decontamination may be an emergency, radiological decontamination is not.[2,9] Radiological contamination can be readily confirmed and localized by passing the probe of the radiation detector (RADIAC or other Geiger-Müller counter) over the entire body. It would be advantageous to cover the probe with a surgical glove to prevent contamination of the probe itself. A person trained in and familiar with radiation equipment can supervise, interpret contamination measurements, and advise the medical staff on the contamination levels.[52–54]

Emergency rescuers and first responders, including medics, who enter high-radiation areas need augmented personal protection and radiation monitoring devices. Initial triage on site may include a hasty decontamination performed on priority casualties who will be sent directly to the MTF for clinical retriage and treatment. This may consist, for example, of removing outer, contaminated clothing and quickly wiping the face and exposed skin while the person awaits transport to the MTF. However, a patient with life-threatening injuries should not be decontaminated if doing so would delay transport. A brief, hasty decontamination can also be performed during transport.

Casualties who have both radiation contamination and wounds must be directed to an MTF or, if one has been established, to a designated medical triage station. The first or second decontamination may occur at the MTF. Personnel providing decontamination at the MTF must protect themselves from most radiation contamination. They do not require augmented protection, as do first responders and emergency rescuers. For emergency treatment and decontamination, adequate protection is provided by standard hospital barrier clothing as used in universal precautions,

which consists of a surgical gown or other protective outer clothing and lightweight surgical apron, gloves, shoe covers, surgical mask, and cap to cover the hair.

Contaminated personnel without injuries, as well as ambulatory casualties with minimal injuries, should not be decontaminated at the MTF, which will be overwhelmed by casualties with significant mechanical and thermal trauma. They should be sent to decontamination sites for self-decontamination, washing their exposed skin and hair (and showering, if possible) after removing and bagging their contaminated clothing. Clothing and footwear should either be replaced or shaken or brushed to remove loose contamination. Families should not be separated, and parents should decontaminate their children. Those not capable of decontaminating themselves should receive assistance.[2,3] However, with overwhelming numbers of contaminated individuals, the decontamination staff will be limited. The decontamination staff is also tasked with using detectors to evaluate decontamination levels. To assist decontamination efforts, the staff should seek volunteers from among those who were not contaminated or who have already been decontaminated.[3] Ideal decontamination sites would be located where there are sources of water for washing and showering, preferably separated by gender, such as those found in school gymnasiums, health clubs, and indoor sports arenas.

External Decontamination

Decontamination of radionuclides is a second priority after the initial resuscitative support of casualties with salvageable life-threatening injuries.[2,9,31,32] For immediate-treatment patients requiring surgery, lavage of contaminated open wounds can be done before and also during surgery. However, aggressive surgery, such as amputation, should not be undertaken to eliminate contamination as long as the contamination poses no serious acute risk to the patient or the medical staff. The surgical damage will far exceed any potential reduction of lifetime risk due to radiation exposure.

Removing outer clothing and shoes and washing exposed skin and hair should eliminate 95% or more of the external radioactive contamination. Regular soap and water is the preferred method to remove external contamination. Casualties entering an MTF must be assumed to be contaminated and must therefore undergo at least simple, hasty decontamination if radiation-monitoring devices are not available. During decontamination in the receiving medical facility, wounds get first priority. Bandages are removed and wounds are decontaminated first and copiously irrigated with normal saline or water; the bandages are then replaced, if appropriate. Stubborn contamination after irrigation may require wound debridement and further irrigation. Burns should be rinsed gently with water and cleared of debris. In patients whose burn wounds cannot be completely decontaminated, most of the contamination will remain in the burn eschar when it sloughs. After wounds, priority is given to the nose, mouth, eyes, and ears.

After outer clothing removal and wound decontamination, intact skin can be decontaminated, if indicated. A wet washcloth with soap and a basin of water may be used to remove a significant amount of superficial contamination. To prevent cross-contamination, wounds and burns can be covered with waterproof dressings before the skin is decontaminated. Abrasions and lacerations are usually relatively easy to decontaminate. Gentle brushing may help remove contamination from the skin, but care should be taken not to irritate or abrade the skin because some contamination can be absorbed though injured skin. Hair (and skin) can be decontaminated with any commercial shampoo. Cutting or clipping the hair or beard (not shaving) can also remove contaminants. Fingernails and toenails should be checked and cut if necessary. Contaminated wastewater can be disposed of without restriction.

After each skin or wound decontamination, the patient should undergo another contamination check with a radiation detector to determine the effectiveness of the decontamination. The goal, which cannot always be reached, is to decontaminate to a level two or three times below the background radiation level. An alternative goal is to stop if subsequent decontamination attempts are ineffective at reducing the count rate by more than 10% to 20% of the prior count rate. At this time, there is no universally accepted threshold of radioactivity (external or internal) above which a person is considered contaminated and below which a person is considered decontaminated.[2,25,32]

Internal Decontamination

Internal contamination is more likely if high levels of contamination are found on the face, particularly at the nostrils. Nasal swabs that show a strong, positive indication of contamination will also indicate the probable inhalation of radioactive particles. However, one may assume that some inhalation has occurred in most patients in the mass casualty phase after a nuclear

detonation, but immediate treatment for internal contamination, in general, is not necessary. Fortunately, the amount of internal contamination is usually a very small fraction of the external contamination, which is generally of greater concern but more easily removed. Therefore, in a nuclear detonation scenario, a radiation dose received from internal contaminants will not be a major concern compared to mechanical or thermal trauma or to the potentially large external radiation dose received from exposure either at the time of detonation or later from fallout.[2] A recent independent review of the issue concluded that internal decontamination will not be a high priority in the immediate aftermath of a nuclear detonation.[55] However, there may be a few special cases that will warrant relatively early treatment. Clinical judgment needs to be exercised as to whether internal decontamination is needed. Internal contamination is minimized by reducing absorption, increasing excretion, or both. Medical management, when it is necessary, depends on the type of isotope. Techniques to be applied may include the following:

- Oral and nasopharyngeal suction.
- Increased oral fluid intake versus IV hydration (and possibly diuretics); this is effective for any isotope, including iodine, phosphorus, and tritium.
- Administration of laxatives (cathartics), such as a biscodyl or phosphate soda enema, or magnesium sulfate to speed gastrointestinal transit time.
- Stomach lavage.
- Administration of antacids, particularly aluminum hydroxide, to reduce absorption.
- Administration of therapeutic agents including blocking or diluting agents, such as potassium iodide for radioactive iodine; mobilizing agents, such as ammonium chloride for radiostrontium; chelating agents, such as calcium or zinc diethylenetriaminepentaacetic acid for plutonium and americium; other specific agents, such as ferric ferrocyanide (Prussian blue), which has proven useful for cesium and thallium internal contamination; and sodium bicarbonate, which is used to prevent kidney toxicity from uranium.

Detailed information on treatment for exposure to a range of radioisotopes is available from the National Council on Radiation Protection and Measurements.[56]

PSYCHOLOGICAL EFFECTS ON MILITARY AND CIVILIAN PERSONNEL

Overwhelming casualties and radiation exposure create stress and fear in both military and civilian

populations. Traditional treatment for combat stress has involved rest for several days in physical proximity to the soldier's unit rather than reassignment and evacuation. Counseling during the rest period involved a positive expectation that soldiers would be able to return to their units. However, this traditional military doctrine is not as practical in the event of a single, geographically localized nuclear detonation as it was during conventional wars of the past century. In modern times, it is evident that nonessential personnel need to be removed from the area of operations. The number of military combat stress casualties depends today, as it did in the past, on the prior training, leadership, and cohesiveness of a unit.[8,9]

There is less cohesiveness and practiced discipline among the civilian population, and a nuclear detonation will result in widespread fear and panic.[2,17] Many will immediately self-evacuate, not realizing that by doing so they may be putting themselves, and their families, at even greater risk. Others, anxious to be checked for contamination (or have their children checked), will flood emergency rooms or tie up communication channels. Reactions to this kind of psychological trauma will produce symptoms ranging from insomnia and anxiety to irrational and aggressive behavior. Occasionally, psychosomatic symptoms that mimic symptoms of exposure to high radiation (eg, nausea, rashes) may be seen in patients who were not significantly exposed.

Firm command and control needs to be established in the civilian sector. Civilian authority will likely request military support. In a mass casualty situation, those who request medical care for themselves or ask to be checked for radiation could be stopped at roadblocks leading to medical facilities, with clearance required to proceed. Otherwise, hospital access and medical treatment for the seriously injured will be severely impeded. The noninjured requiring only radiation checks and those with minor injuries who have external contamination would be diverted to appropriate nonmedical decontamination facilities.[3,42,54–57] These facilities will be staffed with decontamination teams plus several medical personnel to evaluate and handle first aid, triage, and medical problems that might arise. Security personnel will be needed at decontamination sites, triage sites, evacuation sites, hospitals, alternative care sites, and along roads leading to them. A single, unified federal command must be maintained over numerous federal, state, and local entities. The public will respond to strong, effective leadership. People need to believe that leadership decisions are rational; communication to affected populations on the verge of panic must convey reassurance that the leadership is aware of and concerned about radiation effects, that radiation exposure levels will be monitored, and that injuries will be treated. Communication, at the appropriate time, should convey the overall expectation that, based on experience gained from accidents at Chernobyl and Goiânia, most people exposed to contamination will remain asymptomatic and will not suffer severe adverse health effects. The general public needs accurate and timely information and reassurance. In the months that follow the radiation event, treatment needs for those who suffer from posttraumatic stress disorder should be anticipated and planned for.

SUMMARY

The most severe consequence of a nuclear detonation in an urban environment will be the overwhelming surge of casualties. For a 10-kiloton, ground-level nuclear detonation, nearly all deaths, serious injuries, and structural damage in the impact (blast) zone will occur less than 3 miles from the point of detonation. In addition to the predominant thermal and blast injuries, prompt radiation injuries within the blast zone will be caused by radiation instantaneously released at the moment of detonation. Fallout radiation injuries without significant blast or thermal trauma will also be seen in the downwind area outside the impact zone minutes to several hours later. Emergency responders will have radiation-dose measuring devices and operating guidelines to ensure their safety during rescue operations. The death toll, particularly during the first few days, will be high. It can be mitigated in part by effective triage, treatment, and evacuation strategies.

The triage of patients with conventional injuries, radiation-alone injuries, and combined injuries will overwhelm the area's medical resources for days. Patients will first be triaged on the basis of their thermal burns and blast trauma, since these conventional injuries will account for nearly all lethal or immediately life-threatening injuries during the first 72 hours. Patients will receive appropriate treatment for conventional injuries. During that period, assessment of the probable degree of radiation injury will be made based on symptoms, laboratory data, and geographic location relative to both the detonation site and the dangerous fallout zone.

Triage of patients with thermal burns and blast injuries can be based on the military DIME system used in a mass casualty situation: delayed (second priority), immediate (highest priority), minimal (lower priority), and expectant (lowest priority). It is likely that there will be more immediate patients during the first few days than available resources. Among the immediate patients requiring surgery, surgeons will select those with life-threatening conditions who cannot tolerate delay but have a good chance to be saved in a timely fashion without excessive resource use. During the first day, triage priority modifications may occur as information on total body radiation-dose estimates becomes available. Casualties with two or three types of significant injury have a much worse prognosis than those with one significant injury type. Those with more than one life-threatening injury will be classified as expectant rather than immediate.

Distance from ground zero and shielding were the principal factors influencing casualty rates at Hiroshima and Nagasaki. For any given distance from ground zero, the lethality was much higher for those who were outdoors. Unlike Hiroshima in 1945, there are tall buildings in US urban environments that will provide some shielding, so there will not be uniform zones around the detonation point. There may also be some relatively open sectors without tall buildings where the blast, thermal, and radiation effects will be channeled in full force along corridors. Given the important data from the zonal casualty-rate analysis at Hiroshima, current planning in the United States involves a modification of the three Hiroshima blast zones. There will be no precise circular boundaries, but visual evidence of the degree of structural damage will define the operational boundaries of the three blast zones.

Unlike the low-altitude detonations in Japan, a ground-level detonation will result in downwind radioactive fallout. The first public response should be to take shelter, since being outdoors in the dangerous fallout zone during the first day could result in lethal radiation injury. People who were outdoors prior to sheltering will probably be contaminated with radioactive fallout particles. Almost all fallout will be removed by showering and changing clothing. For those requiring medical treatment, decontamination of fallout material should be integrated with medical care in a way that does not interfere with urgent medical care. Immediate treatment for internal contamination, which is generally a very small fraction of the amount of external decontamination, is in general not necessary but will be reserved for special cases.

In the first few days following a nuclear detonation, a scarcity of resources will develop in local healthcare facilities. This will include personnel and medical supplies. In austere conditions, treatment protocols may need to be modified. The overwhelming number of casualties and the radiation exposure will create extreme stress in the affected population and result in the need to address management of posttraumatic stress in the weeks and months following a radiation event.

REFERENCES

1. Mettler FA, Voelz GL. Major radiation exposure—what to expect and how to respond. *N Engl J Med*. 2002;346:1554–1561.

2. National Security Staff Interagency Policy Coordination Subcommittee for Preparedness and Response to Radiological and Nuclear Threats. *Planning Guidance for Response to a Nuclear Detonation*. 2nd ed. Washington, DC: Executive Office of the President; 2010. http://www.hps.org/hsc/documents/Planning_Guidance_for_Response_to_a_Nuclear_Detonation-2nd_Edition_FINAL.pdf. Accessed October 12, 2010.

3. Flynn DF, Goans RE. Nuclear terrorism: triage and medical management of radiation and combined-injury casualties. *Surg Clin N Am*. 2006;86:601–636.

4. Glasstone S, Dolan PJ, eds. *The Effects of Nuclear Weapons*. 3rd ed. Washington, DC: US Government Printing Office; 1977.

5. Glasstone S, ed. *The Effects of Nuclear Weapons*. Revised ed. Washington, DC: US Government Printing Office; 1962.

6. Oughterson AW, Warren S. *Medical Effects of the Atomic Bomb in Japan*. In: *National Nuclear Energy Series, Manhattan Project Technical Section*. Vol 8. New York: NY; McGraw-Hill: 1956.

7. Stein M, Hirsberg A. Medical consequences of terrorism. *Surg Clin North Am*. 1999;79(6):1537–1552.

8. US Department of Defense. *Emergency War Surgery*, 3rd United States Revision. Burris DG, Dougherty PJ, Elliot DC, et al, eds. Washington, DC: US Department of the Army, Borden Institute; 2004.

9. Military Medical Operations, Armed Forces Radiobiology Research Institute. *Medical Management of Radiological Casualties. Online Third Edition (June 2010)*. Bethesda, MD: AFRRI; 2010. AFRRI Serial Publication 10-1. http://www.afrri.usuhs.mil/outreach/pdf/3edmmrchandbook.pdf. Accessed July 27, 2012.

10. *NATO Handbook on Medical Aspects of NBC Defensive Operations*. NATO AMED P-6(B). US Army Field Manual 8-9, US Navy Publication NAVMED P-5059, and US Air Force Pamphlet 161-3. Washington, DC: DA, DN, and USAF; 1995.

11. *NATO Handbook on the Concept of Medical Support in NBC Environments*. NATO AMED P-7(A). Brussels, Belgium: North Atlantic Treaty Organization; 1978.

12. US Department of Defense. *Treatment of Nuclear and Radiological Casualties*. Washington, DC: Departments of the Army, Navy, Air Force, and Commandant, Marine Corps; 2001. Army FM 4-02.283, Navy NTRP 4-02.21, Air Force AFMAN 44-161(1), Marine Corps MCRP 4-11.1B. http://www.globalsecurity.org/wmd/library/policy/army/fm/4-02-283/fm4-02-283.pdf. Accessed October 18, 2010.

13. Alt LA, Forcino CD, Walker RI. Nuclear events and their consequences. In: Walker RI, Cerveny TJ, eds. *Medical Consequences of Nuclear Warfare*. In: Zajtchuk R, Jenkins DP, Bellamy RF, Ingram VM, eds. *Textbooks of Military Medicine*. Washington, DC: Office of the Surgeon General, Department of the Army, Borden Institute; 1989.

14. Ricks RC, Berger MC, Ohara FM. *The Medical Basis for Radiation Accident Preparedness: Clinical Care of Victims*. Boca Raton, FL: CRC Press; 2002.

15. Gusev IA, Guskova AK, and Mettler FA. *Medical Management of Radiation Accidents*. 2nd ed. Boca Raton, FL: CRC Press; 2001.

16. Gonzalez AJ, Lauriston S. Taylor lecture: radiation protection in the aftermath of a terrorist attack involving exposure to ionizing radiation. *Health Phys*. 2005;89(5):418–446.

17. Buddemeier B. Effects of a 10-kt IND detonation on human health and the area health care system—delayed effects of fallout. In: Benjamin GC, McGeary M, McCutchen SR, eds. *Assessing Medical Preparedness to Respond to a Terrorist Nuclear Event: Workshop Report*. Washington, DC: Institute of Medicine of the National Academies, The National Academies Press; 2009: 16–20.

18. Buddemeier B. Improving response to the aftermath of radiological and nuclear terrorism. Publication number LLNL-PRES-404937-rev1. Paper presented at: 2008 Bio-Dose Conference; September 8, 2008; Hanover, NH.

19. Dallas CE, Bell WC. Prediction modeling to determine the adequacy of medical response to urban nuclear attack. *Disaster Med Public Health Prep*. 2007;1(2):80–89.

20. Department of the Army; Department of the Navy; Department of the Air Force; Department of the Coast Guard. *Operations in Chemical, Biological, Radiological, and Nuclear (CBRN) Environments*. Washington, DC: Department of Defense; 2008. Joint Publication 3-11. www.dtic.mil/doctrine/new_pubs/jp3_11.pdf. Accessed August 31, 2010.

21. US Department of Health and Human Services, Centers for Disease Control and Prevention, National Institute for Occupational Safety and Health. *Guidance on Emergency Responder Personal Protective Equipment (PPE) for Response to CBRN Terrorism Incidents*. Atlanta, GA: CDC; 2008. http://www.cdc.gov/niosh/docs/2008-132/pdfs/2008-132.pdf. Accessed August 31, 2010.

22. National Council on Radiation Protection and Measurements. *Key Elements of Preparing Emergency Responders for Nuclear and Radiological Terrorism*. Bethesda, MD: NCRP; 2005. Commentary No. 19.

23. National Council on Radiation Protection and Measurements. *Management of Terrorist Events Involving Radioactive Material*. Bethesda, MD: NCRP; 2001. NCRP Report No. 138.

24. US Department of Homeland Security, Federal Emergency Management Agency. Planning guidance for protection and recovery following radiological dispersal device (RDD) and improvised nuclear device (IND) incidents. *Fed Regist*. 2008;73:45029. http://www.fema.gov/good_guidance/download/10260. Accessed October 18, 2010.

25. Conference of Radiation Control Program Directors, Inc. *Handbook for Responding to a Radiological Dispersal Device. First Responder's Guide—The First 12 Hours*. Frankfort, KY: CRCPD; 2006. http://www.crcpd.org/RDD_handbook/RDD-handbook-forWeb.pdf. Accessed August 31, 2010.

26. Musolino SV, Harper FT. Emergency response guidance for the first 48 hours after an outdoor detonation of an explosive dispersal device. *Health Phys*. 2006;90:377–388.

27. Musolino SV, DeFranco J, Schloeck R. The ALARA principle in the context of a radiological or nuclear emergency. *Health Phys*. 2008;94:109–111.

28. National Research Council of the National Academies. *Health Risks from Exposure to Low Levels of Ionizing Radiation: BEIR VII Phase 2*. Washington, DC: The National Academies Press; 2006.

29. Mettler FA, Upton AC. *Medical Effects of Ionizing Radiation*. Philadelphia, PA: Saunders; 2008.

30. Ricks RC. Data presented at: Annual Meeting of the American Society for Therapeutic Radiology and Oncology; October 19, 2003; Salt Lake City, Utah.

31. MacVittie TJ, Weiss JF, Browne D, eds. Advances in treatment of radiation injuries. In: *Advances in Bioscience*. Vol 94. New York, NY: Pergamon; 1996.

32. Berger ME, Leonard RB, Ricks RC, Wiley AL, Lowry PC, Flynn DF. *Hospital Triage in the First 24 Hours After a Nuclear or Radiological Disaster*. Oak Ridge, TN: Radiation Emergency Assistance Center/Training Site; 2004. http://orise.orau.gov/files/reacts/triage.pdf. Accessed August 31, 2010.

33. Waselenko JK, MacVittie TJ, Blakely WF, et al. Medical management of the acute radiation syndrome: recommendations of the Strategic National Stockpile Radiation Working Group. *Ann Intern Med*. 140(12):1037–1051;2004.

34. US Department of Homeland Security. *Working Group on Radiological Dispersal Devices (RDD) and Preparedness, Medical Preparedness and Response Subgroup Report*. Washington, DC: DHS; 2003. http://www.va.gov/emshg. Accessed September 30, 2010.

35. Goans RE, Waselenko JK. Medical management of radiological casualties. *Health Phys*. 2005;89(5):505–512.

36. Andrews GA. Medical management of accidental total-body irradiation. In: Hubner K, Fry S. *Medical Basis for Radiation Accident Preparedness*. New York, NY: Elsevier; 1980.

37. Goans RE, Holloway EC, Berger ME, Ricks RC. Early dose assessment following severe radiation accidents. *Health Phys*. 1997;72(4):513–518.

38. Goans RE, Holloway EC, Berger ME, Ricks RC. Early dose assessment in criticality accidents. *Health Phys*. 2001;81(4):446–449.

39. Koenig KL, Goans RE, Hatchett RJ, et al. Medical treatment of radiological casualties. *Ann Emerg Med*. 2005;45:643–652.

40. Blakely WF, Salter CA, Prasanna P. Early-response biological dosimetry—recommended countermeasure enhancements for mass-casualty radiological incidents and terrorism. *Health Phys*. 2005;89(5):494–504.

41. Weinstock DM, Case C Jr, Bader JL, et al. Radiologic and nuclear events: contingency planning for hematologists/oncologists. *Blood*. 2008;111(12):5440–5445.

42. Hrdina C, Coleman CN, Bogucki S, et al. The "RTR" medical response system for nuclear and radiological mass-casualty incidents: a functional TRiage-TReatment-TRansport medical response model. *Prehosp Disast Med*. 2009;24(3):167–178.

43. Dainiak N, Waselenko JK, Armitage JO, MacVittie TJ, Farese AM. The hematologist and radiation casualties. *Hematology Am Soc Hematol Educ Program*. 2003;473–496.

44. Bader JL, Nemhauser J, Chang F, et al. Radiation event medical management (REMM): website guidance for health care providers. *Prehosp Emerg Care*. 2008;12(1):1–11.

45. Berger ME, Christensen DM, Lowry PC, Jones OW, Wiley AL. Medical management of radiation injuries: current approaches. *Occup Med*. 2006;56:162–172.

46. Baranov A, Gale RP, Guskova A, et al. Bone marrow transplantation after the Chernobyl nuclear accident. *N Eng J Med*. 1989;321:205–212.

47. Hamza NS, Ghannoum MA, Lazarus HM. Choices aplenty: antifungal prophylaxis in hematopoietic stem cell transplant recipients. *Bone Marrow Transplant*. 2004;34:377–389.

48. Freifeld AG, Bow EJ, Sepkowitz KA, et al. Clinical practice guideline for the use of antimicrobial agents in neutropenic patients with cancer: 2010 update by the Infectious Diseases Society of America. *Clin Infect Dis*. 2011;52(4):e56–e93. http://www.cid.oxfordjournals.org/content/52/4/e56.full. Accessed January 27, 2012.

49. Hospenthal DR, Murray CK, Andersen RC, et al. Guidelines for the prevention of infections associated with combat-related injuries: 2011 update: endorsed by the Infectious Diseases Society of America and the Surgical Infection Society. *J Trauma*. 2011;71(2 Suppl 2):S210–S234.

50. Pizzo PA. Fever in immunocompromised patients. *N Engl J Med*. 1999;341(12):893–899.

51. Radiation Emergency Assistance Center/Training Site (REAC/TS). *Medical Aspects of Radiation Incidents*. Revised 4/19/2011. http://www.orise.orau.gov/reacts. Accessed January 27, 2012.

52. Miller K, Erdman M. Health physics considerations in medical radiation emergencies. *Health Phys*. 2004;87(suppl 2):S19–S24.

53. Smith JM, Ansari A, Harper FT. Hospital management of mass radiological casualties: reassessing exposures from contaminated victims of an exploded radiological dispersal device. *Health Phys*. 2005;89(5):513–520.

54. Miller K, Groff L, Erdman M, King S. Lessons learned in preparing to receive large numbers of contaminated individuals. *Health Phys*. 2005;89(suppl 2):S42–S47.

55. Institute of Medicine of the National Academies. *Assessing Medical Preparedness to Respond to a Terrorist Event—10-Kiloton Nuclear Detonation at Ground Level in an Urban Environment*. Washington, DC: The National Academies Press; 2009. Workshop report.

56. National Council on Radiation Protection and Measurements. *Management of Persons Contaminated with Radionuclides: Handbook*. Bethesda, MD: NCRP; 2009. No. 161.

57. US Department of Health and Human Services, Centers for Disease Control and Prevention. Population monitoring in radiation emergencies: a guide for state and local public health planners. Published August 2007. http://emergency.cdc.gov/radiation/pdf/population-monitoring-guide.pdf. Accessed September 21, 2010.

Chapter 4

TREATMENT OF INTERNAL RADIONUCLIDE CONTAMINATION

JOHN F. KALINICH, PhD[*]

[*]Program Advisor, Internal Contamination and Metal Toxicity Program, Armed Forces Radiobiology Research Institute, Uniformed Services University of the Health Sciences, 8901 Wisconsin Avenue, Building 42, Bethesda, Maryland 20889

INTRODUCTION

A variety of events pose the risk of internal radionuclide contamination. A nuclear detonation will result in the release of over 400 radioactive isotopes.[1] Of these, approximately 40 are considered potential human health hazards because of their long radiological half-lives or their ability to concentrate in critical organ systems. Accidents at or attacks on nuclear reactors can result in internal radionuclide contamination, either through direct exposure to the released isotopes or as a result of radioactive fallout. In noncombat situations, accidents with radioisotopes used in medical and industrial applications can also result in internal radionuclide contamination. In addition, since the terrorist attacks of September 11, 2001, concern about the use of radiological weapons against civilians or military personnel has increased, and these fears are no longer limited to nuclear fission devices delivered by rogue states or terrorist groups. Terrorist use of a radiological dispersal device, or "dirty bomb," is also now a critical concern.[2]

Radionuclide internalization, whether accidentally or from a deliberate attack, is a critical medical situation for which treatment decisions should not be delayed. Although there are a seemingly endless number of radioisotopes, this chapter will focus on those most widely used in medical and industrial applications, as well as those thought to be potential radiological dispersal device components.

Routes of Exposure and Normal Clearance Mechanisms

Radionuclides can be internalized through three major routes: inhalation, ingestion, and wound contamination. Although percutaneous absorption is another potential exposure route, it is only a significant internalization pathway for tritium, or when the epithelial layer of the skin is damaged. Regardless of the route of exposure, several factors govern the eventual health effects induced by the internalized radionuclide. Clearly, the amount of radionuclide internalized plays a major role in the end result of any exposure; equally important, however, are the chemical and physical properties of the radionuclide. These properties include solubility characteristics (particularly in biological fluids), particle size, speciation, and chemical reactivity. The energy and type of radiation (α, β, γ) emitted by the isotope will dictate the damage it has the potential to inflict. For high-energy, short-lived isotopes, the radiological half-life is of concern. More important for longer lived isotopes is the biological half-life; the time it takes, without therapeutic intervention, for the internalized radionuclide to be cleared from the body. The final important issue is the "critical organ," or final deposition site for the radionuclide if it is not cleared from the body. Together, these factors ultimately determine the health effect of the internalized radionuclide, as well as its potential to be therapeutically removed or "decorporated" from the body.

Inhalation is the primary route of exposure for internalized radionuclides, with their ultimate fate depending on the size of the inhaled particles as well as the solubility of the radionuclide. Approximately 25% of inhaled radionuclides are immediately exhaled.[3] Of the remaining 75%, particles less than 5 μm in diameter can reach the alveolar space, while particles greater than 10 μm tend to remain in upper areas of the lung.[4] Once deposited in the lung, the particle's solubility becomes important. Radionuclides such as tritium, phosphorus, and cesium are rapidly solubilized and enter the circulatory system. Less-soluble radionuclides, such as the oxides of plutonium, uranium, cobalt, and americium, will eventually be removed through the process of phagocytosis by the alveolar macrophages. Until that occurs, the radioactive particle will continue to irradiate the surrounding tissue. Research has shown that in most cases, the internalized radionuclide will have both soluble and insoluble components,[5,6] further complicating treatment decisions. Larger inhaled particles, unable to access the alveolar space, will be removed from the lung via mucocilliary clearance. However, many of the particles, once cleared, will be swallowed and thus enter the gastrointestinal (GI) tract.

In addition to swallowing after mucocilliary clearance, radionuclides can be ingested through contaminated food or liquids. Once ingested, absorption of radionuclides will depend on chemical form and solubility. The majority of radionuclides are poorly absorbed by the GI tract. Some exceptions include strontium, tritium, and cesium. The amount of damage inflicted will be determined by the transit time through the GI tract, with the greatest potential for damage occurring in the descending colon prior to the ingested radionuclide being excreted in the feces. GI transit times are affected by a variety of factors, including diet, fluid intake levels, and physical activity, but generally range from 1 to 5 days.[7]

Wound contamination is the final route of exposure to be considered. Wound radionuclide contamination

TABLE 4-1

ISOTOPES OF CONCERN

Element	Isotopes of Concern	Source	Radiation Type	Critical Organ(s)
Americium	^{241}Am	Smoke detectors, fallout	α, γ	Bone, liver, lung
Cesium	^{137}Cs	Radiotherapy units	β, γ	Total body (especially kidney)
Cobalt	^{60}Co	Radiotherapy units, commercial irradiators	β, γ	Total body (especially liver)
Iodine	^{131}I	Fallout, reactor accidents	β, γ	Thyroid
Iridium	^{192}Ir	Radiography source (material testing, brachytherapy)	β, γ	Spleen
Phosphorus	^{32}P	Medical research	β	Bone
Plutonium	^{238}Pu, ^{239}Pu	Nuclear weapons, reactors	α, γ	Bone, liver, lung
Polonium	^{210}Po	Antistatic devices	α	Spleen, kidney
Radium	^{226}Ra	Radioluminescent dials in old equipment	α, β, γ	Bone
Strontium	^{90}Sr	Radioisotope thermoelectric generators, medical uses	β, γ	Bone
Tritium	^{3}H	Medical research	β	Total body
Uranium	^{235}U, ^{238}U	Fuel rods, nuclear weapons, armor-piercing munitions (depleted uranium)	α, β, γ	Kidney, bone

can occur as a result of isotopes entering open wounds (eg, as dust or liquid) or as embedded fragments of a radionuclide. As with other routes of exposure, the physiochemical properties of the radionuclide are of prime importance when determining the effect of the internalized isotope. Research with intramuscularly injected radionuclides has shown that even those considered insoluble can be solubilized in vivo.[8–10] This was shown in studies investigating the health effects of embedded fragments of depleted uranium, where solubilization and urinary excretion of the uranium was found within 48 hours after implantation of the solid metal into the leg muscles of laboratory

rodents.[11] These results point to the complex nature of radionuclide internalization as a result of embedded fragments and the potential difficulties involved in treating them.

Isotopes of Concern

As noted previously, there are hundreds of natural and manufactured radioisotopes that could result in internal contamination. However, in reality, only a handful are likely candidates for internalization due to their widespread use or potential incorporation into radiological dispersal devices (Table 4-1).

ASSESSING CONTAMINATED PERSONNEL

By the time contaminated patients reach a medical care facility, they should have undergone an external decontamination procedure, usually at or near the site of the radiological event; however, it is safer to assume no decontamination has occurred unless told otherwise. Medical staff should work closely with health physics personnel in initially assessing potentially contaminated personnel. While external decontamination is essential to prevent the spread of

radiological contamination, it should not take priority over the initiation of immediate lifesaving measures. If not already completed, external decontamination procedures should be undertaken before assessing the patient for internal radiological contamination. Decontamination procedures decrease external radiation levels, allowing for a more accurate determination of internal radionuclide contamination (methods to determine internal contamination depend on the suspected radionuclide, physical form of the radio-nuclide [ie, liquid, solid, gas], and route of exposure, and are beyond the scope of this chapter). In addition, thorough external decontamination procedures will prevent accidental radionuclide internalization during patient assessment and treatment. Those decontamination procedures need not be exhaustive; simply removing the patient's outer clothing and shoes can reduce external contamination by 90%.[12] Additional decontamination procedures, including washing the skin and hair with soap and water, further decrease external contamination levels; however, open wounds need to be covered to prevent the unintentional internalization of external contamination during decontamination procedures. The logistics involved in establishing a decontamination area are beyond the scope of this chapter, but several excellent sources of information are available.[13–17]

Initial Determination of Radioactive Contamination

Information from the accident or attack scene (preferably in the form of a firsthand account from the patient) will provide the first information on the radioisotopes involved. However, in many cases, the exact isotope and route of exposure will not be known. Although the identity of a radioactive contaminant, especially one that has been internalized, could take days to determine, several simple assessments can determine whether the contaminant is a β or γ emitter, and may also indicate a possible exposure route. Thus, as a preliminary step, a thorough body survey with a Geiger-Müller meter incorporated into the external decontamination procedure is recommended. A general survey may be done when the patient arrives for triage and may be repeated after contaminating clothing has been removed and skin washed. Survey details are generally reported by body area (for more information, see Chapter 3, Triage and Treatment). A Geiger-Müller meter is capable of detecting β- and γ-emitting isotopes, but not those emitting α particles. The first scan should be made with the shield of the Geiger-Müeller meter open to detect the presence and location of β and γ contamination. The second scan should be conducted with the shield closed. Results from this scan will indicate what proportion of the contamination is due to γ-emitting isotopes alone. Radioactive contamination by α emitters should also be determined. However, because of the difficulties involved with such measurements, these procedures require the assistance of experienced personnel. Special consideration should be given to the mouth and nasal regions, as well as to the areas around wounds. In addition to a body survey, swabs of each

nostril should be taken, stored in sealed tubes to prevent unintentional contamination, and analyzed by health physics staff for radioactive contamination to help identify the potential contaminant and indicate whether clinically significant inhalation exposure has occurred.

Evaluating Contaminated Patients

After a patient has been identified by health physics staff as being internally contaminated, the next step is to positively identify the contaminants so that the body burden (the total amount of a substance in an individual's body) and dose estimates can be calculated. It should not be assumed that there is only a single radionuclide present unless proven by radioanalysis. Measuring and identifying external patient contamination is the first step in this process and should have been initiated during the decontamination procedure. Swabs, including nasal, obtained during decontamination; fluids used to cleanse wounds (as much as can reasonably be collected by personnel using standard precautions and personal protective equipment); tissue and fluid samples from wound debridement; and wound dressings (the number of which and the time period covered depend on radioanalytical results obtained by health physics staff) should all be analyzed for radiation contamination using appropriate radioanalytical techniques.[18] Urine and fecal samples should also be collected, depending on the identity and form of the nuclide and the recommendations of the health physics staff, and analyzed to provide an indication of the excretion pattern of the internalized radionuclide. Although this information can be used to calculate body burden, it is only an estimate of the amount of internal contamination present. More sensitive in-vivo measurements provide a more accurate assessment of dose. For example, whole-body counters can be used to measure radiation given off by the body; however, these are only useful for radionuclides that emit γ rays.

Treatment Decisions

If internal radionuclide contamination is likely and a tentative identification of the isotope and extent of contamination can be made, treatment decisions must follow. Most treatment protocols for internal radionuclide contamination carry some risk; therefore, it is imperative that, prior to initiation, the potential risk of the treatment be weighed against the possible benefit. In most cases, the benefits of treatment far outweigh the risks, and potential treatment risks can usually be successfully managed.

TREATING INTERNAL RADIONUCLIDE CONTAMINATION

The first step in dealing with internal radionuclide contamination is to remove sources of potential contamination. As discussed above, external decontamination procedures are vital in reducing the risk of additional internal contamination events. Isotope-specific pharmacological treatments can begin once thorough external decontamination is performed. Agents used to treat internal radionuclide contamination can be loosely grouped into four categories: uptake-reducing agents, blocking or diluting agents, mobilizing agents, and chelating agents.[19] These are not mutually exclusive groupings; the action of many compounds can span two or more of the categories. More importantly, no single compound works for all radionuclides, illustrating the need for competent radioanalytical support to identify the radiological contaminant. (Table 4-2)

Uptake-Reducing Agents

One of the keys to a successful treatment outcome is to reduce or eliminate the uptake of internalized radionuclides before they can reach the critical organ. Simple procedures, such as irrigation of the nasal passages and mouth, should not be overlooked as treatment options. For exposure due to ingestion, emetics (eg, ipecac) and laxatives or purgatives (eg, castor oil) can be considered in order to reduce the time the radionuclide spends in the GI tract.

Ion exchangers can also be used to reduce radionuclide uptake in the GI tract. Ferric hexacyanoferrate (Prussian blue) is approved by the US Food and Drug Administration (FDA) for the treatment of internal cesium and thallium contamination. This insoluble compound is taken orally but is not absorbed by the GI tract. Once in the GI tract, it binds preferentially to cesium and thallium (radioactive and nonradioactive forms) with very high affinity. This changes and increases the rate of elimination from primarily urinary to fecal. Other ion exchangers and absorption compounds that may be useful in reducing the uptake of ingested radionuclides are sodium polystyrene sulfonate and activated charcoal. Although both compounds are used for other indications, neither is FDA-approved specifically for treating internalized radionuclides. Oral administration of calcium- and aluminum-containing antacids to decrease the GI uptake of radioactive strontium and radium has also been suggested.[20,21]

Blocking or Diluting Agents

The terms "blocking" or "diluting" agent can, in most cases, be used interchangeably. These compounds reduce the uptake of a radionuclide by saturating binding sites with a stable, nonradioactive element, thereby diluting the deleterious effect of the radioisotope. For example, potassium iodide is the FDA-recommended treatment to prevent radioactive iodine from being sequestered in the thyroid. Speed is essential when administering potassium iodide; delay in treatment (> 4 hours postexposure) results in a greater uptake of radioactive iodine in the thyroid, lessening this treatment's effectiveness. Nonradioactive strontium compounds may also be used to block the uptake of radioactive strontium. In addition, elements with chemical properties similar to the internalized radionuclide are often used as blocking agents. For example, calcium, and to a lesser extent phosphorus, can be used to block uptake of radioactive strontium. Isotopic dilution techniques are also included in this category. For example, internal tritium contamination may be treated by forcing fluids to reduce the time the isotope remains in the body.

Mobilizing Agents

Mobilizing agents are compounds that help release deposited radionuclides by increasing the natural rate of elimination. One example is ammonium chloride, which, when given orally, results in acidification of the blood and increased elimination of internalized radiostrontium. Sodium bicarbonate, given orally or intravenously, is used to increase urinary pH; such increases in alkalinity are useful in preventing the deposition of internalized uranium as it passes through the kidney.

Chelating Agents

A chelating agent is a compound that binds with a metal to form a stable, preferably less toxic, complex that facilitates excretion of the metal.[22] Chelating agents such as ethylenediaminetetraacetic acid (EDTA), desferrioxamine, dimercaptosuccinic acid (succimer), D-penicillamine, and 2,3-dimercaptopropanol (dimercaprol, British anti-Lewisite) have been used for many years as antidotes for acute heavy metal poisoning. In some cases, laboratory research has indicated that these compounds may also be useful in chelating radionuclides; however, chelation therapy can have a number of undesired side effects. Many chelating agents are chemically toxic and lack specificity for the target metal. This can lead to the depletion of metals essential for normal homeostasis. For example, EDTA, a compound often recommended for chelating lead and mercury, can also decrease metabolic calcium to dangerously low levels. Chelating agents can also have the unintended side effect of redistributing toxic metals to previously uncontaminated tissues. For example, the chelator 2,3-dimercaptopropanol, once tested as an antidote for arsenic poisoning, was subsequently shown to move arsenic into the brain, an area that arsenic alone would not have been able to penetrate.[23] In

some cases, chelation has been shown to enhance the toxicity of a metal. EDTA readily chelates iron, but it does so in a manner that permits the iron to catalyze reactions that result in oxidative stress, leading to greater damage than if chelation therapy had not been used.[24] Despite the potential pitfalls with the use of chelating agents, they represent the most promising avenue of therapeutic intervention in decorporating

TABLE 4-2

INTERNAL RADIONUCLIDE CONTAMINATION TREATMENT OPTIONS[*]

Targeted Radionuclide	Compound(s)	Dosage[1,2]
Americium	DTPA (calcium and zinc salts)[†]	Adults: IV 1 g in 5 mL IV push over 3–4 min, or IV infusion over 30 min, diluted in 250 mL of dextrose (5% in water), lactated Ringer's, or normal saline
		Children (< 12 y): 14 mg/kg IV as above, not to exceed 1 g
Cesium	Prussian blue[†]	Adults: 3 g three times daily orally
		Children (2–12 y): 1 g three times daily orally
Curium	DTPA (calcium and zinc salts)[†]	See americium
Iodine	Potassium iodide[†]	Adults: 130 mg/day orally
		Children (3–18 y): 65 mg/day orally
		Infants (1 mo–3 y): 32 mg/day orally
		Neonates (birth–1 mo): 16 mg/day orally
Phosphorus	Phosphate, dibasic potassium, and sodium salts	Adults: 1–2 tablets (250 mg phosphorus per tablet) orally four times per day with a full glass of water each time, with meals and at bedtime
		Children (> 4 y): 1 tablet orally 4 times daily
Plutonium	DTPA (calcium and zinc salts)[†]	See americium
Polonium	2,3-Dimercaptopropanol	Deep IM injection only, 2.5 mg/kg four times a day for 2 days, then twice a day on day 3, then daily for 5–10 days
Radium	Ammonium chloride	Ammonium chloride: 1 g three times daily for up to 6 days
	Calcium carbonate	Calcium carbonate: 0.5–1.0 g orally twice per day
	Calcium gluconate	Calcium gluconate: 10 g orally
	Sodium alginate	Sodium alginate: 5 g orally twice per day for 1 day, then 1 g four times daily with water
Strontium	Aluminum compounds (hydroxide, phosphate)	Aluminum hydroxide: 60–100 mL orally once for adults; children: 50 mg/kg, not to exceed adult dose
	Ammonium chloride	Ammonium chloride, calcium carbonate, calcium gluconate, sodium alginate: see radium
	Calcium carbonate	
	Calcium gluconate	
	Sodium alginate	
Thallium	Prussian blue[†]	See cesium
Uranium	Sodium bicarbonate	Isotonic sodium bicarbonate, 250 mL slow IV infusion or 2 bicarbonate tablets orally every 4 h until urine pH reaches 8–9; continue for 3 days

DTPA: diethylenetriamine pentaacetic acid
IM: intramuscular
IV: intravenous
[*]Always take into account the possibility of essential metal depletion when initiating treatment. This list contains potential treatment options and should in no way be considered exhaustive.
[†]Approved for use by the US Food and Drug Administration.
Data sources: (1) National Council on Radiation Protection and Measurements. *Management of Persons Contaminated with Radionuclides.* Bethesda, MD: National Council on Radiation Protection and Measurements; 2009. NCRP Report 161. (2) Armed Forces Radiobiology Research Institute. Medical management of radiological casualties. 3rd ed. Bethesda, MD: AFRRI; June 2010. AFRRI Special Publication 10-1. http://www.usuhs.mil/afrri/outreach/pdf/3edmmrchandbook.pdf. Accessed March 17, 2011.

internal radionuclide contamination.

Two formulations of a chelating agent have been approved by the FDA for the treatment of internal contamination with plutonium, americium, and curium. The calcium (Ca) and zinc (Zn) salts of diethylenetriamine pentaacetic acid (DTPA) were approved for use in 2004. Ca-DTPA has been shown to be almost 10 times more effective than Zn-DTPA at chelating the transuranics (plutonium, americium, and curium) when given early after radionuclide exposure. However, this advantage is lost by 24 hours after exposure, when Ca-DTPA and Zn-DTPA are equally effective chelating agents. Because of this property, and the fact that Ca-DTPA has more adverse side effects than Zn-DTPA, standard practice is to start with Ca-DTPA for initial chelation therapy and switch to less-toxic Zn-DTPA to continue more protracted therapy regimens. In either case, depletion of essential trace metals should be monitored and mineral replacements given as needed.

Although not FDA-approved for treating internal radionuclide contamination, the off-label use of D-penicillamine for cobalt and iridium contamination, EDTA for cobalt, and dimercaprol for polonium should be considered in the absence of other options.[25]

Treating Contaminated Wounds

Radionuclides internalized as a result of wound contamination are eliminated in the same way as those internalized via other exposure pathways. In most cases, thorough irrigation and cleaning of the wound is sufficient. In some situations, adding a chelating agent to the irrigation solution facilitates radionuclide removal from the wound site. For wound contamination with plutonium, americium, or curium, standard chelation therapy with Ca-DTPA and Zn-DTPA should be initiated.

Wounds containing embedded radioactive fragments pose a unique treatment dilemma. In many of these situations, treatment with chelating agents is not indicated because of the potential to solubilize excessive amounts of metal from the embedded fragment and distribute it throughout the body. In these cases, it may be necessary to surgically remove the embedded fragment. Special precautions may be required depending on the radionuclide, including protective shielding for the surgical staff. Surgically removed fragments should be placed in lead containers and appropriately shielded. The facility's health physics staff is essential in helping deal with these situations in the safest manner possible.

SUMMARY

Radiological contamination remains a threat to civilians and military personnel alike. Because radionuclides may be internalized through inhalation, ingestion, and wound contamination, treatment methods vary, and each treatment option carries with it some risk. Internal radionuclide contamination treatment procedures are currently an area of much research, particularly in the field of chelating agents.[26–28] It is important that healthcare professionals are aware of treatment advances (please refer to the references for additional information[29–31]).

REFERENCES

1. National Council on Radiation Protection and Measurements. *Radiological Factors Affecting Decision-Making in a Nuclear Attack*. Bethesda, MD: NCRP; 1974. NCRP Report 42.

2. Conklin WC, Liotta PL. Radiological threat assessment and the federal response plan—a gap analysis. *Health Phys*. 2005;89:457–470.

3. Bates DV, Fish BR, Hatch TF, Mercer TT, Morrow PE. Deposition and retention models for internal dosimetry of the human respiratory tract. Task group on lung dynamics. *Health Phys*. 1966;12:173–207.

4. Morrow PE, Gibb FR, Gazioglu KM. A study of particulate clearance from the human lungs. *Am Rev Respir Dis*. 1967;96:1209–1221.

5. Muggenburg BA, Mewhinney JA, Griffith WC, et al. Dose-response relationships for bone cancers from plutonium in dogs and people. *Health Phys*. 1983;44(suppl 1):529–535.

6. Harrison JD, Muirhead CR. Quantitative comparisons of cancer induction in humans by internally deposited radionuclides and external radiation. *Int J Radiat Biol*. 2003;79:1–13.

7. Eve IS. A review of the physiology of the gastrointestinal tract in relation to radiation doses from radioactive materials. *Health Phys*. 1966;12:131–161.

8. Bistline RW, Watters RL, Lebel JL. A study of translocation dynamics of plutonium and americium from simulated puncture wounds in beagle dogs. *Health Phys*. 1972;22:829–831.

9. Lloyd RD, Atherton DR, Mays CW, McFarland SS, Williams JL. The early excretion, retention and distribution of injected curium citrate in beagles. *Health Phys*. 1974;27:61–67.

10. Dagle GE, Lebel JL, Phemister RD, Watters RL, Gomez LS. Translocation kinetics of plutonium oxide from the popliteal lymph nodes of beagles. *Health Phys*. 1975;28:395–398.

11. Pellmar TC, Fuciarelli AF, Ejnik JW, et al. Distribution of uranium in rats implanted with depleted uranium pellets. *Toxicol Sci*. 1999;49:29–39.

12. Koenig KL, Goans RE, Hatchett RJ, et al. Medical treatment of radiological casualties: current concepts. *Ann Emerg Med*. 2005;45:643–652.

13. National Council on Radiation Protection and Measurements. *Management of Persons Contaminated With Radionuclides*. Bethesda, MD: NCRP; 2009. NCRP Report 161.

14. International Atomic Energy Agency. *Rapid Monitoring of Large Groups of Internally Contaminated People Following a Radiation Accident*. Vienna, Austria: Radiation Safety Section, IAEA; 1994. IAEA-TECDOC-746.

15. National Council on Radiation Protection and Measurements. *Management of Terroristic Events Involving Radioactive Material*. Bethesda, MD: NCRP; 2001. NCRP Report 138.

16. Mettler FA Jr. Medical resources and requirements for responding to radiological terrorism. *Health Phys*. 2005;89:488–493.

17. Smith JM, Ansari A, Harper FT. Hospital management of mass radiological casualties: reassessing exposures from contaminated victims of an exploded radiological dispersal device. *Health Phys*. 2005;89:513–520.

18. National Council on Radiation Protection and Measurements. *Use of Bioassay Procedures for Assessment of Internal Radionuclide Deposition*. Bethesda, MD: NCRP; 1987. NCRP Report 87.

19. Waller EA, Stodilka RZ, Leach K, Prud'homme-Lalonde L. *Literature Survey on Decorporation of Radionuclides From the Human Body*. Ottawa, Canada: Defence Research and Development Canada; 2002. DRDC Technical Memorandum TM2002-042.

20. Durakovic A. Internal contamination with medically significant radionuclides. In: Conklin JJ, Walker, RI, eds. *Military Radiobiology*. Orlando, FL: Academic Press; 1987: Chap 13.

21. Jarrett DG, Sedlak RG, Dickerson WE, Reeves GI. Medical treatment of radiation injuries—current US status. *Radiat Meas*. 2007;42:1063–1074.

22. Andersen O. Chemical and biological considerations in the treatment of metal intoxications by chelating agents. *Mini Rev Med Chem*. 2004;4:11–21.

23. Hoover TD, Aposhian HV. BAL increases the arsenic-74 content of rabbit brain. *Toxicol Appl Pharmacol*. 1983;70:160–162.

24. Singh S, Khodr H, Taylor MI, Hider RC. Therapeutic iron chelators and their potential side-effects. *Biochem Soc Symp*. 1995;61:127–137.

25. Marcus CS. Administration of decorporation drugs to treat internal radionuclide contamination. *RSO Magazine*. 2004;9:9–15.

26. Fukuda S. Chelating agents used for plutonium and uranium removal in radiation emergency medicine. *Curr Med Chem*. 2005;12:2765–2770.

27. US Department of Health and Human Services, Food and Drug Administration, Center for Drug Evaluation and Research. *Guidance for Industry: Internal Radioactive Contamination, Development of Decorporation Agents*. Rockville, MD: FDA; 2006.

28. Durbin PW, Lauriston S. Taylor lecture: the quest for therapeutic actinide chelators. *Health Phys*. 2008;95:465–492.

29. Armed Forces Radiobiology Research Institute. *Medical Management of Radiological Casualties*. 3rd ed. Bethesda, MD: AFRRI; June 2010. http://www.usuhs.mil/afrri/outreach/pdf/3edmmrchandbook.pdf. Accessed March 17, 2011.

30. US Department of Health and Human Services. Radiation emergency medical management Web site. http://www.remm.nlm.gov. Accessed March 17, 2011.

31. US Department of Energy. Radiation Emergency Assistance Center/Training Site (REAC/TS) Web site. http://orise.orau.gov/reacts. Accessed March 17, 2011.

Chapter 5

THERAPY FOR BACTERIAL INFECTIONS FOLLOWING IONIZING RADIATION INJURY

THOMAS B. ELLIOTT, PhD,[*] AND G. DAVID LEDNEY, PhD[†]

[*]Research Microbiologist, Scientific Research Department, Radiation and Combined Injury Infection Group, Uniformed Services University of the Health Sciences, 8901 Wisconsin Avenue, Building 42, National Naval Medical Center, Bethesda, Maryland 20889
[†]Research Biologist, Scientific Research Department, Radiation and Combined Injury Infection Group, Uniformed Services University of the Health Sciences, 8901 Wisconsin Avenue, Building 42, National Naval Medical Center, Bethesda, Maryland 20889

INTRODUCTION

Infectious diseases have historically caused more casualties than battle injuries. Nuclear, biological, and chemical weapons would cause a large number of casualties either during military operations or from terrorist events. Combinations of biological and nuclear weapons could be synergistic, so that injury severity would be much greater than from either weapons or infectious agents alone. Irradiation diminishes innate immune responses, particularly the inflammatory response, without which systemic infections among large numbers of casualties may become difficult to treat effectively and may not respond to antimicrobial regimens used in usual clinical practice. In many cases, partial-body irradiation could allow some undamaged hematopoietic and intestinal stem cells to repopulate those tissues; however, traumatic injury when combined with irradiation further complicates infection management. This chapter reviews the current state of knowledge since the last *Textbook of Military Medicine* on this topic and other presentations (Exhibit 5-1),[1] including laboratory investigations that illustrate essential principles and factors, about the available preventive and therapeutic measures against bacterial infections to decrease mortality and ameliorate synergistic combined insults, which are caused by endogenous and exogenous microorganisms and can occur during operations following exposure to ionizing radiation.

Factors that predispose individuals to irradiation-induced infections were described by Walker.[1] The innate immune and inflammatory responses are impaired following irradiation. Numbers of circulating neutrophilic granulocytes as well as lymphocytes diminish and hematopoietic tissue (ie, bone marrow) is damaged by radiation. Neutropenia provides a valuable marker to indicate increased susceptibility to bacterial infections and is used as a clinical indicator to begin antimicrobial therapy.[2–4]

Bacterial infections are a major cause of morbidity and mortality in humans and laboratory animals that receive whole-body doses of ionizing radiation in a range that causes hematopoietic failure. Hematopoiesis and numbers of circulating blood leukocytes and thrombocytes are reduced within several days after irradiation.[5] Innate immune responses that protect against infection are therefore depressed[1] and hemorrhage occurs easily in tissues. The course of recovery from hematopoietic failure in laboratory animals differs from that seen in humans; the course of manifest illness in laboratory animals occurs within several days to a few weeks,[6,7] whereas the course in humans occurs between a few weeks to a few months following exposure.[5]

Fundamental research in radiation biology is essential and must be performed in laboratory animals because such studies may not be performed in humans. Prophylactic or therapeutic regimens must be evaluated in at least two suitable animal species (in place of a human clinical study) to satisfy the requirements of the US Food and Drug Administration (FDA). Laboratory animal models provide a scientific basis for comparing controlled variables of the complex cellular and molecular interactions of metabolism and immune responses in vivo.[8] They allow sufficient numbers of animals and trials to evaluate variables and ensure statistical validity. Results are generally reproducible and can often be extrapolated to humans.[9] The laboratory mouse provides a principal model for studies of infectious diseases and antimicrobial agents, including mechanism of action, pharmacokinetics, pharmacodynamics, efficacy, and toxicity.[9,10] The mouse mimics the human response to antimicrobial agents, although mice have a higher metabolic rate than humans. Andes and Craig[11–13] established guidelines for correlating efficacy between mice and humans. Further, the laboratory mouse is colonized by genera and species of intestinal facultative and anaerobic microorganisms similar to those found in humans.[14–16] The intestinal microbial ecosystem establishes and maintains functional stability despite constant challenges to the compositional sta-

---

EXHIBIT 5-1

RECOMMENDED READING

Browne D, Weiss JF, MacVittie TJ, Pillai MV, eds. *Treatment of Radiation Injuries*. New York, NY: Plenum Press; 1990.

Ledney GD, Madonna GS, McChesney DG, Elliott TB, Brook I. Complications of combined injury: radiation damage and skin wound trauma in mouse models. In: Browne D, Weiss JF, MacVittie TJ, Pillai MV, eds. *Treatment of Radiation Injuries*. New York, NY: Plenum Press; 1990: 153–164.

Walker RI, Gruber DF, MacVittie TJ, Conklin JJ, eds. *The Pathophysiology of Combined Injury and Trauma: Radiation, Burn, and Trauma*. Baltimore, MD: University Park Press; 1985.

---

bility. Factors that challenge the microbial community include continuous turnover of the epithelium and mucus layer, a system that is open to the external environment, peristaltic activity that ensures constant exposure to dietary macromolecules, gastrointestinal secretions, and exogenous bacteria. The irradiated mouse provides a unique model for testing safety, efficacy, and immunogenicity of potential therapeutic drugs in immunodepressed animals because effects of irradiation are prolonged compared to only a few days following drug-induced immunosuppression.

Neutropenia and thrombocytopenia have long been recognized as significant complications and risk factors of serious infections, particularly sepsis, following irradiation. Neutropenia is used as an indicator for initiating antimicrobial therapy, whereas thrombocytopenia was shown to be an independent prognostic indicator of mortality only in patients with sepsis in an intensive care unit.[17] In irradiated laboratory animals (eg, mice), circulating leukocytes drop precipitously within 2 days to barely detectable numbers, begin to recover gradually after approximately 15 days, and approach normal levels in 28 days or longer.[7] The number of thrombocytes in mice decreases after 5 days and begins to recover within 10 to 12 days. In humans, lymphocytes decrease promptly, neutrophils decline over several days, thrombocytes begin to decrease after approximately 8 days, and hematopoiesis begins to recover after 30 days.[5]

Profound neutropenia ($< 1.0 \times 10^5$ neutrophilic granulocytes/mL, or 100 neutrophils/μL), particularly if the duration is more than 7 days, is the greatest risk factor for infection. Other factors that will affect the efficacy of treatment include phagocytic and bactericidal function of granulocytes and macrophages, changes in the endogenous microbial flora, endemic microorganisms in the local environment, changes in defensive barriers, and general health status (for example, combat personnel are likely to be nutritionally and physically stressed). Secondary fungal infections could also occur as the duration of neutropenia increases.

Since the end of the Cold War in the early 1990s, concerns about nuclear disasters have not diminished; rather they have shifted to emphasize the low-dose acute and low-dose–rate chronic irradiation scenarios of nuclear accidents, tactical situations, and terrorist activities. During 1995–1996, a North Atlantic Treaty Organization working group considered the range of gamma photon radiation between 0.25 and 1.5 Gy acceptable for conducting military operations. The US Army Groundfire 95 Low Level Radiation Exposure Issues Workshop examined options for soldiers deployed as part of peacekeeping or humanitarian assistance missions. The dose range of radiation between 0.70 and 3.0 Gy was considered to produce effects of immediate military relevance. Significant risk was acknowledged to range from 0.25 to 0.70 Gy. The North Atlantic Treaty Organization standardization agreement 2083, Commander's Guide on the Effects from Nuclear Radiation Exposure During War, states the doses and probable tactical effects on groups. A dose of 0.75 Gy up to 1.25 Gy will induce probable initial tactical effects up to 5% latent ineffectiveness, which is "the casualty criterion defined as the lowest dose at which personnel will (*a*) become combat ineffective (less than 25% capable) at any time within 6 weeks post exposure followed by death or recovery, or (*b*) become performance degraded (ie, 25–75% capable) within 3 hours after exposure and remain so until death or recovery."[18] An exposed group would be considered combat effective and would not require medical care after 1 day following a dose ranging from 0.75 to 1.25 Gy. However, following doses greater than 1.25 Gy, groups probably would not be able to perform complex tasks and sustained efforts would be hampered.

Such radiation doses are not associated with neutron irradiation, which occurs during detonation of a nuclear weapon. In the latter case, those persons who would be in the zone of survivability from the heat and blast effects would be exposed to neutrons as well as gamma photons. The approximate $LD_{50/30}$ (the dose of radiation required to kill 50% of the test population within 30 days) in humans for uncomplicated prompt irradiation is generally accepted as approximately 4.5 Gy gamma photons with basic clinical support or 3.0 Gy without clinical support, whereas the $LD_{50/30}$ in $B6D2F_1$/J female mice in our laboratory in the Armed Forces Radiobiology Research Institute is 9.4 Gy, or approximately twice the human value. The LD_{50} (median lethal dose) decreases with combined injury, and the LD_{50} increases as the dose rate decreases, such as in a fallout field.[19]

Lethal doses of ionizing radiation induce systemic infections that are caused by endogenous or exogenous microorganisms. Endogenous infections arise from facultative microorganisms that translocate from the upper and lower intestinal tract, which is normally colonized predominantly by anaerobic bacteria and lesser numbers of facultative bacteria. The anaerobic bacteria ordinarily provide colonization resistance against pathogenic exogenous microorganisms. On the other hand, nonlethal doses of ionizing radiation enhance susceptibility to exogenous bacterial infections acquired from the environment and enhance mortality, as well.

ETIOLOGY OF INFECTIONS

A predominant number of casualties in Hiroshima and Nagasaki in August 1945 who were beyond the range for blast and heat injuries and who suffered gamma radiation injury with associated fever and pronounced leukopenia developed overwhelming infections that became septicemias. Estimates of the mortality rate from irradiation varied widely in subsequent reports of those two major events. Representative autopsy reports of victims following the atomic bombings showed that oropharyngitis was most frequently seen among the various infections, with necrotizing tonsillitis in a majority of cases, followed by infections of the large intestinal tissue, esophagus, bronchus, lungs, uterus, and urinary tract. These sites were considered the portal of entry for generalized infection (ie, septicemia and bacteremia, in many cases).[20] However, no definitive incidence or specific causes of infection were described. Following the accident at the Chernobyl, Ukraine, power station on April 26, 1986, 500 individuals were hospitalized. Over 100 received doses of radiation greater than 1 Gy. Over 90% of hospitalized victims survived. Although reports did not provide incidence of, causes of, or specific therapy for infections during the first month after the event, *Staphylococcus* species were reported to be the most frequent cause of septicemias.[21] Antimicrobial selective decontamination of the intestinal flora with sulfamethoxazole/trimethoprim and nystatin was used to reduce the chance of infection. Systemic antimicrobial therapy with two aminoglycosides, three cephalosporins, or two semisynthetic penicillins was used in febrile, granulocytopenic patients. Antifungal amphotericin B was used when fever persisted for more than 1 week, and antiviral acyclovir was used when herpes simplex virus was activated.

The kinds of microorganisms that cause infections depend on the quality and dose of radiation in each case. Gram-positive, nonsporulating rods and enterococci tend to predominate in the ileum of laboratory mice that are given moderately lethal doses (10–12 Gy) of gamma photon radiation, whereas facultative gram-negative rods of the family Enterobacteriaceae predominate in mice that are given equivalent lethal doses of mixed-field (gamma and neutron) radiation (6–7 Gy, where the ratio of neutron dose to total dose of neutrons plus gamma photons is 0.67).[22,23] Polymicrobial septicemias occur after lethal doses of radiation. The recovery of bacteria from the blood of mice correlated to changes that occurred in the gastrointestinal flora following exposure to ionizing radiations. Following lethal doses of gamma radiation (10 Gy), numbers of facultative and anaerobic bacteria in the ileum of

experimental C3HeB/FeJ mice decreased beginning 2 days after irradiation.[24] This decline reached a nadir between 5 and 7 days after irradiation. Mortality began 7 to 9 days after irradiation and correlated with an increase in the number of Enterobacteriaceae in the intestinal flora, while the numbers of anaerobic bacteria remained low. Endogenous *Escherichia coli* and *Proteus mirabilis* appeared in the blood, spleens, and livers of the animals. Anaerobic bacteria, which comprise approximately 90% of intestinal microflora, provide colonization resistance against invading facultative bacteria. With decreased numbers of anaerobic bacteria following lethal doses of radiation, the facultative bacteria, including Enterobacteriaceae, have the opportunity to fill the niche normally filled by the anaerobic bacteria and then, when intestinal tissue is injured by radiation, the bacteria translocate through the lymphatics into the blood. It appears likely that the selective translocation of bacteria is related to the greater injury to intestinal tissues by neutrons compared with injury caused by gamma photons based on the detailed findings of Lawrence and Tennant, who compared injuries with neutrons and X-rays.[25] Predominantly gram-negative sepsis followed lethal mixed-field (n/[n+γ] = 0.67) irradiation, whereas predominantly gram-positive sepsis followed lethal ^{60}Co-gamma-photon irradiation in mice.[26]

Wound and burn infections are more severe in the irradiated than in the nonirradiated host. The number of organisms in these infections is greater than in a nonirradiated host, and antimicrobial agents have a limited role in preventing systemic complications. In laboratory animals, wounds or burns that are infected with exogenous bacteria develop life-threatening infections after nonlethal irradiation, even with antimicrobial therapy.[27] Polymicrobial infections are common, as demonstrated by the findings of the following experiment. In 1957, swine were placed behind sheets of glass at measured distances from ground zero of a nuclear detonation, including at 4,430 ft (Station 6), 4,770 ft (Station 7), and 5,320 ft (Station 8).[28] Bacteria were isolated from wound, blood, and fecal specimens from each animal at these three stations. The number of wound cultures that demonstrated growth of bacteria decreased with time on day 1 (44%), day 2 (22%), day 3 (11%), and day 5 or later (4%). A greater number of "aerobic gram-positive" microorganisms were isolated (10^4 to > 10^6), which increased with time, than "coliform" bacteria (< 10^3 to 10^5), which decreased with time. The predominant bacteria isolated from wounds included *Micrococcus pyogenes* var *albus* (*Staphylococcus epidermidis*), *M pyogenes* var *aureus* (*Staphylococcus aureus*), β-hemolytic *Streptococcus* (several species of *Streptococcus* are known to produce complete hemolysis of red blood cells in culture media), "coliforms" (lactose-fermenting Enterobacteriaceae, such as *Escherichia* species, *Enterobacter* species, *Klebsiella* species, etc), *Streptococcus faecalis* (*Enterococcus faecalis*), and α-hemolytic *Streptococcus* (numerous species). *Clostridium* species and *Proteus vulgaris* appeared in low numbers of wounds. The predominant microorganism found in blood cultures was *Staphylococcus albus* (*S epidermidis*) at the three stations.

Consequently, the choice of antimicrobial agents depends on the quality and dose of radiation and the microorganisms that cause the ensuing infection. Prompt laboratory identification of the microorganisms that cause the infection is imperative to ensure effectiveness of the carefully selected therapeutic agents. Early isolation and identification of resident microorganisms with antimicrobial susceptibility assessment from the orophyarynx, rectum, and axilla of casualties would be valuable to compare with those isolated later, when casualties develop subsequent systemic infection, and to provide optimal antimicrobial therapy based on the pharmacodynamic parameters of the selected drugs. Such a preliminary study was performed in nonhuman primates (*Macaca mulatta*) before irradiation[29] in preparation for subsequent studies after irradiation. Knowledge of predominant endemic microorganisms in a geographical region where a conflict could occur would also aid in planning appropriate treatments.

Endogenous Bacterial Infections

Sepsis

Following lethal doses of radiation, sepsis is a complex consequence of depressed hematopoiesis, immunosuppression, and mucosal damage, as well as injury to cells of the intestines and lungs. Bacteria translocate principally from the intestinal lumen but also from other mucous membranes or wounds into local and regional lymphatics, causing sepsis, multiple organ failure, and death. Following nonlethal irradiation, susceptibility to exogenous infection is increased, which can progress to sepsis, but bacterial translocation from endogenous sources does not generally occur after sublethal irradiation. Trauma and physical exercise stress also increase bacterial translocation from the intestines and could contribute to increased infections after nonlethal irradiation. Sepsis is characterized by uncontrolled host inflammatory responses to bacterial infection, including overproduction of pro-inflammatory cytokines as the syndrome progresses toward multiple organ failure.[30,31] Despite improved

antimicrobial agents and clinical support, mortality from sepsis in intensive care units has remained at 35% to 45% for more than a half century.[32]

In clinical practice, severe systemic infections caused by gram-negative bacteria are generally treated with aminoglycosides combined with β-lactam antibiotics. From 1989 until recently, vancomycin was reserved to treat severe infections caused by antibiotic-resistant, gram-positive bacteria in an immunocompromised host. Effective therapy can be provided by single agents, including piperacillin/tazobactam, carbapenems or fourth-generation cephalosporins, or a combination of penicillin and gentamicin with or without vancomycin, depending on the microorganisms that cause the specific infection.

Selective decontamination of the digestive tract with antimicrobial agents is an infection-control strategy that can prevent infection in an immunocompromised host.[33] Four objectives of selective decontamination using four component protocols (compared to conventional therapy for sepsis)[34] include the following: (1) treat the primary endogenous infection with a systemic parenteral antimicrobial agent; (2) prevent a secondary endogenous infection by microorganisms acquired during hospitalization with enteral, nonabsorbable agents; (3) prevent exogenous infection through a rigorous hygiene protocol; and (4) perform surveillance cultures of the intestinal tract to detect potential exogenous microorganisms that have been acquired. This evidence-based medical intervention significantly reduces morbidity and mortality, prevents the emergence of resistant microorganisms, and is cost effective.[35]

Following irradiation, the concept of selective decontamination can be adapted, but the antimicrobial agents are chosen to inhibit Enterobacteriaceae and spare the indigenous anaerobic bacteria. 4-Fluoroquinolones possess high bactericidal activity against most gram-negative bacteria in vitro.[36] These agents can be given orally, are relatively free of serious side effects, and are used for selective decontamination of the intestinal tract to prevent sepsis in neutropenic, immunocompromised hosts. Except for norfloxacin, the quinolones are readily absorbed, so not only do they reduce the number of facultative enteric bacteria in the intestinal lumen without suppressing anaerobic bacteria, they also eliminate facultative microorganisms that might spread systemically. Other agents that are nonabsorbable include polymyxin B and neomycin. These agents are useful for selective decontamination, but they would be toxic if they were absorbed through injured intestinal mucosa.

To be optimal, selective decontamination should be initiated to anticipate and prevent the translocation of intestinal bacteria following irradiation. Time of initiation of selective decontamination, as for systemic antimicrobial therapy, is not definitively established but will depend on timing of thrombocytopenia and neutropenia as measurable indicators of susceptibility, dose and quality of radiation, source and extent of infection, and the extent of trauma, burns, or other physical injuries.

Polymicrobial Infections

Polymicrobial sepsis following lethal doses of ionizing radiation or wound infections can occur following irradiation that is associated with trauma. Such infections are enhanced because of depressed innate immune responses and translocation from the intestinal tract.

Effective management of polymicrobial infections in an irradiated host is complex.[37] It is imperative to prevent translocation of intestinal bacteria that cause sepsis, multiple organ failure, and death. Translocation of facultative and aerobic intestinal bacteria can be increased by suppressing the indigenous anaerobic intestinal flora, which normally provides colonization resistance against potential invading bacteria, particularly gram-negative aerobic and facultative microorganisms.[24] Effective therapy can be achieved by using antimicrobial agents, which eliminate the microorganisms that cause the local or systemic infection and yet possess minimal inhibitory activity against strictly anaerobic bacteria in the intestinal tract.[38] For example, in experimentally irradiated mice, metronidazole enhanced mortality because it reduced the anaerobic intestinal bacteria. On one hand, successful management of intraabdominal and other polymicrobial infections (eg, *E coli* and *Bacteroides fragilis*) requires administration of antimicrobial agents that are effective against both microorganisms.[39] However, in irradiated hosts, adverse effects can be associated with the use of an antimicrobial agent that is effective against anaerobic bacteria. When the numbers of intestinal anaerobic bacteria are reduced, Enterobacteriaceae may increase in number, translocate, and cause sepsis.[24,40]

Ofloxacin and metronidazole efficacy was evaluated in mice given 8.0 or 8.5 Gy ^{60}Co gamma-photon radiation[40] (levofloxacin is the active racemic isomer of ofloxacin). Metronidazole (50 mg/kg) or ofloxacin (40 mg/kg), administered intramuscularly in divided doses every 12 hours, was initiated 48 hours after irradiation for 21 days. After 8.0 Gy, 40% of saline-control and 90% of ofloxacin-treated mice survived at 30 days, whereas no mice treated with metronidazole survived after 16 days ($P < 0.05$). After 8.5 Gy, all saline-treated control mice were dead by day 25 but all metronida-

zole-treated mice were dead by day 9 ($P < 0.05$), and 50% of ofloxacin-treated mice survived 30 days.

Use of clindamycin may also have similar adverse effects following irradiation. Clindamycin is active against most aerobic and anaerobic gram-positive cocci as well as gram-negative anaerobic bacilli, but has poor activity against most gram-negative facultative aerobes and *Enterococcus* strains.[41] In sublethally irradiated experimental mice that were challenged on day 4 with *Bacillus anthracis* Sterne spores intratracheally, a polymicrobial sepsis ensued.[42] Twice-daily, subcutaneous antimicrobial therapy with ciprofloxacin (50 mg/kg), clindamycin (200 mg/kg), or a combination was started 24 hours after bacterial challenge and continued for 21 days.[43] Ciprofloxacin and clindamycin separately improved 45-day survival 77% and 86% ($P < 0.001$), respectively, compared to saline-treated controls (4%), but combination therapy decreased survival to 45% compared to clindamycin alone ($P < 0.01$). In this study, the combination of clindamycin and ciprofloxacin was used to broaden the antimicrobial spectrum of therapy and increase survival. An earlier study in healthy human volunteers did not detect adverse interactions between ciprofloxacin and clindamycin, nor any changes in the pharmacokinetics of ciprofloxacin when combined with clindamycin.[44] This approach, however, revealed an adverse interaction between clindamycin and ciprofloxacin, particularly in gamma-irradiated animals, that reduced survival significantly.

Exogenous Bacterial Infections

Nonlethal doses of ionizing radiation sufficiently depress innate immune responses to increase susceptibility to exogenous bacterial infections, so that small numbers of bacteria can cause an enhanced infection that becomes life threatening,[7,8,42,45] as seen in human patients who are given whole-body radiation treatment prior to bone marrow transplantation.[46] During the 2- to 4-week period of profound neutropenia after irradiation, sources of infection include the patient's own microflora, particularly *S epidermidis*. Microorganisms, including *Pseudomonas aeruginosa* and *Klebsiella pneumoniae*, are frequently isolated in immunocompromised patients or those who have been exposed to ionizing radiation (therapeutically or accidentally). Known microorganisms are used as indicators to demonstrate susceptibility and to evaluate essential factors of effective therapy, including route of infection, route of administration of antimicrobial agents, and duration of therapy.

When *K pneumoniae* is inoculated subcutaneously into experimental mice 3 or 4 days after nonlethal irradiation, the bacterial $LD_{50/30}$ decreases from approximately 4×10^6 colony-forming units (CFUs) in nonirradiated animals to 2×10^2 CFUs in irradiated mice that are given 7.0 Gy gamma photons (γ) or 3.5 Gy mixed-field neutrons (n) and gamma (γ) radiation [$\gamma/(n+\gamma) = 0.64$].[45,47] These are nonlethal doses of radiation in mice. When ceftriaxone was started 1 day after bacterial challenge and given subcutaneously once daily for 10 days, 60% to 70% of mice survived.[48]

Similarly, when 10^8 CFUs *K pneumoniae* were inoculated per os into mice 2 days after 8.0 Gy ^{60}Co gamma-photon radiation, the quinolones (ofloxacin, pefloxacin, and ciprofloxacin), when given orally starting 1 day after bacterial challenge, reduced colonization of the ileum from 57% in controls to 13% in treated animals ($P < 0.005$).[38] Survival increased from 25% in controls to 70% to 85% in treated mice (keeping in mind that levofloxacin is the active racemic isomer of ofloxacin). When 10^7 CFUs *P aeruginosa* were inoculated per os, oral ofloxacin reduced colonization of the ileum from 86% to 17% and survival increased from 20% in controls to 95% in treated animals ($P < 0.005$).[38,49,50]

Duration of antimicrobial therapy and eradication of infection are other factors to consider in the irradiated host. In one laboratory study, mice were given 8.0 Gy ^{60}Co gamma-photon radiation.[51] A dose of 10^8 CFUs *K pneumoniae* was given orally 4 days after irradiation and therapy with ofloxacin was started 1 day later. One group of 20 mice was given ofloxacin for 7 days,

one group for 21 days, and one group was untreated. The optimal duration of therapy with ofloxacin for *K pneumoniae* infection was found to be 21 days (90% survival), compared to 7 days (55% survival). On the fourteenth day after irradiation, *K pneumoniae* was isolated in the ileum of 7 of 9 mice that had received ofloxacin for 7 days and 5 of 6 untreated mice, but no *K pneumoniae* was found in the ileum of mice that were treated for 9 days with ofloxacin ($P < 0.05$). Also, *K pneumoniae* was isolated from the livers of 4 of 6 untreated mice, in 4 of 9 that had received 7 days of ofloxacin, and in none of the mice that had received 9 days of ofloxacin ($P < 0.05$). A 21-day course of therapy would provide protection in humans during the period of greatest risk for infection until the innate immune responses recover and circulating neutrophilic granulocytes begin to approach normal numbers.[51,52]

Fungal and Viral Infections

In addition to bacterial infections, it is important to be aware that fungi may cause life-threatening infection if leukopenia is prolonged after irradiation for more than 14 days. Further, herpes simplex virus was activated in many victims of the Chernobyl accident. The viral infections responded well to acyclovir. However, appropriate preventive and therapeutic approaches to fungal and viral infections are beyond the scope of this chapter.

PROPHYLACTIC METHODS FOR PREVENTING INFECTIONS

Primary or recent booster vaccinations against common endemic and epidemic infectious agents are likely to continue providing protection if immunity relies on circulating antibodies. Vaccinations that induce cell-mediated responses by lymphocytes and that are administered before irradiation, however, may provide inadequate immunity following even low, nonlethal doses of ionizing radiation because the number of circulating lymphocytes decreases rapidly. Further, recovery of the number of lymphocytes is likely to be too slow to respond adequately to a vaccine. Because the number of lymphocytes is diminished after irradiation, any vaccination soon after irradiation is unlikely to provide adequate immunity. In particular, the use of live, active, or attenuated vaccines is contraindicated because these agents could induce life-threatening infection if given within a few weeks before or soon after exposure to ionizing radiation.

Methods that prevent exposure to potential pathogenic microorganisms should be initiated early in the care of medical casualties who have received moderate to severe doses of ionizing radiation, whether

in the field or hospital. Such methods include disinfecting water, appropriately cooking foods, frequent hand washing, use of medical or dental gloves, and air filtration. Selective decontamination of aerobic and facultative intestinal bacteria, while preserving anaerobic flora, can reduce bacterial translocation of facultative and aerobic bacteria, a major source of endogenous bacterial infections. Puncturing skin with needles or using intravenous catheters should be avoided, if possible, because bacteria can be inserted into the injection site and microbial biofilms can easily develop on catheters in situ and become sources of infection. Alimentary feeding will stimulate and maintain the integrity of the intestinal tract as well as provide adequate nutrition. The ingestion of probiotics that are selected species and strains of microorganisms, particularly *Lactobacillus* species used for preparing food products (eg, yogurt), may help prevent endemic gastrointestinal infections, but scientific evaluations are limited and need further investigation to substantiate their efficacy and lack of virulence in immunocompromised hosts.

THERAPEUTIC AGENTS

Antimicrobial agents are the mainstay for therapeutic management of bacterial infections. Cidal antimicrobial agents rather than inhibitory agents offer the best treatment after irradiation because of decreased innate immune responses, which are required for efficacy of inhibitory, or bacteriostatic, antimicrobial agents. Nonspecific and specific immunomodulatory agents also show propensity to improve the outcome of infections after irradiation, but such substances remain under investigation. Use of single agents, either an antimicrobial or an immunomodulator, is not likely to provide effective therapy after irradiation, based on experimental evidence. Prompt therapeutic interventions that would enhance the innate immune responses in a natural manner as well as eliminate pathogenic microorganisms would be a critical requirement to improve chances of survival from infections after irradiation.

Antimicrobial Agents

Careful selection of antimicrobial agents depends on knowledge of both quality and dose of ionizing radiation as well as antimicrobial susceptibility of the microorganisms that cause infection, particularly for polymicrobial sepsis. A radiation event becomes a distinct milestone for measuring time of onset of signs and symptoms and initiation of therapeutic modalities. Time of initiation and duration of antimicrobial therapy depend on the timing of thrombocytopenia and neutropenia as measurable indicators of susceptibility, as well as on dose and quality of radiation, source and extent of infection, and the extent of trauma, burns, or other physical injuries. Experimentally irradiated animals require antimicrobial support during the period when they are most vulnerable to polymicrobial infection (between 7 and 25 days after irradiation, or between approximately 2 and 25 days after combined injury). Inappropriate choice of antimicrobial agents and dosage can lead to failure to eradicate the infection. Bacterial resistance and adverse effects of therapeutic agents can complicate therapy even further.

The dose and interval of administration for each antimicrobial agent depend on the particular pharmacokinetics and pharmacodynamics. The pharmacokinetic and pharmacodynamic parameters are unique for each antimicrobial agent and may vary following irradiation compared with those in nonirradiated patients, perhaps even more so following combined injury. Consequently, antimicrobial dosage regimens that would be appropriate and effective in nonirradiated persons may need to be adjusted to achieve a satisfactory outcome in ir-

radiated persons based on preliminary research data from laboratory animals (Elliott TB, unpublished data). The concentration of the selected antimicrobial agent at the site of infection should exceed the minimum inhibitory concentration for the specific microorganisms for at least 40% of the dosing interval for β-lactam antibiotics.[13] For aminoglycosides and quinolones, the maximum concentration or the area under the concentration-time curve relative to the minimum inhibitory concentration predicts their efficacy.

High doses of one or more broad-spectrum antimicrobial agents should be continued until the number of neutrophilic granulocytes has recovered to at least 5.0×10^8 cells/L (500 cells/μL) and the patient is afebrile for 24 hours.[2–4,36,53] Aminoglycosides should be avoided because of toxicities associated with this class of agents. Regimen adjustments should be based on specific laboratory findings, including identification of microbial species and antimicrobial susceptibilities. When antimicrobial-resistant, gram-positive bacteria, such as *Enterococcus* species, are isolated from a patient, vancomycin, linezolid, or daptomycin should be included in the regimen.

Alternative dosing regimens are designed and adjusted based on pharmacokinetic parameters to improve eradication of infection and clinical outcome. The desired microbiological outcome is indicated by eradication or prevention of infection and the desired clinical outcome is survival or, at least, extension of survival time to allow time for additional interventions to enhance recovery of radiation-injured proliferative tissues. Evaluation of pharmacokinetics and pharmacodynamics provides a basis for developing alternative strategies to achieve a successful microbiological outcome for radiation-induced sepsis. Adjusting some of the variable principal factors of traditional dosing regimens (dose, route, duration, frequency of administration, period of greatest risk, emergence of antimicrobial-resistant microorganisms, and combination therapy) could improve survival outcome as well.[54] Particularly for concentration-dependent agents, increasing dose and dose rate would likely improve the rate of bacteria elimination; however, that adjustment alone will not suffice following lethal irradiation. The duration of treatment could be limited to the period of greatest risk. Frequent drug administration further irritates radiation-injured soft tissues and can cause inadvertent bleeding because of thrombocytopenia. Therefore, reducing administration frequency to once daily would alleviate intermittent injury to soft tissues. Since efficacy of the quinolones is concentration-dependent, a higher dose once daily might improve survival as well as eradicate infection.[55] This latter strategy might also alleviate some of the adverse consequences of administering aminoglycosides parenterally following irradiation, since aminoglycosides have been shown to provide efficacy when given once daily for serious infections in neutropenic patients,[55,56] but should be based on pharmacodynamic end points and individualized pharmacokinetic assessment in critically ill surgical patients.[57]

Delivering Therapeutic Agents

Oral

Oral administration of therapeutic agents is optimal and preferred because this route avoids local bleeding and introducing bacteria at the injection site, is noninvasive, and is especially practical for treating large numbers of casualties. However, using this route of administration depends on the patient's ability to tolerate oral administration (irradiation can induce emesis), the presence of intestinal motility, and absorption of the selected drug from the intestine, which might be altered by irradiation, depending on the quality or dose of radiation. Drugs administered by this route can alter the composition of the intestinal microflora, so oral administration should be used with caution. Oral delivery might be more appropriate in persons who receive low doses of radiation that would cause minimum disturbance to intestinal tissue.

Intravenous

The intravenous route provides immediate, therapeutic concentrations of antimicrobial agents systemically. An intravenous injection could introduce skin or environmental microorganisms directly into the blood, which could be dangerous because of reduced host resistance to infections after irradiation. Because microorganisms form a biofilm on intravenous catheters, which remain in situ for several days, the biofilm provides a nidus for infection. Intravenous delivery might be more appropriate for those who receive high, lethal doses of radiation that cause injury to intestinal tissue and alter absorption of oral drugs. Strict aseptic maintenance at the insertion site of an intravenous catheter is required to prevent a local infection that could become systemic and local bleeding because of thrombocytopenia.

Subcutaneous

The subcutaneous route also provides direct introduction of therapeutic agents, but absorption depends on adequate local circulation in capillaries.

Subcutaneous drug administration could be deleterious because multiple daily injections are required that would introduce skin or environmental microorganisms into those who have reduced resistance to infection after irradiation. Further, subcutaneous bleeding can occur because of thrombocytopenia. Survival was lower in experimental, sublethally irradiated mice that were given only daily injections of saline or water as a control vehicle than in mice that were given no injections after irradiation.[51] However, this risk can be reduced by cleaning injection sites with iodine solution and rinsing with 70% ethanol three times before injection.

Intramuscular

Similar to the subcutaneous route, the intramuscular route depends on adequate local circulation but is contraindicated because excessive bleeding is a major consequence due to thrombocytopenia.

Topical

Antimicrobial salves or lotions have been shown to reduce mortality from infections in experimental irradiated animals that have sustained combined injury from burns or wounds.[58,59] Although local absorption may provide sufficient therapeutic concentrations in injured tissues, absorption is inadequate to achieve therapeutic concentrations systemically and in deep tissue.

Antimicrobial Agents Available for Managing Serious Infections After Irradiation

Three important principles were established in a mouse model that impact efficacious antimicrobial therapy after radiation exposure. First, irradiation increases the probability of translocation of intestinal bacteria.[23] Second, the management of a polymicrobial infection after lethal irradiation is complex and requires the use of antimicrobial agents effective against both gram-positive and gram-negative facultative bacteria, which readily develop antimicrobial resistance.[36] Third, killing anaerobic intestinal bacteria, which are required to maintain colonization resistance against pathogenic bacteria,[33] enhances mortality after lethal irradiation.[24] Further, bactericidal activity is required against infections after irradiation. Bacteristatic agents require phagocytic cells, including granulocytes and macrophages, to be effective against microorganisms; however, the innate immune responses are greatly diminished within a few days after irradiation. The fundamental principles for selecting the most appropriate antimicrobial agents in the following classes have been recommended for managing post-irradiation infection.[36] Conventional dosing regimens for antimicrobial agents are readily available[60] but some dosage regimens should be adjusted for irradiated neutropenic casualties.

Penicillins

Penicillin G remains the drug of choice to control many microorganisms that do not produce β-lactamases, including streptococci, community isolates of *S aureus*, and nonresistant, anaerobic, gram-negative bacilli. However, penicillin G would not be used in neutropenic patients because of the prevalence of antimicrobial resistance among microorganisms in the general population. A β-lactamase–producing strain could "shield" penicillin-susceptible microorganisms from the antibacterial activity of penicillin in a mixed infection. Combinations of a penicillin-class agent plus a β-lactamase inhibitor can provide effective therapy against some penicillin-resistant bacteria.

Cephalosporins

Cephalosporin activity against aerobic and facultative gram-positive and gram-negative bacteria and *Bacteroides* species varies. Cefoxitin, a second-generation cephalosporin, is the most active cephalosporin against β-lactamase–producing *Bacteroides* species. Third-generation cephalosporins have improved activity against the family Enterobacteriaceae. Ceftazidime and cefepime are cephalosporins that are effective against *P aeruginosa*. However, extended spectrum β-lactamases confer resistance among microorganisms against extended-spectrum cephalosporins and monobactams. Consequently, their use in neutropenic patients is limited.

Carbapenems

Carbapenems are bactericidal against methicillin-resistant staphylococci and are resistant to most β-lactamases. Imipenem, a thienamycin antibiotic, coupled with cilastatin, and meropenem have a broad spectrum of antibacterial activity against strictly anaerobic bacteria and gram-negative and gram-positive facultative bacteria.

Metronidazole

This synthetic antimicrobial agent has exceptional activity against anaerobic bacteria only. Metronidazole should be used with caution after irradiation because its activity can be deleterious in an immunocompro-mised host. Metronidazole suppresses the indigenous intestinal anaerobic flora following irradiation so that Enterobacteriaceae can grow unimpeded, translocate from the intestinal tract, and cause sepsis.[24]

Clindamycin

This semisynthetic antibiotic has a broad spectrum of activity against anaerobic bacteria and gram-positive cocci. It also inhibits production of toxins by *Clostridium* species and *Streptococcus pyogenes*. It is indicated in the therapy of serious infections caused by *S pyogenes* as well as anaerobic bacteria.

Aminoglycosides

This class of antibiotics is the major means of controlling gram-negative enteric bacterial infections. These drugs are bactericidal against gram-negative bacilli. However, many gram-negative enteric bacteria exhibit resistance to aminoglycosides. Use of gentamicin, tobramycin, and amikacin is limited because of nephrotoxicity and ototoxicity. They are not effective against anaerobic bacteria or aerobic bacteria in an anaerobic environment.

Quinolones

The 4-fluoroquinolones are active against Enterobacteriaceae, *S aureus*, and other facultative and aerobic bacteria. They are bactericidal and primarily used to inhibit gram-negative bacteria. Ciprofloxacin is the most effective agent in this class against *P aeruginosa*. With increasing use of quinolones, resistance of *P aeruginosa* and Enterobacteriaceae has increased against these drugs. Ciprofloxacin and levofloxacin are included in the Strategic National Stockpile for use against infections following mass casualty events. Newer quinolones, such as moxifloxacin and gatifloxacin, are effective against gram-positive facultative cocci, including *Streptococcus pneumoniae*, as well as gram-negative bacilli. Ciprofloxacin and moxifloxacin were shown to ameliorate leukopenia and neutropenia in immunocompromised mice.[61] The quinolones are not as toxic as aminoglycosides and the older members do not inhibit anaerobic bacteria. However, one quinolone, pefloxacin, was found to decrease bone marrow progenitor cells and overall survival in nonlethally irradiated mice.[62]

Vancomycin

After 1989, vancomycin was reserved as the treatment of last resort for infections caused by antimicrobial-resistant, gram-positive bacteria, especially

Enterococcus faecium, S aureus, and *S pneumoniae.* However, resistance to vancomycin has emerged in recent years. This drug is bactericidal against gram-positive bacteria. Recommendations for use of vancomycin can be found in the current literature.[2,63]

Oxazolidinones

The oxazolidinones are represented by linezolid, the first member of this class of synthetic drugs to be approved by the FDA in April 2000. Linezolid is reserved for treating infections associated with vancomycin-resistant *E faecium,* including bloodstream infection, hospital-acquired pneumonia, and complicated skin and skin structure infections, including cases due to methicillin-resistant *S aureus.* In addition, this drug may be used to treat community-acquired pneumonia and uncomplicated skin and skin structure infections. Linezolid is bacteriostatic against enterococci and staphylococci. It is bactericidal against the majority of strains of streptococci.

Streptogramins

Quinupristin and dalfopristin are two semisynthetic derivatives of pristinamycin I and IIa, respectively. They are combined in a single formulation that is indicated for the treatment of patients with serious or life-threatening infections associated with vancomycin-resistant *E faecium* bacteremia or complicated skin and skin structure infections caused by *S aureus* (methicillin susceptible) or *S pyogenes.* Quinupristin/ dalfopristin formulation is bacteriostatic against *E faecium* but not *E faecalis,* and bactericidal against strains of methicillin-susceptible staphylococci. Because it is bacteriostatic against *E faecium,* phagocytic leukocytes are required for clearance. Therefore, this drug may not be effective against *E faecium* in individuals who are neutropenic.

Synergistic Combinations of Antimicrobial Agents

To be effective in an immunocompromised host, antimicrobial agents must be bactericidal because the innate immune response is not reliable for clearing infectious agents. Synergism has been demonstrated with aminoglycosides together with penicillin or vancomycin against enterococci, α-hemolytic streptococci, and *Prevotella melaninogenica (Bacteroides melaninogenicus);* nafcillin against *S aureus;* ticarcillin against *P aeruginosa;* cephalosporins against *K pneumoniae;* ampicillin against lactose-fermenting Enterobacteriaceae; and clindamycin or metronidazole against *B fragilis.*

Biological Response Modifiers and Immunomodulating Agents

Prompt therapeutic interventions that enhance the innate immune responses in a natural manner would be a critical requirement for improving survival from infection after irradiation. There are specific and nonspecific immunomodulating agents that have potential therapeutic value for treating infections in individuals who are immunocompromised due to ionizing radiation. The proinflammatory cytokines are key components of the initial host response to an infection. Experimental evidence has shown that cytokines and chemokines improve survival of irradiated animals.[64–68] Cytokines and chemokines have specific receptors on specific types of cells with specific consequences.

Nonspecific immunomodulating agents, such as those used as adjuvants for vaccines, also improved survival in animals that were given either lethal doses of ionizing radiation or nonlethal doses of radiation followed by challenge with nonlethal doses of bacteria. The optimal nonspecific immunomodulating agent would stimulate a natural cascade of the remaining innate immune responses in the irradiated host and could facilitate an earlier recovery. Drugs that have been evaluated against bacterial infections in irradiated animals include synthetic trehalose dicorynomycolate,[58,59,69] β-1,3-glucan,[70] 3D-monophosphoryl lipid A,[69,71] and 5-androstenediol.[72,73] Sufficient numbers of progenitor stem cells, which support the innate immune response, may remain viable in the bone marrow, perhaps because they are in a nonvulnerable phase of the cell cycle at the time of irradiation, particularly after partial-body irradiation. Further, these progenitor cells could be stimulated and revived to respond to an invading microorganism or a foreign antigen, such as occurs during infection or following transplantation of exogenous tissue. Some nonspecific immunomodulators can cause adverse side effects, such as granulomas or liver fibrosis caused by synthetic trehalose dicorynomycolate, but such nonlethal effects might be outweighed by their benefits to reduce mortality and improve recovery.

Specific immunomodulating agents, in particular the cytokines, granulocyte colony-stimulating factor (G-CSF), interleukin-1β, and interleukin-11 improved survival in lethally irradiated animals.[74–76] However, use of cytokines or their inhibitors for treating sepsis in animal models may not yet reflect a similar effect in humans in clinical trials.[30] They are generally provided as recombinant molecules and must be injected daily or on alternate days, but G-CSF conjugated with methionine (filgrastim) or polyethylene glycol (pegfilgrastim) is more stable, with a longer half-life than G-CSF, and can be injected once subcutaneously. Timing of administration relative to irradiation and bacterial challenge is consequential as well. For example, interleukin-1β increases survival from infection with *K pneumoniae* when given after nonlethal irradiation and several days before bacterial challenge, but also decreases survival when given during the course of infection (Elliott TB, unpublished data).

COMBINED THERAPY: IMMUNOMODULATING AND ANTIMICROBIAL AGENTS

Combined therapy overcomes the limitations of treating infections in irradiated persons with either antimicrobial agents or immunomodulating agents alone. A nonspecific immunomodulating agent, given once within 24 hours after irradiation, stimulates a natural cascade of the remaining innate immune responses while the antimicrobial agent attacks the microorganisms that cause the spreading infection. The value of nonspecific immunomodulators for treating infections has been demonstrated in irradiated animals, as noted above. Combined therapy with a broad-spectrum antimicrobial agent improved the outcome even more than the immunomodulator alone against a higher infecting challenge dose of bacteria.

Combining specific immunomodulators, such as chemokines and cytokines, together with antimicrobial therapy has also been investigated for efficacy. The results and conclusions of various studies are inconclusive. Further, disadvantages include multiple daily injections following irradiation, as well as consequential bleeding, increased risk of introducing bacteria, and high financial cost. Further studies are needed to evaluate combination therapies following whole-body irradiation.

FUTURE CONSIDERATIONS

Drug Delivery

Timed release of antimicrobial agents (oral, subcutaneous, or topical) to maintain a concentration above the minimum inhibitory concentration could further improve therapeutic efficacy following irradiation. Also, transdermal drug delivery by microneedle array on patches is likely to offer an alternative method to subcutaneous inoculation of therapeutic drugs. The microneedle array might be contraindicated for use in the immunocompromised host because multiple skin punctures could introduce skin and environmental microorganisms.

Antimicrobial Vaccines and Drugs

There is a continuing need for innovative vaccines and antimicrobial agents to provide unequivocal protection against resistant infectious agents at reasonable cost. Recent advances include development of newer generations of older antimicrobial agents, dual-action synergistic antimicrobial agents, and antimicrobial peptides.

Immunomodulators

Dosage, timing intervals, and routes of delivery of specific cytokines may soon be sufficiently practical for application in irradiated victims. Combinations of cytokine molecules show promise in experiments in laboratory animals to reduce toxicity and improve efficacy, particularly in febrile and neutropenic individuals. The inflammatory response to sepsis is complex. A combination of agents targeted at multiple pathways offers optimal chances for a successful outcome in each patient.[30]

CURRENT RECOMMENDATIONS FOR MILITARY USE OR NATIONAL DISASTERS

Based on current knowledge and practice, recommendations can be made to prevent or treat infections that occur following irradiation. These recommendations are based on drugs currently approved for human use by the FDA, including vaccines and antimicrobial agents used for treating immunocompromised or neutropenic patients or those that have been shown to be efficacious in laboratory models of infection in whole-body-irradiated animals. The FDA has not approved biological response modifiers and immunomodulators, which are currently being studied in laboratory animals, for treating infections in humans. The 1997, 2002, and 2010 guidelines for the use of antimicrobial agents in neutropenic patients [2,3,53] offer the best consensus opinion for treating infections in victims of irradiation. Nevertheless, the irradiated host may present specific and unique challenges for effective therapy and improved outcome.

Infection is best prevented by prior vaccination for known endemic or epidemic infectious agents. Therapeutic vaccinations given within several weeks after irradiation are not likely to immunize because of lymphopenia. Attenuated vaccines are contraindicated because attenuated infectious agents could cause enhanced, life-threatening infection after irradiation.

After nonlethal irradiation, therapy for infection, even in the absence of physical injuries, is best achieved by either early initiation of antimicrobial therapy for demonstrated infection by endogenous or exogenous infectious agents, including known exposure to a biological warfare agent, or selective decontamination of the intestinal tract with antimicrobial agents against endogenous microorganisms. After lethal irradiation, broad-spectrum antimicrobial therapy should be started when the absolute number of neutrophilic cells decreases below 500 cells/μL and the number of thrombocytes decreases below 50,000 cells/μL in anticipation of endogenous bacterial translocation. Neutropenia and thrombocytopenia should be monitored.

Individuals should be monitored continually for signs and symptoms of infection for at least 21 days (up to 40 days in some cases). When signs or symptoms of infection do appear, antimicrobial therapy should be promptly initiated and continued for at least 14 and up to 21 days when there is no known exposure to a specific infectious agent, although the optimal duration of therapy is not definitively established. When physical injuries, such as trauma or burns, occur in addition to irradiation, antimicrobial therapeutic agents, both topical and systemic, should be promptly initiated and continued until wounds close, which occurs more slowly than normally after irradiation. When exposure to a known infectious agent, such as an opportunistic microorganism or a biological attack agent, occurs within 7 days after irradiation, specific, recommended antimicrobial therapy should be promptly initiated and continued for 21 days. However, specifically for *B anthracis* infections, penicillin G or ciprofloxacin should be given for 6 weeks. Casualties who develop infections should be promptly transported to a hospital to ensure optimal supportive care.

Under controlled hygienic conditions (eg, in a hospital), parenteral therapy with a carbapenem and ceftazidime, with or without vancomycin, is recommended. The site of intravenous catheterization must be kept meticulously aseptic. However, in cases of mass casualties in which resources are inadequate, quinolones are recommended. Quinolones in particular offer advantages for effective antimicrobial therapy of bacterial infections after irradiation. Quinolones can be administered either orally or parenterally. They provide a broad spectrum of antimicrobial activity, principally against facultative gram-negative bacteria, with minimal activity against strictly anaerobic bacteria in the intestinal tract, thereby preserving colonization resistance against pathogenic microorganisms.

When either nonspecific or specific immunomodulators are approved for use in humans against infections, they may offer further advantages in combination with antimicrobial agents for improving the outcome of infections after irradiation by enhancing and advancing recovery of innate immune responses.

SUMMARY

Nuclear weapons will cause combined injuries from wounds, burns, or blunt trauma together with ionizing radiation. Severe bacterial infections will also occur from endogenous and exogenous sources. Injury severity will be much greater than from either weapon or infectious agent alone. A comprehensive therapeutic regimen will be required to effectively treat these complex injuries. This chapter reviews the current state of knowledge and experimental research about the preventive and therapeutic measures available to diminish casualty numbers and ameliorate synergistic combined insults. Nevertheless, the irradiated host may present specific challenges for effective therapy and improved outcome. Bacterial, especially polymicrobial, infections are difficult to treat effectively in those who receive whole-body ionizing radiation because the innate immune responses are diminished. In general, antimicrobial agents alone cannot be expected to assure survival greater than 40% to 60%. Parenteral therapy, which can be monitored, is recommended for hospitalized patients, but oral administration would be more expedient for mass casualties. Quinolones appear to offer the broadest therapeutic application for infections after irradiation. Use of nonspecific or specific biological response modifiers or immunomodulators could improve outcome, but they are either not approved for human use or their efficacy has not been demonstrated in irradiated humans or experimental models of infection in irradiated animals. Further studies are needed to develop more efficacious drugs, particularly nonspecific immunomodulators, cytokines, and chemokines in irradiated animals.

Acknowledgement

We are fortunate for expert reviews of the manuscript and recommendations offered by I Brook, MD, CDR, MC, US Navy (Retired), infectious disease physician and expert on principles of antimicrobial therapy following irradiation. We are also particularly grateful for the excellent technical and scientific contributions of RA Harding, MM Moore, and GS Madonna in the experimental research studies summarized in this review.

REFERENCES

1. Walker RI. Infectious complications of radiation injury. In: Walker RI, Cerveny TJ, eds. *Medical Consequences of Nuclear Warfare*. In: Zajtchuk R, Jenkins DP, Bellamy RF, Ingram VM, eds. *Textbook of Military Medicine*. Washington, DC: Department of the Army, Office of the Surgeon General, Borden Institute; 1989:67–83.

2. Freifeld AG, Bow EJ, Sepkowitz KA, et al. Clinical practice guideline for the use of antimicrobial agents in neutropenic patients with cancer: 2010 update by the Infectious Diseases Society of America. *Clin Infect Dis* 2011;52(4):e56–e93.

3. Hughes WT, Armstrong D, Bodey GP, et al. 1997 guidelines for the use of antimicrobial agents in neutropenic patients with unexplained fever. Infectious Diseases Society of America. *Clin Infect Dis.* 1997;25(3):551–573.

4. Waselenko JK, MacVittie TJ, Blakely WF, et al. Medical management of the acute radiation syndrome: Recommendations of the Strategic National Stockpile Radiation Working Group. *Ann Intern Med.* 2004;140(12):1037–1051.

5. Cerveny TJ, MacVittie TJ, Young RW. Acute radiation syndrome in humans. In: Walker RI, Cerveny TJ, eds. *Medical Consequences of Nuclear Warfare*. In: Zajtchuk R, Jenkins DP, Bellamy RF, Ingram VM, eds. *Textbook of Military Medicine*. Washington, DC: Department of the Army, Office of the Surgeon General, Borden Institute 1989:15–36.

6. Cronkite EP. The hemorrhagic syndrome of acute ionizing radiation illness produced in goats and swine by exposure to the atomic bomb at Bikini, 1946. *Blood.* 1950;5:32–45.

7. Elliott TB, Brook I, Stiefel SM. Quantitative study of wound infection in irradiated mice. *Int J Radiat Biol.* 1990; 58:341–350.

8. Brook I, Elliott TB, Ledney GD. Infection after ionizing irradiation. In: Zak O, Sande MA, eds. *Handbook of Animal Models of Infection: Experimental Models in Antimicrobial Chemotherapy*. San Diego, CA: Academic Press; 1999: 151–161.

9. Reinhard JF. Pharmacological screening. In: Foster HL, Small JD, Fox JG, eds. *The Mouse in Biomedical Research Experimental Biology and Oncology*. Vol IV. New York, NY: Academic Press; 1982: 313–327.

10. Madden DL, Fujiwara K. Selected bacterial diseases. In: Foster HL, Small JD, Fox JG, eds. *The Mouse in Biomedical Research Experimental Biology and Oncology*. Vol IV. New York, NY: Academic Press; 1982: 257–270.

11. Andes DR, Craig WA. Pharmacodynamics of fluoroquinolones in experimental models of endocarditis. *Clin Infect Dis.* 1998;27:47–50.

12. Andes DR, Craig WA. Pharmacodynamics of the new fluoroquinolone gatifloxacin in murine thigh and lung infection models. *Antimicrob Agents Chemother.* 2002;46(6):1665–1670.

13. Craig WA. Pharmacokinetic/pharmacodynamic parameters: rationale for antibacterial dosing of mice and men. *Clin Infect Dis.* 1998;26:1–12.

14. Falk PG, Hooper LV, Midtvedt T, Gordon JI. Creating and maintaining the gastrointestinal ecosystem: what we know and need to know from gnotobiology. *Microbiol Molec Biol Rev.* 1998;62(4):1157–1170.

15. Fritz TE, Brennan PC, Giolitto JA, Flynn RJ. Interrelations between X-irradiation and the intestinal flora of mice. In: Sullivan MF, ed. *Gastrointestinal Radiation Injury, Symposium, Richland, Washington, September 25-28, 1966*. New York, NY: Excerpta Medica; 1968: 279–291.

16. Schaedler RW, Orcutt RP. Gastrointestinal microflora. In: Foster HL, Small JD, Fox JG, eds. *The Mouse in Biomedical Research Normative Biology, Immunology, and Husbandry.* Vol III. New York, NY: Academic Press; 1983: 327–345.

17. Lee KH, Hui KP, Tan WC. Thrombocytopenia in sepsis: a predictor of mortality in the intensive care unit. *Singapore Med J.* 1993;34(3):245–246.

18. North Atlantic Treaty Organization Military Committee Joint Standardization Board. *Standardization Agreement. Commander's Guide on the Effects From Nuclear Radiation Exposure During War.* 7th ed. Brussels, Belgium: NATO Standardization Agency; 2009. STANAG 2083.

19. US Departments of the Army, Navy, and Air Force. *NATO Handbook on the Medical Aspects of NBC Defensive Operations.* Washington, DC: DA; 1996. AMedP-6(B), Army Field Manual 8-9, Chap 6. http://www.dtic.mil/cgi-bin/GetTRDoc?AD=ADA434662. Accessed August 2, 2012.

20. The Committee for the Compilation of Materials on Damage Caused by the Atomic Bombs in Hiroshima and Nagasaki. *Hiroshima and Nagasaki: The Physical, Medical, and Social Effects of the Atomic Bombings.* New York, NY: Basic Books, Inc; 1981.

21. Bebeshko V, Belyi D, Kovalenko A, Gergel O. *Health Consequences in the Chernobyl Emergency Workers Surviving After Confirmed Acute Radiation Sickness.* Vienna, Austria: International Atomic Energy Agency; 2002. IAEA-TECDOC-1300.

22. Brook I, Tom SP, Ledney GD. Quinolone and glycopeptide therapy for infection in mouse following exposure to mixed-field neutron-gamma-photon radiation. *Int J Radiat Biol.* 1993;64(6):771–777.

23. Elliott TB, Ledney GD, Harding RA, et al. Mixed-field neutrons and γ photons induce different changes in ileal bacteria and correlated sepsis in mice. *Int J Radiat Biol.* 1995;68:311–320.

24. Brook I, Walker RI, MacVittie TJ. Effect of antimicrobial therapy on bowel flora and bacterial infection in irradiated mice. *Int J Radiat Biol Relat Stud Phys Chem Med.* 1988;53:709–716.

25. Lawrence JH, Tennant R. The comparative effects of neutrons and X-rays on the whole body. *J Exp Med.* 1937;66:667–688.

26. Ledney GD, Elliott TB, Landauer MR, et al. Survival of irradiated mice treated with WR-151327, synthetic trehalose dicorynomycolate, or ofloxacin. *Adv Space Res.* 1994;14:583–586.

27. Ledney GD, Elliott TB. Combined injury: factors with potential to impact radiation dose assessments. *Health Phys.* 2010;98(2):145–152.

28. McDonnel GM, Crosby WH, Tessmer CF, et al. *Effects of Nuclear Detonations on a Large Biological Specimen (Swine), Operation Plumbbob, Project 4.1.* Sandia Base, Albuquerque, New Mexico: Defense Atomic Support Agency; 1961. WT-1428.

29. Carrier CA, Elliott TB, Ledney GD. Resident bacteria in a mixed population of rhesus macaque (*Macaca mulatta*) monkeys: a prevalence study. *J Med Primatol.* 2009;38(6):397–403.

30. Aoki N, Xing Z. Use of cytokines in infection. *Expert Opin Emerg Drugs.* 2004;9(2):223–236.

31. Zanotti S, Kumar A, Kumar A. Cytokine modulation in sepsis and septic shock. *Expert Opin Investig Drugs.* 2002;11(8):1061–1075.

32. Opal SM, Cohen J. Clinical gram-positive sepsis: does it fundamentally differ from gram-negative bacterial sepsis? *Crit Care Med.* 1999;27(8):1608–1616.

33. van der Waaij D. The last epidemic: selective decontamination in the control of mortality among radiation victims. *Scand J Infect Dis Suppl.* 1982;36:141–149.

34. Silvestri L, van Saene HKF, Milanese M, Gregori D, Gullo A. Selective decontamination of the digestive tract reduces bacterial bloodstream infection and mortality in critically ill patients. Systematic review of randomized, controlled trials. *J Hosp Infect.* 2007;65(3):187–203.

35. Silvestri L, Mannucci F, van Saene HKF. Selective decontamination of the digestive tract: a life saver. *J Hosp Infect.* 2000;45(3):185–190.

36. Brook I, Elliott TB, Ledney GD, Shoemaker MO, Knudson GB. Management of postirradiation infection: lessons learned from animal models. *Mil Med.* 2004;169(3):194–197.

37. Brook I. Use of antibiotics in the management of postirradiation wound infection and sepsis. *Radiat Res.* 1988;115(1):1–25.

38. Brook I, Ledney GD. Quinolone therapy in the management of infection after irradiation. *Crit Rev Microbiol.* 1992;18:235–246.

39. Brook I. Management of infection following intra-abdominal trauma. *Ann Emerg Med.* 1988;17(6):626–632.

40. Brook I, Ledney GD. Effect of antimicrobial therapy on the gastrointestinal bacterial flora, infection and mortality in mice exposed to different doses of irradiation. *J Antimicrob Chemother.* 1994;33:63–72.

41. Falagas ME, Gorbach SL. Clindamycin and metronidazole. *Med Clin North Am.* 1995;79(4):845–867.

42. Brook I, Elliott TB, Harding RA, et al. Susceptibility of irradiated mice to *Bacillus anthracis* Sterne by the intratracheal route of infection. *J Med Microbiol.* 2001;50:702–711.

43. Brook I, Germana A, Giraldo DE, et al. Clindamycin and quinolone therapy for *Bacillus anthracis* Sterne infection in ^{60}Co-gamma-photon-irradiated and sham-irradiated mice. *J Antimicrob Chemother.* 2005;56(6):1074–1080.

44. Boeckh M, Lode H, Deppermann KM, et al. Pharmacokinetics and serum bactericidal activities of quinolones in combination with clindamycin, metronidazole, and ornidazole. *Antimicrob Agents Chemother.* 1990;34(12):2407–2414.

45. McChesney DG, Ledney GD, Madonna GS. Trehalose dimycolate enhances survival of fission neutron-irradiated mice and *Klebsiella pneumoniae*-challenged irradiated mice. *Radiat Res.* 1990;121(1):71–75.

46. Engelhard D, Marks MI, Good RA. Infections in bone marrow transplant recipients. *J Pediatr.* 1986;108(3):335–346.

47. Ledney GD, Elliott TB, Harding RA, Jackson WE III, Inal CE, Landauer MR. WR-151327 increases resistance to *Klebsiella pneumoniae* infection in mixed-field- and γ-photon irradiated mice. *Int J Radiat Biol.* 2000;76:261–271.

48. Madonna GS, Ledney GD, Elliott TB, et al. Trehalose dimycolate enhances resistance to infection in neutropenic animals. *Infect Immun.* 1989;57:2495–2501.

49. Brook I, Ledney GD. Oral ofloxacin therapy of *Pseudomonas aeruginosa* sepsis in mice after irradiation. *Antimicrob Agents Chemother.* 1990;34(7):1387–1389.

50. Brook I, Ledney GD. Oral aminoglycoside and ofloxacin therapy in the prevention of gram-negative sepsis after irradiation. *J Infect Dis.* 1991;164(5):917–921.

51. Brook I, Ledney GD. Short and long courses of ofloxacin therapy of *Klebsiella pneumoniae* sepsis following irradiation. *Radiat Res.* 1992;130(1):61–64.

52. Brook I, Elliott TB, Ledney GD, Knudson GB. Management of postirradiation sepsis. *Mil Med.* 2002;167 (Suppl 1):105–106.

53. Hughes WT, Armstrong D, Bodey GP, et al. 2002 Guidelines for the use of antimicrobial agents in neutropenic patients with cancer. *Clin Infect Dis.* 2002;34:730–751.

54. Rubenstein E, Zhanel GG. Forum: Anti-infective research and development—problems, challenges, and solutions. The hospital physician. *Lancet Infect Dis.* 2007;7:69–70.

55. Lortholary O, Lefort A, Tod M, Chomat A-M, Darras-Joly C, Cordonnier C. Pharmacodynamics and pharmacokinetics of antibacterial drugs in the management of febrile neutropenia. *Lancet Infect Dis.* 2008;8(10):612–620.

56. Roberts JA, Lipman J. Pharmacokinetic issues for antibiotics in the critically ill patient. *Crit Care Med*. 2009;37(3):840–851; quiz 859.

57. Mueller EW, Boucher BA. The use of extended-interval aminoglycoside dosing strategies for the treatment of moderate-to-severe infections encountered in critically ill surgical patients. *Surg Infect (Larchmt)*. 2009;10(6):563–570.

58. Ledney GD, Madonna GS, Moore MM, Elliott TB, Brook I. Synthetic trehalose dicorynomycolate and antimicrobials increase survival from sepsis in mice immunocompromised by radiation and trauma. *J Med*. 1992;23:253–264.

59. Madonna GS, Ledney GD, Moore MM, Elliott TB, Brook I. Treatment of mice with sepsis following irradiation and trauma with antibiotics and synthetic trehalose dicorynomycolate (S-TDCM). *J Trauma*. 1991;31:316–325.

60. Bartlett JG. Preparations and recommended dosing regimens for antimicrobial agents. In: Bartlett JG, ed. *2005-6 Pocket Book of Infectious Disease Therapy*. 13th ed. Philadelphia, PA: Lippincott Williams & Wilkins; 2005: 1–17.

61. Shalit I, Kletter Y, Halperin D, et al. Immunomodulatory effects of moxifloxacin in comparison to ciprofloxacin and G-CSF in a murine model of cyclophosphamide-induced leukopenia. *Eur J Haematol*. 2001;66:287–296.

62. Patchen ML, Brook I, Elliott TB, Jackson WE. Adverse effects of pefloxacin in irradiated C3H/HeN mice: correction with glucan therapy. *Antimicrob Agents Chemother*. 1993;37(9):1882–1889.

63. Rybak M, Lomaestro B, Rotschafer JC, et al. Therapeutic monitoring of vancomycin in adult patients: a consensus review of the American Society of Health-System Pharmacists, the Infectious Diseases Society of America, and the Society of Infectious Diseases Pharmacists. *Am J Health-Syst Pharm*. 2009;66:82–98.

64. Degre M. Interferons and other cytokines in bacterial infections. *J Interferon Cytokine Res*. 1996;16(6):417–426.

65. Neta R. Modulation with cytokines of radiation injury: suggested mechanisms of action. *Environ Health Perspect*. 1997;105(Suppl 6):1463–1465.

66. Neta R, Oppenheim JJ, Schreiber RD, Chizzonite R, Ledney GD, MacVittie TJ. Role of cytokines (interleukin 1, tumor necrosis factor, and transforming growth factor beta) in natural and lipopolysaccharide-enhanced radioresistance. *J Exp Med*. 1991;173(5):1177–1182.

67. Neta R, Oppenheim JJ, Wang JM, Snapper CM, Moorman MA, Dubois CM. Synergy of IL-1 and stem cell factor in radioprotection of mice is associated with IL-1 up-regulation of mRNA and protein expression for c-kit on bone marrow cells. *J Immunol*. 1994;153(4):1536–1543.

68. Neta R, Perlstein R, Vogel SN, Ledney GD, Abrams J. Role of interleukin 6 (IL-6) in protection from lethal irradiation and in endocrine responses to IL-1 and tumor necrosis factor. *J Exp Med*. 1992;175(3):689–694.

69. Peterson VM, Adamovicz JJ, Elliott TB, et al. Gene expression of hematoregulatory cytokines is elevated endogenously following sublethal gamma-irradiation and is differentially enhanced by therapeutic administration of biological response modifiers. *J Immunol*. 1994;153:2321–2330.

70. Patchen ML. Immunomodulators and cytokines: their use in the mitigation of radiation-induced hemopoietic injury. In: Bump EA, Malaker K, eds. *Radioprotectors: Chemical, Biological, and Clinical Perspectives*. Boca Raton, Florida: CRC Press; 1998:213–236.

71. Snyder SL, Walden TL, Patchen ML, MacVittie TJ, Fuchs P. Radioprotective properties of detoxified lipid A from *Salmonella minnesota* R595. *Radiat Res*. 1986;107(1):107–114.

72. Whitnall MH, Elliott TB, Landauer MR, et al. *In vivo* protection against gamma-irradiation with 5-androstenediol. *Exp Biol Med (Maywood)*. 2001;226(7):625–627.

73. Whitnall MH, Elliott TB, Landauer MR, et al. Protection against gamma-irradiation with 5-androstenediol. *Mil Med*. 2002;167(2 Suppl):64–65.

74. MacVittie TJ, Monroy RL, Patchen ML, Souza LM. Therapeutic use of recombinant human G-CSF (rhG-CSF) in a canine model of sublethal and lethal whole-body irradiation. *Int J Radiat Biol.* 1990;57(4):723–736.

75. Neta R, Oppenheim JJ. Cytokines in therapy of radiation injury. *Blood.* 1988;72(3):1093–1095.

76. Redlich CA, Gao X, Rockwell S, Kelley M, Elias JA. IL-11 enhances survival and decreases TNF production after radiation-induced thoracic injury. *J Immunol.* 1996;157(4):1705–1710.

Chapter 6

EARLY-PHASE BIOLOGICAL DOSIMETRY

WILLIAM F. BLAKELY, PhD[*]

[*]Senior Scientist and Biodosimetry Research Program Advisor, Biological Dosimetry Research Group, Scientific Research Department, Armed Forces Radiobiology Research Institute, Uniformed Services University of the Health Sciences, Bethesda, Maryland 20889; Adjunct Assistant Professor, Preventive Medicine and Biometrics Department, Uniformed Services University of the Health Sciences, Bethesda, Maryland

INTRODUCTION

Biological dosimetry is radiation dose or injury assessment using clinical signs and symptoms, including bioindicators from the hematological, gastrointestinal (GI), cerebrovascular, and cutaneous systems; radiation biomarkers (ie, chromosome aberrations measured in mitogen-stimulated peripheral blood lymphocytes), and other available biodosimetry approaches.[1] Alternative biodosimetry assessment methods can include measuring absorbed dose in solid matrix materials (ie, teeth enamel, bone, nail clippings) from suspected exposed individuals. For example, absorbed dose derived from free radicals detected in enamel from extracted teeth from an individual can be measured using electron paramagnetic resonance (EPR), and is considered by many to be a component of biophysical or biological dosimetry. Confirming individual internal contamination by measuring radioactivity from radionuclides in biological samples (ie, urine, blood, feces, etc), which is commonly referred to as a "radiation bioassay," and using radioactivity detectors to measure radionuclide contamination after clothing removal and washing are also commonly included in radiation exposure assessment. In-depth descriptions of radiation bioassays are beyond the scope of this chapter; hence, further discussions will be limited to recording of the type, amount, and body position of radionuclide contamination. Tissues and organs (ie, parotid gland, GI tissues, bone marrow, etc) exhibit cell and tissue injury at various times after radiation exposure, resulting in leakage of organ-specific components into blood that is often excreted in urine. The levels of these organ-specific biomarkers measured in blood plasma or urine have been used to augment clinical signs and symptoms of radiation dose and injury assessment. Proteomic biodosimetry and other selective emerging radiation exposure diagnostic technologies that show promise to provide triage and clinical biodosimetry applications will be described.[2,3]

Multiple parameter biological dosimetry is generally used to assess the severity of acute radiation syndrome or sickness (ARS), which is typically characterized into three phases in individuals suspected of exposure to life-threatening radiation doses: (1) initial or prodromal, (2) latent, and (3) manifest (or obvious) illness. The time to onset and severity for these three phases are influenced by radiation dose, quality (ie, gamma rays versus neutrons), dose rate, and the individual's sensitivity to radiation (Table 6-1).

The primary purpose of early-response biodosimetry following suspected radiation overexposure is to rapidly provide first responders and medical providers scientifically sound diagnostic radiation injury and dose assessment to support treatment decisions.[4] Assessing clinical signs and symptoms associated with the severity of organ-specific (ie, hematological, GI, cerebrovascular, and cutaneous) ARS, as developed and advocated by Professor TM Fliedner (Ulm, Germany), is essential for victim triage.[5,6] The risk of death from life-threatening radiation exposure depends on the level of medical care available (Figure 6-1 a).[4] The US Strategic National Stockpile Radiation Working Group recommended a treatment approach using both the organ-specific clinical signs and symptoms (based on the Medical Treatment Protocols for Radiation Accident Victims diagnostic system) and biological dosimetry (ie, time to onset of nausea and vomiting, decline in absolute lymphocyte counts over several hours to days after exposure, and appearance of chromosome aberrations [ie, dicentrics and rings]).[7] In the case of a mass casualty radiation emergency, this working group recommended cytokine, antibiotic, and stem-cell transplant therapies (Figure 6-1 b). The working group also encouraged cytokine therapy to be initiated 24 hours after radiation exposure, based on the preclinical studies by MacVittie and colleagues.[8] This will likely necessitate an initial reliance on diagnostic information based on early bioindicators of radiation

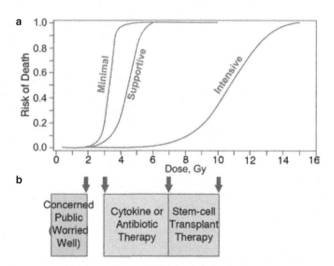

Figure 6-1. (a) The effects of medical care levels on the risk of death as a function of radiation dose.

(b) Various medical treatment support approaches at dose windows recommended by the US Strategic National Stockpile Radiation Working Group.

Data source: Waselenko JK, MacVittie TJ, Blakely WF, et al. Medical management of the acute radiation syndrome: recommendations of the Strategic National Stockpile Working Group. *Ann Intern Med.* 2004;140(12):1037–1051.

TABLE 6-1

ACUTE RADIATION SYNDROME IN HEALTHY ADULTS: WHOLE-BODY IRRADIATION FROM ACUTE PHOTON EQUIVALENT DOSES*

		Survivability					
		Highly Survivable		Survivable to Lethal		Lethal	
		Degree of ARS					
		Mild		Moderate to Severe	Very Severe	Lethal	
		Dose Range					
Phase of Syndrome	Characteristic	0–100 cGy	100–200 cGy	200–600 cGy	600–800 cGy	800–3,000 cGy	> 3,000 cGy
Prodromal phase	Vomiting:	NA	5%–50%	50%–100%	75%–100%	98%–100%	100%
	Time of onset:		3–6 h	1–6 h	< 2 h	< 1 h	< 1 h
	Duration:		< 24 h	< 24 h	< 48 h	< 48 h	< 48 h
	Lymphocyte count (cells/mm³)	NA	< 1,400 at 4 days	< 1,400 at 48 h	< 1,000 at 24 h	< 800 at 24 h	NA
	CNS function	No impairment		Routine task performance; cognitive impairment for 6–20 h	Simple and routine task performance; cognitive impairment for > 24 h	Transient incapacitation	
Latent phase	Duration, days	NA	7–15	0–21	0–2	0–2	
	Granulocytes (cells/mm³)	NA	> 2	1–2	≤ 0.5	≤ 0.1	
	Diarrhea	None		Rare	Appears on days 6–9	Appears on days 4–5	
	Epilation	None		Moderate, beginning on days 11–21	Complete earlier than day 11	Complete earlier than day 10	
	Latency period, days	NA	21–35	8–28	7 or less	None	
Manifest (obvious) illness	Signs and symptoms	None	Moderate leukopenia	Severe leukopenia, purpura, hemorrhage, pneumonia, hair loss after 300 rad (cGy)		Severe diarrhea, fever, electrolyte disturbance	Convulsions, ataxia, tremor, lethargy
	Lymphocyte count (cells/mm³)	NA	0.8–1.0	0.1–0.8		0–0.1	
	Platelet count (cells/mm³)	NA	60–100	15–60		< 20	
	Time of onset	NA	> 2 wk	2 days–2 wk		0–2 days	
	Critical period	NA	None	4–6 wk		5–14 days	1–48 h
	Principal organ system	None	Hematopoietic	Hematopoietic and gastrointestinal		Gastrointestinal (mucosal surfaces)	CNS
Hospitalization	%	0%	< 5%	90%	100%	100%	100%
	Duration		45–60 days	60–90 days	90+ days	2 wk	2 days
Fatality	NA	0%	0%	0%–80%	80%–100%	98–100%	
Time of death	NA	NA	NA	3–12 wk		1–2 wk	1–2 days

(**Table 6-1** *continues*)

Table 6-1 *continued*

ARS: acute radiation syndrome; CNS: central nervous system; NA: not applicable
*Tabulated data for fatality incidence assumes no treatment.
Data source: Armed Forces Radiobiology Research Institute. *AFRRI Pocket Guide: Emergency Radiation Medicine Response.* Bethesda, MD: AFRRI; September 2008. www.usuhs.mil/afrri/outreach/pdf/AFRRI-Pocket-Guide.pdf. Accessed March 23, 2011.

dose, which will then be replaced by bioindicators of the severity of ARS response as the clinical case evolves.

The accepted generic multiparameter and early-response approach is described in Exhibit 6-1.[1,9] Effective medical management of a suspected acute radiation overexposure incident necessitates recording dynamic medical data, measuring appropriate radiation bioassays, and estimating dose from dosimeters and radioactivity assessments to provide diagnostic information to the treating physician and a dose assessment for personnel radiation protection records.

An additional purpose for biodosimetry is to support a quality radiation protection program by documenting the levels of radiation exposure for individuals suspected or known to be overexposed to radiation. Historically, a major activity in these effects is retrospective biodosimetry, which entails an assessment of radiation exposure long (ie, months to years) after the exposure. In these cases, dose assessment by biodosimetry methods has typically been limited to use of persistent radiation biomarkers supplemented by alternative physical dose reconstruction methodologies.[10] Dose assessments by retrospective dosimetry are commonly used to contribute to radiation epidemiology studies.

MEDICAL RECORDING

Medical recording is essential for effectively diagnosing and managing radiation at the incident scene as well as during transport to and while at the medical treatment facility. Medical recording guidance concerning radiation casualty management is available from the International Atomic Energy Agency.[11] The Armed Forces Radiobiology Research Institute (AFRRI) has approached this requirement using medical recording forms in annotatable portable document format (PDF) and medical recording and dose-assessment software (Figure 6-2).

Medical recording for radiation incidents should be consistent with an "all hazards" approach used by first responders. AFRRI's Adult/Pediatric Field Medical Record (AFRRI Form 330) provides a medical record template in a convenient, 1-page form for gathering emergency medical information in the field. It is applicable to both adult and pediatric cases (Attachment 1). The AFRRI Biodosimetry Worksheet (AFRRI Form 331) represents a comprehensive data entry worksheet, recently expanded from 4 to 6 pages to accommodate a modified version of the Medical Treatment Protocols

---

EXHIBIT 6-1

BIODOSIMETRY: GENERAL GUIDANCE FOR EARLY-PHASE RESPONSE*

Actions needed in suspected overexposures:

- Perform measurements and bioassay, if appropriate, to determine radioactivity contamination.
- Observe and record prodromal signs and symptoms.
- Obtain complete blood count with white blood cell differential immediately, then every 6 hours for 2 to 3 days, and then twice a day for 4 days.
- Record physical dosimetry measurements, if available.
- Contact a qualified laboratory to evaluate performance of chromosome aberration cytogenetic bioassay for dose assessment.
- Consider other opportunistic dosimetry approaches, as available.

*Lifesaving measures should be given higher priority than biodosimetry assessment. The sequence of actions can be modified depending on the radiation exposure scenario.

Biodosimetry Tools Supporting Medical Recording

www.afrri.usuhs.mil/outreach/biodostools.htm

Medical Recording Forms

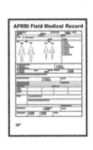 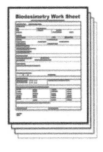 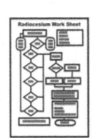

Software Program for Collection of Radiation Exposure Medical Data

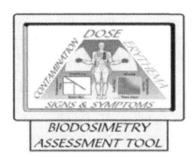

First-Responder Radiological Assessment Triage (FRAT)

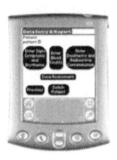 

Expert panel weighted triage dose based on currently available biodosimetric indices

Outreach Distribution

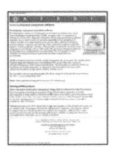 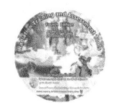

Military Medicine Operations CDROM

Figure 6-2. Armed Forces Radiobiology Research Institute's biological dosimetry tools supporting medical recording. Courtesy of: Armed Forces Radiobiology Research Institute, Bethesda, MD.

for Radiation Accident Victims ARS severity scoring system. It provides a place to record the facts about a case of radiation exposure, including the source and type of radiation, the extent of exposure, relevant biosimetry diagnostic information, and the nature of the resulting injuries. The form is applicable to both adult and pediatric cases (Attachment 2).

The Biodosimetry Assessment Tool (BAT) program (version 1.0) for Windows XP (Microsoft Corporation, Redmond, WA) was developed by AFRRI scientists as a tool to record and deliver diagnostic information (clinical signs and symptoms, physical dosimetry, etc) to healthcare providers responsible for managing radiation casualties.[1,12–15] It is designed primarily for early use after a radiation incident and permits collection, integration, and archiving of data obtained from patients suspected or known to be exposed to ionizing radiation. Relevant data is collected via struc-

tured templates and user-friendly software, enabling the generation of diagnostic indices for developing a multiparameter dose assessment. The BAT program is not a substitute for treatment decisions by physicians and other trained healthcare professionals. Additional clinical parameters (ie, infection, treatments, etc) useful for casualty management are also assessed. The resulting display of patient diagnostic information provides treating healthcare providers with concise and relevant information on which to base clinical decisions. This information can be archived for further use in radiation protection management. An integrated, interactive, human body map makes it possible to record radionuclides detected by an appropriate radiation-detection device. BAT is distributed online upon review of a download request application (available at http://www.afrri.usuhs.mil). An alternative version of BAT (eBAT) with more secure data handling is distributed by Medical Communications for Combat Casualty Care (www.mc4.army.mil/index.asp).

The First-Responders Radiological Assessment Triage (FRAT) program enables first responders to triage suspected radiation casualties based on the initial, or prodromal, features listed in the *AFRRI Pocket Guide: Emergency Radiation Medicine Response*.[16,17] FRAT is being developed initially for the Palm operating system (Palm, Inc, Sunnyvale, CA) and may eventually be available for other devices using other operating systems (eg, Windows). With minimum text entry, FRAT will record signs and symptoms, blood lymphocyte counts, and dosimetry data. The program will assess multiparameter triage dose or exposure without an assigned dose, or it will indicate that there is no evidence of overexposure. Additional FRAT output features include triage dose-specific messages addressing reliability and diagnostic information, hospitalization estimations, and mortality projections. The FRAT utility provides a triage dose estimate based on multiple-parameter, weighted, dose-assessment indices.

INTERNAL CONTAMINATION AND PHYSICAL DOSIMETRY

An individual's location relative to a radiation source, as well as internal contamination of radionuclides, if applicable, can contribute to radiation exposure assessment. The location of radionuclide contamination on the body, internal contamination information, dose estimation based on location, and dose based on personal dosimeters, if available, should be recorded by first responders and medical personnel (Figure 6-3).[1,9] The BAT application provides templates for recording these and other relevant parameters (eg, location and activity of radiation source, patient location relative to radiation source, etc) that can contribute to medical management and dose reconstruction. Metallic (or other) fragment samples should be collected for isotope classification, as appropriate, for identifying the radiation exposure scenario. In addition, biologi-

RECORD BODY LOCATION*

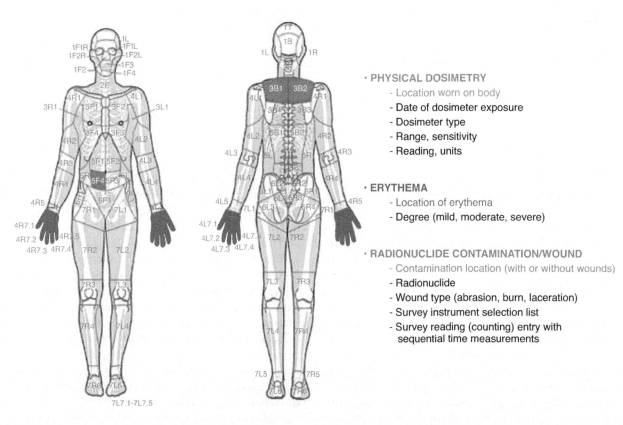

- **PHYSICAL DOSIMETRY**
  - Location worn on body
  - Date of dosimeter exposure
  - Dosimeter type
  - Range, sensitivity
  - Reading, units

- **ERYTHEMA**
  - Location of erythema
  - Degree (mild, moderate, severe)

- **RADIONUCLIDE CONTAMINATION/WOUND**
  - Contamination location (with or without wounds)
  - Radionuclide
  - Wound type (abrasion, burn, laceration)
  - Survey instrument selection list
  - Survey reading (counting) entry with sequential time measurements

Figure 6-3. Illustration of a record and recommended data collection for body location of physical dosimeters, presence of radiation-induced erythema, and radionuclide contamination in an exposed individual.

cal samples (ie, urinalysis, fecal, wound, swabs from body orifices) should also be collected for determining the committed dose. Protocols for biological sample collection for radiation bioassays and information for estimating dose based on location are described by Alexander and colleagues.[9] AFRRI's FRAT application uses information from physical dosimeters and radionuclide contamination that remains after clothing removal and washing as evidence for radiation exposure in a triage dose assessment algorithm.

PRODROMAL SIGNS AND SYMPTOMS

The prodromal response to exposure to ionizing radiation is characterized by a dose-dependent expression of a constellation of signs and symptoms, including the following:

- nausea,
- vomiting,
- headache,
- fever,
- tachycardia,
- fatigue,
- weakness,
- abdominal pain,
- parotid pain, and
- erythema.[18]

The time to onset and severity of early prodromal phase signs and symptoms can provide some valuable information regarding the absorbed "dose range." The FRAT application integrates these early-phase radioresponses to provide a triage dose assessment. Progressive increases in radiation dose result in an increased percentage of both the incidence and the constellation of prodromal signs and symptoms.

The appearance of acute symptoms, such as vomiting, is directly dependent on the radiation dose to an overexposed individual and contributes to the multiparameter diagnostic index (Table 6-2) used for assessing dose.[18] Data used to develop algorithms for dose predictions based on onset of vomiting used in the BAT and FRAT applications were drawn from the work of Anno et al[18] and Goans et al.[19–21] Following photon and criticality incident exposures, the BAT program can be used to record prodromal symptoms and assess dose-prediction models for time to onset of vomiting.[12–14] An acute photon exposure dose of 2 Gy would cause about 50% of individuals to exhibit emesis approximately 4.6 hours post-irradiation. However, since potential confounders (influenza epidemic, etc) can also induce similar symptoms, caution is warranted when using selective prodromal symptoms alone to assess dose and efficiently treat the radiation incident victim. For example, the incidence of psychogenic vomiting would likely be elevated during stressful events, such as a radiological mass casualty incident. Prodromal symptoms cannot be ignored but should be recorded and medically managed.

The location and time course of radiation-induced cutaneous injury should also be recorded (see Figure 6-3). Reddening of the skin, or initial erythema, is generally seen within a few hours to a few days following exposure to a high radiation dose (> 2 Gy) and lasts for only a day or two. Diagnostic information about local partial versus whole-body injury can be gleaned by observing if selected body regions exhibit erythema; these observations can later help define the boundary of the radiation exposure area when skin grafts are necessary. The AFRRI Biodosimetry Worksheet (Attachment 2) and BAT program provide data templates for this purpose. The time course for the skin's erythema response to radiation is biphasic. This type of skin reaction is largely due to capillary dilation caused by the release of histamine-like substances. Erythema increases during the first week following exposure and then generally subsides during the second week. It may return 2 to 3 weeks after the initial insult and last up to 30 days, and additional changes, such as desquamation, bullae formation, or even skin sloughing, may follow, all of which make even a crude estimation of radiation dose problematic.

HEMATOLOGICAL BIOINDICATORS

Hematological responses are early response biomarkers for radiation dose assessment. Data derived from radiation accidents registries contribute to the development of dose and injury severity assessment models.[5,18,19,22–25] Fliedner advocates the use of blood cell changes after whole-body radiation exposures as reliable bioindicators of injury and critical aids to planning therapeutic treatments.[5,22] Immediately following exposure, a complete blood cell count with white-cell differential should be obtained, then repeated three times a day for the next 2 to 3 days, and then twice a day for the following 3 to 6 days. The combined use of early-phase lymphocyte depletion, rise and then fall in neutrophils, and increases in the ratio of neutrophils to lymphocytes provides a hematology profile to identify individuals with potentially severe bone marrow ARS.

TABLE 6-2

BIODOSIMETRY BASED ON ACUTE PHOTON-EQUIVALENT EXPOSURES[*]

Dose Estimate (Gy)	Individuals Who Vomit (%)[†]	Time to Onset of Vomiting (h)	Absolute Lymphocyte Count ($\times 10^9$/L)[‡] (day)						Lymphocyte Depletion Rate (rate constant)	Relative Increase in Serum Amylase Activity at 1 Day Compared to Normal	Number of Dicentrics[§]	
			0.5	1	2	4	6	8			Per 50 Metaphases	Per 1,000 Metaphases
0	NA	NA	**2.45**	**2.45**	**2.45**	**2.45**	**2.45**	**2.45**	NA	1	0.05–0.1	1–2
1	19	>10.0	**2.30**	**2.16**	**1.90**	**1.48**	1.15	0.89	0.126	2	4	88
2	35	4.63	**2.16**	**1.90**	**1.48**	0.89	0.54	0.33	0.252	4	12	234
3	54	2.62	**2.03**	**1.68**	1.15	0.54	0.25	0.12	0.378	6	22	439
4	72	1.74	**1.90**	**1.48**	0.89	0.33	0.12	0.044	0.504	10	35	703
5	86	1.27	**1.79**	1.31	0.69	0.20	0.06	0.020	0.63	13	51	1034
6	94	0.99	**1.68**	1.15	0.54	0.12	0.03	0.006	0.756	15	ND	ND
7	98	0.79	**1.58**	1.01	0.42	0.072	0.012	0.002	0.881	16.5	ND	ND
8	99	0.66	**1.48**	0.89	0.33	0.044	0.006	< .001	1.01	17.5	ND	ND
9	100	0.56	1.39	0.79	0.25	0.030	0.003	< .001	1.13	18	ND	ND
10	100	0.48	1.31	0.70	0.20	0.020	0.001	< .001	1.26	18.5	ND	ND

[*]Depicted above are the most useful elements of biodosimetry. Dose range is based on acute photon-equivalent exposures. Two or more determinations of blood lymphocyte counts are made to predict a rate constant, which is used to estimate exposure dose. The final column represents the current "gold standard," which requires several days before results are known. Colony-stimulating factor therapy should be initiated when onset of vomiting, lymphocyte depletion kinetics, or serum amylase suggests an exposure dose for which treatment is recommended. Therapy may be discontinued if results from chromosome dicentrics analysis indicate lower estimate of whole-body dose.
[†]Cumulative percentage of individuals with vomiting.
[‡]Normal range: 1.4–3.5 x 10^9/L. Numbers in bold fall within this range.
[§]Number of dicentric chromosomes in human peripheral blood.
NA: not applicable; ND: not done
Data sources: (1) Blakely WF. Early biodosimetry response: recommendations for mass-casualty radiation accidents and terrorism. Paper presented at: Refresher Course for the 12th International Congress of the International Radiation Protection Association; October 19–24, 2008; Buenos Aires, Argentina. (2) Waselenko JK, MacVittie TJ, Blakely WF, et al. Medical management of the acute radiation syndrome: recommendations of the Strategic National Stockpile Working Group. *Ann Intern Med*. 2004;140(12):1037–1051. (3) Sandgren DJ, Salter CA, Levine IH, Ross JA, Lillis-Hearne PK, Blakely WF. Biodosimetry Assessment Tool (BAT) software-dose prediction algorithm. *Health Phys*. 2010;99(Suppl 5):S171–S183. (4) Waselenko JK, MacVittie TJ, Blakely WF, et al. Medical management of the acute radiation syndrome: recommendations of the Strategic National Stockpile Working Group. *Ann Intern Med*. 2004;140(12):1037–1051. (5) Chen IW, Kereiakes JG, Silberstein EB, Aron BS, Saenger EL. Radiation-induced change in serum and urinary amylase levels in man. *Radiat Res*. 1973;54:141–151.

At later times (> 10 days) after radiation exposure, progressive depletions of peripheral blood platelets and neutrophil counts below baseline levels are indicative of a higher radiation dose and severity of injury.

Lymphocyte cell counts and lymphocyte depletion kinetics can provide early-phase dose assessment predictions that fall in the equivalent photon dose range of 1 to 10 Gy for up to 10 days after radiation exposure (see Table 6-2). Decline of approximately 50% in peripheral blood lymphocyte counts over 12 hours that also fall below normal vales (1.4×10^9/L) is indicative of a potential severe radiation overexposure.[4,7] Caution is warranted in the use of lymphocyte cell counts that fall in the normal range for radiation dose predictions. Goans and colleagues introduced lymphocyte-depletion kinetic models for dose estimates based on human radiation accident registry data for whole-body, acute gamma exposures and, more recently, for criticality accidents.[19–21] The BAT program permits the recording of peripheral blood lymphocyte counts and then converts them into dose predictions using lymphocyte depletion kinetic models based on consensus data from radiation accidents registries.[18–21,23,24]

Fliedner and colleagues reported consensus results for the early rise (granulocytosis) and subsequent fall (granulocytopenia) in peripheral blood granulocyte cell counts following exposure to ionizing radiation.[5,22,25] Recently Zhang and colleagues proposed monitoring the ratio of neutrophils (major subset of granulocytes) to lymphocytes early after radiation exposure as a more practical, multifactorial, prognostic radiation indicator.[26] These hematological changes are proposed as prognostic indices to identify severely irradiated individuals indicative of partial or complete failure of the blood-forming system.[5,7] Decreased normal peripheral blood lymphocyte and neutrophil baseline counts, however, are seen in certain populations (eg, people of African and Middle Eastern descent).[27,28] Diagnostic use of hematopoietic cell count for radiation exposure assessment requires comparison of results with appropriate baseline level controls.

In a radiological mass-casualty incident, it may not be practical to perform repeated serial blood cell counts on multiple individuals. In this case it may be difficult to catch the early transitory rise in neutrophils (or granulocytes) early after radiation exposure. As initially recommended by Zhang and colleagues (based on the analysis of human accident registry results and later confirmed by Blakely and colleagues using nonhuman, primate radiation models), the early-phase decrease in lymphocytes (ie, 12 hours to 10 days after irradiation) and increase in the ratio of neutrophils to lymphocytes (ie, 1 to 3 days after irradiation) early after radiation exposure can aid in identifying individuals with life-threatening radiation overexposures.[26,29,30]

EMERGING TRIAGE DIAGNOSTIC APPROACHES

Several provisional and emerging approaches have been considered as methods to provide triage, clinical, and definitive dose assessment. For a review of these and other established dose assessment methods, see reports by Blakely et al,[1] Turteltaub et al,[3] and Alexander et al.[9]

EPR-based detection of free radicals is a well accepted and validated method for measuring dose to dental enamel from tooth biopsy and has recently been extended to measure absorbed dose from teeth in vivo and nail clippings ex vivo.[2,9,31,32] Provisional protocols for sample collection of nail clippings are established.[9] There are ongoing efforts to establish diagnostic technologies for in-vivo EPR from teeth.[9] Biophysical dose assessment using in-vivo EPR from teeth, along with ex-vivo EPR from nail-clipping samples from the extremities would contribute to mapping partial-body exposures and allow an estimate of regional (head, extremities) radiation exposure, and could point to bone-marrow sparing.[33]

Blood biochemical markers of radiation exposure have also been advocated for use in early triage of radiation casualties.[17,34–36] An increase in serum amylase activity (hyperamylasemia) from the irradiation of salivary tissue has been proposed as a biochemical measure of early radiation effects.[37,38] Several studies have also advocated its use as a candidate biochemical dosimeter in humans.[17,39–43] A few hours after irradiation injury, cells in the salivary glands show acute inflammation and degenerative changes resulting in increases in serum amylase activity. Histochemical, isozyme analysis, and partial-body exposure studies confirm that the increase in serum amylase activity originated from the salivary glands. Serum amylase activity increases occur early after head and neck irradiation of humans and generally show peak values between 18 and 30 hours after exposure, returning to normal levels within a few days.[42,44] Sigmoidal dose-dependent increases in early (1 day) hyperamylasemia are supported by radioiodine therapy, radiotherapy, and from limited data from three individuals exposed in a criticality accident.[37,39–47] Significant interindividual variations are reported in dose-response studies, which represent a potential major confounder for use of serum amylase activity alone as a reliable biodosimeter.[38,44,46,47] This interindividual variation in biochemical response is not unexpected, since it is well known that the radiation level causing irreversible failure of the hematopoietic system varies among individuals and may reflect genetic and physiological differences and relative differences in the radiosensitivity of hematopoietic stem and progenitor cells as well as radiation exposure parameters (ie, partial-body exposures, shielding, dose rate, etc).[48,49]

Radiation causes injury to various tissues and organs, resulting in time- and dose-dependent increases in tissue- and organ-specific proteins in blood. These blood plasma proteins are bioindicators for radiation injury of relevant ARS organ systems (ie, bone marrow, GI system) as well as early bioindicators of absorbed dose (Tables 6-3 and 6-4). Ideally, a panel of radiation protein biomarkers from distinctly different pathways and tissue sources would provide the necessary radiation specificity and sensitivity for clinical and definitive radiation diagnosis and to overcome potential confounders (ie, elevated amylase activity due to salivary gland infection; elevated C-reactive protein due to chronic inflammation, including rheumatoid conditions, autoimmune diseases, and heart attacks; and increases in neutrophil counts due to severe septicemia).

TABLE 6-3

CANDIDATE RADIATION BIOMARKERS AND FUNCTIONAL TESTS FROM VARIOUS TISSUE SYSTEM AND ORGANS

Tissue System/Organ	Candidate Radiation Biomarker	Candidate Radiation Bioindicator or Functional Test	Radiation Pathology
Gastrointestinal/Digestive			
Parotid salivary gland	Amylase activity	↑ serum or urinary amylase activity	Mucositis[1–5]
Small intestine	Citrulline, neurotension, and gastrin hormones	↓ serum or plasma citrulline, neurotensin, or gastrin; ↑ sugar concentration ratios using dual-sugar permeability test measured in serum	GI ARS subsyndrome[6–9]
Liver	CRP, SAA; oxysterol 7a-hydroxycholesterol	↑ serum or plasma CRP or SAA; ↑ plasma oxysterol 7a-hydroxycholesterol	ARS subsyndrome; hepatic tissue radiation injury[3,10–18]
Hemopoietic			
Bone marrow	Flt-3L, IL-6, G-CSF	↑ serum or plasma Flt-3L	Bone marrow ARS subsyndrome[6,16,18–23]
Cutaneous			
Skin	Cytokines (IL-1, IL-6, tumor necrosis factor, GM-CSF, TGF-β, intracellular adhesion molecule, MMP	↑ IL-1, IL-6, GM-CSF, TGF-β, intracellular adhesion molecule, and MMP measured from skin tissues	Cutaneous ARS subsyndrome[24–28]
Respiratory			
Lung	Oxysterol 27-hydrocholesterol	↑ plasma oxysterol 27-hydrocholesterol	Respiratory ARS subsyndrome[15]
Cerebrovascular/Central Nervous			
All	Oxysteril 24S-hydroxycholesterol	↑ plasma oxysteril 24S-hydroxycholesterol	Cerebrovascular ARS subyndrome[15]

ARS: acute radiation syndrome; CRP: C-reactive protein; Flt-3L: FMS-like tyrosine kinase 3 ligand; G-CSF: granulocyte colony-stimulating factor; GM-CSF: granulocyte-macrophage colony-stimulating factor; GI: gastrointestinal; IL: interleukin; MMP: matrix metalloproteinases; SAA: serum amyloid A; TGF-β: transforming growth factor β

(1) Blakely WF, King GL, Ossetrova NI, Port M. Molecular biomarkers of acute radiation syndrome and radiation injury. In: Blakely WF, Duffy F, Edwards K, Janiak MK, eds. *Radiation Bioeffects and Countermeasures*. North Atlantic Treaty Organization, Research and Technology Organization, Human Factors and Medicine: Neuilly-sur-Seine, France; 2011. Chapter 5. Technical Report-099, RTO-TR-HFM-099, AC/323(HFM-099) TP/356. Available at: http://www.rto.nato.int. (2) Chen IW, Kereiakes JG, Silberstein EB, Aron BS, Saenger EL. Radiation-induced change in serum and urinary amylase levels in man. *Radiat Res*. 1973;54:141–151. (3) Blakely WF, Ossetrova NI, Manglapus GL, et al. Amylase and blood cell-count hematological radiation-injury biomarkers in a rhesus monkey radiation model—use of multiparameter and integrated biological dosimetry. *Radiat Meas*. 2007;42(6–7):1164–1170. (4) Blakely WF, Ossetrova NI, Whitnall MH, et al. Multiple parameter radiation injury assessment using a nonhuman primate radiation model—biodosimetry applications. *Health Phys*. 2010;98:153–159. (5) Hofmann R, Schreiber GA, Willich N, Westhaus R, Bögi KW. Increased serum amylase in patients as a probable bioindicator for radiation exposure. *Strahlenther Onkol*. 1990;166(10):688–695. (6) Becciolini A, Porciani S, Lanini A, Balzi M, Faroani P. Proposal for biochemical dosimeter for prolonged space flights. *Phys Med*. 2001;17(Suppl 1):185–186. (7) Bertho JM, Roy L, Souidi M, et al. New biological indicators to evaluate and monitor radiation-induced damage: an accident case report. *Radiat Res*. 2008;169:543–550. (8) Lutgens LC, Deutz NE, Gueulette J, et al. Citrulline: a physiologic marker enabling quantitation and monitoring of epithelial radiation-induced small bowel damage. *Int J Radiat Oncol Biol Phys*. 2003;57:1067–1074. (9) Lutgens LC, Deutz N, Granzier-Peeters M. Plasma citrulline concentration: a surrogate end point for radiation-induced mucosal atrophy of the small bowel. A feasibility study in 23 patients. *Int J Radiat Oncol Biol Phys*. 2004;60:275–285. (10)

(**Table 6-3** *continues*)

Table 6-3 *continued*

Vigneulle RM, Rao S, Fasano A, MacVittie TJ. Structural and functional alterations of the gastrointestinal tract following radiation-induced injury in the rhesus monkey. *Dig Dis Sci.* 2002;47:1480–1491. (11) Dublineau I, Dudoignon N, Monti P, et al. Screening of a large panel of gastrointestinal peptide plasma levels is not adapted for the evaluation of digestive damage following irradiation. *Can J Physiol Pharmacol.* 2004:82:103–113. (12) Mal'tsev VN, Strel'nikov VA, Ivanov AA. C-reactive protein in the blood serum as an indicator of the severity of radiation lesion [in Russian]. *Dokl Akad Nauk SSSR.* 1978;239:750–752. (13) Mal'tsev VN, Ivanov AA, Mikhaĭlov VF, Mazurik VK. The individual prognosis of the gravity and of the outcome of acute radiation disease based on immunological indexes [in Russian]. *Radiats Biol Radioecol.* 2006;46(2):152–158. (14) Goltry KL, Epperly MW, Greenberger JS. Induction of serum amyloid A inflammatory response genes in irradiated bone marrow cells. *Radiat Res.* 1998;149:570–578. (15) Koc M, Taysi S, Sezen O, Bakan N. Levels of some acute-phase proteins in the serum of patients with cancer during radiotherapy. *Biol Pharm Bull.* 2003;26(10):1494–1497. (16) Roy L, Berthro JM, Souidi M, Vozenin MC, Voisin P, Benderitter M. Biochemical approach to prediction of multiple organ dysfunction syndrome. *BJR Suppl.* 2005;27:146–151. (17) Ossetrova NI, Farese AM, MacVittie TJ, Manglapus GL, Blakely WF. The use of discriminant analysis for evaluation of early-response multiple biomarkers of radiation exposure using non-human primate 6-Gy whole-body radiation model. *Radiat Meas.* 2007;42:1158–1163. (18) Ossetrova NI, Sandgren DJ, Gallego S, Blakely WF. Combined approach of hematological biomarkers and plasma protein SAA for improvement of radiation dose assessment in triage biodosimetry applications. *Health Phys.* 2010;98:204–208. (19) Ossetrova NI, Blakely WF. Multiple blood-proteins approach for early-response exposure assessment using an in vivo murine radiation model. *Int J Radiat Biol.* 2009;85(10):837–850. (20) Bertho JM, Roy L. A rapid multiparametric method for victim triage in cases of accidental protracted irradiation or delayed analysis. *Br J Radiol.* 2009;82:764–770. (21) Bertho JM, Demarquay C, Frick J, et al. Level of Flt3-ligand in plasma: a possible new bio-indicator for radiation-induced aplasia. *Int J Radiat Biol.* 2001;77(6):703–712. (22) Beetz A, Messer G, Oppel T, van Beuningen D, Peter RU, Kind P. Induction of interleukin 6 by ionizing radiation in a human epithelial cell line: control by corticosteroids. *Int J Radiat Biol.* 1997;72:3–43. (23) Gartel AL, Tyner AL. The role of the cyclin-dependent kinase inhibitor p21 in apoptosis. *Mol Cancer Ther.* 2002;1:639–649. (24) Bellido T, O'Brien CA, Roberson PK, Manolagas SC. Transcriptional activation of the p21 (WAF1, CIP1, SDI1) gene by interleukin-6 type cytokines. A prerequisite for their pro-differentiating and anti-apoptotic effects on human osteoblastic cells. *J Biol Chem.* 1998;273:21137–21144. (25) Martin M, Vozenin MC, Gault N, Crechet F, Pfarr CM, Lefaix JL. Coactivation of AP-1 activity and TGF-β1 gene expression in the stress response of normal skin cells to ionizing radiation. *Oncogene.* 1997;15:981–989. (26) Ulrich D, Noah EM, von Heimburg D, Pallua N. TIMP-1, MMP-2, MMP-9, and PIIINP as serum markers for skin fibrosis in patients following severe burn trauma. *Plast Reconstr Surg.* 2003;111:1423–1431. (27) Liu W, Ding I, Chen K, et al. Interleukin 1β(IL1B) signaling is a critical component of radiation-induced skin fibrosis. *Radiat Res.* 2006;165:181–191. (28) Müller K, Meineke V. Radiation-induced alterations in cytokine production by skin cells. *Exp Hematol.* 2007;35:96–104. (29) Guipaud O, Holler V, Buard V, et al. Time-course analysis of mouse serum proteome changes following exposure of the skin to ionizing radiation. *Proteomics.* 2007;7:3992–4002.

TABLE 6-4

SELECT RADIATION-RESPONSIVE, BLOOD-BASED, PROTEOMIC, METABOLOMIC, AND HEMATOLOGIC BIOMARKERS

Proposed Blood or Serum Biomarker	Pathways	Dose Range (Gy)				Time Window for Meaningful Diagnostics
		Rodent Studies	Nonhuman Primate Studies	Human Radiation Therapy	Human Radiation Accidents	
Salivary α-amylase activity	Parotid gland tissue injury	NA	0–8.5 Gy	0.5–10 Gy	3.5, 8, and 18 Gy (Tokaimura)	12–36 h; peaks at 24 h[1-5]
IL-6, G-CSF	Immunostimulatory effects on bone marrow cells	1–7 Gy	6.5 Gy	NA	1–10 Gy	Phase 1: 4–48 h Phase 2: 3–8 d[6-11]
Flt-3 ligand	Bone marrow aplasia	1–7 Gy	1–14 Gy	NA	0.25–4.5 Gy	24 h–10 d[12,13]
CRP, SAA	Acute phase reaction	1–7 Gy (SAA)	1–14 Gy (CRP)	1–20 Gy (CRP)	1–10 Gy (CRP)	Phase 1: 6 h–4 d Phase 2: 5–14 d[2,6-8,14-17]
Citrulline	Small bowel epithelial injury	1–14 Gy	Not done	1–20 Gy (2-Gy daily fractions)	~ 4.5 Gy	> 24 h[12,17,18]
Lymphocytes, neutrophils, and ratio of neutrophils to lymphoyctes	Hematopoietic tissue injury	1–7 Gy	1–8.5 Gy	1–20 Gy	0–30 Gy	2 h–8 d[7,19-22]

(**Table 6-4** *continues*)

Table 6-4 *continued*

CRP: C-reactive protein; Flt-3: FMS-like tyrosine kinase 3; G-CSF: granulocyte colony-stimulating factor; IL: interleukin; NA: not applicable; SAA: serum amyloid A

(1) Blakely WF, Ossetrova NI, Manglapus GL, et al. Amylase and blood cell-count hematological radiation-injury biomarkers in a rhesus monkey radiation model—use of multiparameter and integrated biological dosimetry. *Radiat Meas.* 2007;42(6–7):1164–1170. (2) Hofmann R, Schreiber GA, Willich N, Westhaus R, Bögi KW. Increased serum amylase in patients as a probable bioindicator for radiation exposure. *Strahlenther Onkol.* 1990;166(10):688–695. (3) Dubray B, Girinski T, Thames HD, et al. Post-irradiation hyperamylasemia as a biological dosimetry. *Radiother Oncol.* 1992;24(1):21–26. (4) Becciolini A, Porciani S, Lanini A, Balzi M, Faroani P. Proposal for biochemical dosimeter for prolonged space flights. *Phys Med.* 2001;17(Suppl 1):185–186. (5) Ossetrova NI, Farese AM, MacVittie TJ, Manglapus GL, Blakely WF. The use of discriminant analysis for evaluation of early-response multiple biomarkers of radiation exposure using non-human primate 6-Gy whole-body radiation model. *Radiat Meas.* 2007;42:1158–1163. (6) Ossetrova NI, Sandgren DJ, Gallego S, Blakely WF. Combined approach of hematological biomarkers and plasma protein SAA for improvement of radiation dose assessment in triage biodosimetry applications. *Health Phys.* 2010;98:204–208. (7) Ossetrova NI, Blakely WF. Multiple blood-proteins approach for early-response exposure assessment using an in vivo murine radiation model. *Int J Radiat Biol.* 2009;85(10):837–850. (8) Beetz A, Messer G, Oppel T, van Beuningen D, Peter RU, Kind P. Induction of interleukin 6 by ionizing radiation in a human epithelial cell line: control by corticosteroids. *Int J Radiat Biol.* 1997;72:3–43. (9) Gartel AL, Tyner AL. The role of the cyclin-dependent kinase inhibitor p21 in apoptosis. *Mol Cancer Ther.* 2002;1:639–649. (10) Bellido T, O'Brien CA, Roberson PK, Manolagas SC. Transcriptional activation of the p21 (WAF1, CIP1, SDI1) gene by interleukin-6 type cytokines. A prerequisite for their pro-differentiating and anti-apoptotic effects on human osteoblastic cells. *J Biol Chem.* 1998;273:21137–21144. (11) Bertho JM, Roy L, Souidi M, et al. New biological indicators to evaluate and monitor radiation-induced damage: an accident case report. *Radiat Res.* 2008;169:543–550. (12) Bertho JM, Demarquay C, Frick J, et al. Level of Flt3-ligand in plasma: a possible new bio-indicator for radiation-induced aplasia. *Int J Radiat Biol.* 2001;77(6):703–712. (13) Blakely WF, Ossetrova NI, Whitnall MH, et al. Multiple parameter radiation injury assessment using a nonhuman primate radiation model—biodosimetry applications. *Health Phys.* 2010;98:153–159. (14) Mal'tsev VN, Strel'nikov VA, Ivanov AA. C-reactive protein in the blood serum as an indicator of the severity of radiation lesion [in Russian]. *Dokl Akad Nauk SSSR.* 1978;239:750–752. (15) Mal'tsev VN, Ivanov AA, Mikhaĭlov VF, Mazurik VK. The individual prognosis of the gravity and of the outcome of acute radiation disease based on immunological indexes [in Russian]. *Radiats Biol Radioecol.* 2006;46(2):152–158. (16) Goltry KL, Epperly MW, Greenberger JS. Induction of serum amyloid A inflammatory response genes in irradiated bone marrow cells. *Radiat Res.* 1998;149:570–578. (17) Lutgens LC, Deutz NE, Gueulette J, et al. Citrulline: a physiologic marker enabling quantitation and monitoring of epithelial radiation-induced small bowel damage. *Int J Radiat Oncol Biol Phys.* 2003;57:1067–1074. (18) Lutgens LC, Deutz N, Granzier-Peeters M. Plasma citrulline concentration: a surrogate end point for radiation-induced mucosal atrophy of the small bowel. A feasibility study in 23 patients. *Int J Radiat Oncol Biol Phys.* 2004;60:275–285. (19) Blakely WF, Salter CA, Prasanna PG. Early-response biological dosimetry—recommended countermeasure enhancements for mass-casualty radiological incidents and terrorism. *Health Phys.* 2005;89(5):494–504. (20) Blakely WF, Ossetrova NI, Manglapus GL, et al. Amylase and blood cell-count hematological radiation-injury biomarkers in a rhesus monkey radiation model—use of multiparameter and integrated biological dosimetry. *Radiat Meas.* 2007;42(6–7):1164–1170. (21) Goans RE, Holloway EC, Berger ME, Ricks RC. Early dose assessment following severe radiation accidents. *Health Phys.* 1997;72(4):513–518. (22) Gus'kova AK, Baranov AE, Gusev IA. Acute radiation sickness: underlying principles and assessment. In: Gusev AE, Gus'kova AK, Mettler FA Jr, eds. *Medical Management of Radiation Accidents.* Boca Raton, FL: CRC Press; 2001: 33–51.

Data source: Blakely WF, King GL, Ossetrova NI, Port M. Molecular biomarkers of acute radiation syndrome and radiation injury. In: Blakely WF, Duffy F, Edwards K, Janiak MK, eds. *Radiation Bioeffects and Countermeasures.* North Atlantic Treaty Organization, Research and Technology Organization, Human Factors and Medicine: Neuilly-sur-Seine, France; 2011. Chapter 5. Technical Report-099, RTO-TR-HFM-099, AC/323(HFM-099)TP/356. Available at: http://www.rto.nato.int.

CYTOGENETIC BIODOSIMETRY

Multiple cytogenetic chromosome aberration assays (Figure 6-4) are useful for biodosimetry because no single assay is sufficiently robust for all potential radiation scenarios, including early-phase acute-exposures, partial-body exposures, and retrospective or prior exposure (eg, biosampling years after exposure). Applications involving triage cytogenetics are also useful for radiological mass casualty events. Various parameters and radiation scenarios are applicable to these assays (Table 6-5). The metaphase-spread dicentric (and ring) chromosome aberration assay is commonly applied in the early

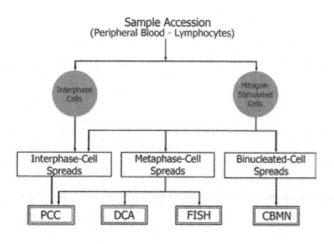

Figure 6-4. Schematic for sample accession of peripheral blood lymphocytes for various cytogenetic chromosome aberration assays (premature chromosome condensation assay, metaphase-spread dicentric [and ring] chromosome aberration assay, metaphase-spread fluorescence in situ hybridization translocation assay, and cytokinesis-blocked micronuclei assay) used for radiation dose assessment.

TABLE 6-5

COMPARISON OF CYTOGENETIC CHROMOSOME ABERRATION ASSAYS

Cytogenetic Chromosome Aberration Assays	Typical Aberrations Scored for Biodosimetry Applications	Typical Radiation Scenario Applications	Photon Equivalent, Acute Dose Range (Gy) for Whole-Body Dose Assessment	Useful for Partial-Body Exposure Applications?	Useful for Triage Dose Assessment?	Standardization of Assay
Premature chromosome condensation assay	Excess chromosome fragments; dicentrics* (and rings); translocations*	Acute (including high doses)	0.2–20	Yes	Yes	NA
Dicentric (and Ring) chromosome aberration assay	Dicentrics (and rings)	Low-level; acute; protracted; prior exposure	0.1–5	Yes	Yes	ISO standard for reference assay (1,000 metaphase spreads or 40 dicentrics); ISO standard for triage assay (20–50 metaphase spreads [pending])
Fluorescent in situ hybridization translocation chromosome aberration (translocation) assay	Dicentrics* (and rings); translocations*	Protracted; prior exposure	0.25–4	NA	NA	NA
Cytokinesis block micronucleus assay	Micronuclei	Acute	0.3–5	NA	Yes	ISO standard for reference assay (pending)

ISO: International Organization of Standardization; NA: not applicable
*Specific chromosome aberrations typically detected by use of centromeric and whole-chromosome specific deoxyribonucleic acid hybridization probes.
Data source: Rojas-Palma C, Liland A, Jerstad AN, et al, eds. *TMT Handbook. Triage, Monitoring and Treatment of People Exposed to Ionizing Radiation Following a Malevolent Act.* Osteras, Hedmark, Norway: Norweigan Radiation Protection Agency; 2009. http://www.tmthandbook. org/index.php?option=com_frontpage&Itemid=1. Accessed March 24, 2011.

phase after radiation exposure. The metaphase-spread fluorescence in situ hybridization translocation assay is typically used in retrospective biodosimetry studies. Variations of the premature chromosome condensation assay are useful for dose assessment at high doses and after partial-body exposures. The cytokinesis-blocked micronuclei assay has been advocated for use in radiological mass casualty events.

Reference laboratories and standards are established to perform dose assessment by cytogenetics.[50,51] Experts from these laboratories apply the appropriate cytogenetic chromosome aberration assay depending on the specific radiation scenarios encountered and for which they are qualified to perform. Cytogenetic biodosimetry networks, which are composed of expert laboratories from various nations, provide assistance to nations that do not have a reference cytogenetic biodosimetry laboratory or when the needs exceed their capabilities.[50]

113

TABLE 6–6

ACUTE–PHASE PATIENT ASSESSMENT METHODS: APPLICATION FOR VARIOUS EXPOSURE SCENARIOS

Assessment Method*	Application for Internal Contamination Assessment	Application for ARS Severity Assessment	Application for Partial–Body Dose Assessment	Applicable for Triage Assessment	Triage Dose (Gy) to Select for Priority Cytogenetic Triage Analysis	ARS Response Category Level to Select for Priority Cytogenetic Triage Analysis[†]	Application for Retrospective Assessment
Direct recording of location history	Yes	NA	Yes	Yes	3–7	NA	Yes
Direct observation of clinical signs and symptoms	NA	Yes	Yes	Yes	3–7	1–4	Yes
Personal monitoring (direct, noninvasive)							
In-vivo EPR	NA	NA	Yes	Yes	3–7	NA	Yes
Portable handheld meters (triage/ screening)	Yes	NA	Yes	Yes	NA	NA	NA
Portal monitors (triage/screening)	Yes	NA	NA	Yes	NA	NA	NA
Whole-body counting	Yes	NA	NA	Yes	Yes	NA	Yes
Personal monitoring (indirect, invasive)							
Blood chemistry (amylase activity, C-reactive protein)	No	NA	Yes	Yes	3–7	No	Yes
CBC and differential/lymphocyte count	No	Yes	No	Yes	3–7	1–4	Yes
In-vitro EPR (eg, nails)	No	No	Yes	Yes	3–7	NA	Yes
Nasal swab	Yes	No	Yes	Yes	NA	NA	Yes
Stool sample	Yes	No	No	Yes	NA	NA	Yes
Urine sample (spot; 24 h)	Yes	No	No	Yes	NA	NA	Yes
Cytogenetics (eg, 20–50 metaphase triage; 1,000 metaphase analysis)	NA	Yes	Yes (indirect)	Yes	3–7	NA	Yes
Area monitoring							
Dosimetry results (eg, TLDs, aerial measurements) combined with personal location information	NA	No	No	Yes	3–7	NA	Yes

(**Table 6-6** *continues*)

Table 6-6 *continued*

ARS: acute radiation syndrome; CBC: complete blood count; EPR: electron paramagnetic resonance; TLD: thermoluminescent dosimeter
*Personal and area monitoring methods are listed in alphabetical order; their location in the table does not infer priority or preference.
†Response category levels reflect graded severity levels of ARS from mild sublethal (1) to very severe acute lethality (4).
Data sources: (1) Alexander GA, Swartz HM, Amundson SA, et al. BiodosEPR-2006 Meeting: acute dosimetry consensus committee recommendations on biodosimetry applications in events involving uses of radiation by terrorists and radiation accidents. *Radiat Meas.* 2007;42:972–996. (2) Waselenko JK, MacVittie TJ, Blakely WF, et al. Medical management of the acute radiation syndrome: recommendations of the Strategic National Stockpile Working Group. *Ann Intern Med.* 2004;140(12):1037–1051

SUMMARY

Radiation dose or injury assessment is based on multiple biodosimetry-based assays and other physical and biophysical dosimetry approaches. Various dose assessment methodologies are typically used for different radiation scenarios and dose-assessment applications (Table 6-6). The accepted generic multiparameter and early-response approach includes measuring radionuclide contamination and monitoring the exposed individual; observing and recording prodromal signs and symptoms; obtaining complete blood counts with white blood cell differential; sampling blood for the chromosome-aberration cytogenetic bioassay using the "gold standard" dicentric assay (translocation assay for long times after exposure) for dose assessment; bioassay sampling, if appropriate, to determine radioactivity contamination; and using other available dosimetry approaches.

In the event of a radiological mass casualty incident, local, national, and international resources need to be integrated to provide suitable dose assessment and medical triage and diagnoses.[4] This capability should be broadly based and include (*a*) training and equipping local responders with tools and knowledge to provide early radiological triage, (*b*) establishing radiological teams capable of rapidly deploying and providing specialized dose assessment capabilities (ie, radiation screening and radiobioassay sampling, hematology, etc), and (*c*) access to reach-back expert reference laboratories (eg, cytogenetic biodosimetry, radiation bioassay, EPR dose assessment). This multifaceted capability needs to be integrated into a biodosimetry "concept of operations" for use in a mass casualty radiological emergency.[4] Ongoing research efforts to identify and validate candidate screening and triage assays should ultimately contribute toward approved, regulated biodosimetry devices or diagnostic tests integrated into local, national, and international radioprotection programs.

Acknowledgment

The author acknowledges contributions by research collaborators, including Drs Natalia I Ossetrova and Gregory L. King (AFRRI) and Dr Ronald Goans (MJW Corp, Amherst NY) for their sustained scientific interactions. The author wishes to thank Ira H Levine and David J Sandgren for their assistance and collaboration, and AFRRI's editorial staff for their expert assistance. The author also thanks CPT John P Madrid (AFRRI), Dr William E Dickerson (Bethesda, MD), and CDR John E Gilstad (AFRRI) for critical review of this chapter.

REFERENCES

1. Blakely WF, Salter CA, Prasanna PG. Early-response biological dosimetry—recommended countermeasure enhancements for mass-casualty radiological incidents and terrorism. *Health Phys.* 2005;89(5):494–504.

2. Pellmar TC, Rockwell S; Radiological/Nuclear Threat Countermeasures Working Group. Priority list of research areas for radiological nuclear threat countermeasures. *Radiat Res.* 2005;163(1):115–123.

3. Turteltaub KW, Hartman-Siantar C, Easterly C, Blakely W. *Technology Assessment and Roadmap for the Emergency Radiation Dose Assessment Program.* Washington, DC: US Department of Homeland Security, Radiological and Nuclear Countermeasures Program; 2005. https://e-reports-ext.llnl.gov/pdf/325832.pdf. Accessed October 19, 2012.

4. Blakely WF. Early biodosimetry response: recommendations for mass-casualty radiation accidents and terrorism. Paper presented at: Refresher Course for the 12th International Congress of the International Radiation Protection Association; October 19–24, 2008; Buenos Aires, Argentina. http://www.irpa12.org.ar/PDF/RC/RC_12_fullpaper.pdf. Accessed March 23, 2011.

5. Fliedner TM, Friesecke I, Beyrer K, eds. *Medical Management of Radiation Accidents: Manual on the Acute Radiation Syndrome*. London, England: British Institute of Radiology; 2001: 1–66.

6. Fliedner TM, Graessle D, Meineke V, Dörr H. Pathophysiological principles underlying the blood cell concentration responses used to assess the severity of effect after accidental whole-body radiation exposure: an essential basis for an evidence-based clinical triage. *Exp Hematol*. 2007;35:8–16.

7. Waselenko JK, MacVittie TJ, Blakely WF, et al. Medical management of the acute radiation syndrome: recommendations of the Strategic National Stockpile Working Group. *Ann Intern Med*. 2004;140(12):1037–1051.

8. MacVittie TJ, Farese AM, Jackson W III. Defining the full therapeutic potential of recombinant growth factors in the post radiation-accident environment: the effect of supportive care plus administration of G-CSF. *Health Phys*. 2005;89(5):546–455.

9. Alexander GA, Swartz HM, Amundson SA, et al. BiodosEPR-2006 Meeting: acute dosimetry consensus committee recommendations on biodosimetry applications in events involving uses of radiation by terrorists and radiation accidents. *Radiat Meas*. 2007;42:972–996.

10. Simon SL, Bailiff I, Bouville A, et al. BiodosEPR-2006 consensus committee report on biodosimetric methods to evaluate radiation doses at long times after exposure. *Radiat Meas*. 2007;42:948–971.

11. International Atomic Energy Agency; World Health Organization. *Generic Procedures for Medical Response During a Nuclear or Radiological Emergency*. Vienna, Austria: IAEA; 2005. EPR-MEDICAL 2005.

12. Sine RC, Levine IH, Jackson WE, et al. Biodosimetry Assessment Tool: a postexposure software application for management of radiation accidents. *Mil Med*. 2001;166(12):85–87.

13. Salter CA, Levine IH, Jackson WE, Prasanna PGS, Salomon K, Blakely WF. Biodosimetry tools supporting the recording of medical information during radiation casualty incidents. In: Brodsky A, Johnson RH Jr, Goans RE. *Public Protection from Nuclear, Chemical, and Biological Terrorism: Health Physics Society 2004 Summer School*. Madison, WI: Medical Physics Publishing; 2004: 481–488.

14. Salter CA, Levine IH, Jackson WE, et al. Medical recording tools for biodosimetry in radiation incidents. In: The proceedings of the NATO Human Factors and Medicine Panel Research Task Group 099 Meeting, "Radiation Bioeffects and Countermeasures"; June 21–23, 2005; Bethesda, MD. AFRRI CD 05–2.

15. Waller E, Millage K, Blakely WF, et al. Overview of hazard assessment and emergency planning software of use to RN first responders. *Health Phys*. 2009;97(2):145–156.

16. Armed Forces Radiobiology Research Institute. *AFRRI Pocket Guide: Emergency Radiation Medicine Response*. Bethesda, MD: AFRRI; September 2008. www.usuhs.mil/afrri/outreach/pdf/AFRRI-Pocket-Guide.pdf. Accessed March 23, 2011.

17. Blakely WF, Ossetrova NI, Manglapus GL, et al. Amylase and blood cell-count hematological radiation-injury biomarkers in a rhesus monkey radiation model—use of multiparameter and integrated biological dosimetry. *Radiat Meas*. 2007;42(6–7):1164–1170.

18. Anno GH, Baum SJ, Withers HR, Young RW. Symptomatology of acute radiation effects in humans after exposure to doses of 0.5–30 Gy. *Health Phys*. 1989;56:821–838.

19. Goans RE, Holloway EC, Berger ME, Ricks RC. Early dose assessment following severe radiation accidents. *Health Phys*. 1997;72(4):513–518.

20. Goans RE, Holloway EC, Berger ME, Ricks RC. Early dose assessment in criticality accidents. *Health Phys.* 2001;81(4):46–49.

21. Goans RE. Clinical care of the radiation-accident patient: patient presentation, assessment, and initial diagnosis. In: Ricks RC, Berger ME, O'Hara FM Jr, eds. *The Medical Basis for Radiation-Accident Preparedness: The Clinical Care of Victims. Proceedings of the Fourth International REAC/TS Conference on the Medical Basis for Radiation-Accident Preparedness, March 2001, Orlando, Florida.* Boca Raton, FL: The Parthenon Publishing Group; 2002: 11–22.

22. Fliedner TM. Nuclear terrorism: the role of hematology in coping with its health consequences. *Curr Opin Hematol.* 2006;13(6):436–444.

23. Gus'kova AK, Baranov AE, Gusev IA. Acute radiation sickness: underlying principles and assessment. In: Gusev AE, Gus'kova AK, Mettler FA Jr, eds. *Medical Management of Radiation Accidents.* Boca Raton, FL: CRC Press; 2001: 33–51.

24. Sandgren DJ, Salter CA, Levine IH, Ross JA, Lillis-Hearne PK, Blakely WF. Biodosimetry Assessment Tool (BAT) software-dose prediction algorithm. *Health Phys.* 2010;99(Suppl 5):S171–S183.

25. Graessle DH, Hofer EP, Lehn F, Fliedner TM. Classification of the individual medical severeness of radiation accidents within short time. In: The 10th Japanese–German Seminar, Nonlinear Problems in Dynamical Systems—Theory and Applications; September 30–October 3, 2002; Hakui, Ishikawa, Japan.

26. Zhang A, Azizova TV, Wald N, Day R. Changes of ratio of peripheral neutrophils and lymphocytes after radiation exposure may serve as a prognostic indicator of accident severity. In: *Final Program, 49th Annual Meeting of the Health Physics Society, July 11–15, 2004, Washington, DC.* McLean, VA: Health Physics Society; 2004. Abstract. http://hps.org/documents/49finalprogram.pdf. Accessed February 1, 2012.

27. Bertho JM, Roy L, Souidi M, et al. New biological indicators to evaluate and monitor radiation-induced damage: an accident case report. *Radiat Res.* 2008;169:543–550.

28. Bertho JM, Roy L. A rapid multiparametric method for victim triage in cases of accidental protracted irradiation or delayed analysis. *Br J Radiol.* 2009;82:764–770.

29. Blakely WF, Ossetrova NI, Manglapus GL, et al. Amylase and blood cell-count hematological radiation-injury biomarkers in a rhesus monkey radiation model—use of multiparameter and integrated biological dosimetry. *Radiat Meas.* 2007;42(6–7):1164–1170.

30. Blakely WF, Ossetrova NI, Whitnall MH, et al. Multiple parameter radiation injury assessment using a nonhuman primate radiation model—biodosimetry applications. *Health Phys.* 2010;98:153–159.

31. International Commission on Radiation Units and Measurements. *Retrospective Assessment of Exposures to Ionizing Radiation (Report 68).* Bethesda, MD: ICRU; 2002.

32. International Atomic Energy Association. *Use of Electron Paramagnetic Resonance Dosimetry With Tooth Enamel for Retrospective Dose Assessment TECDOC-1331.* Vienna, Austria: IAEA; 2002.

33. Prasanna PG, Blakely WF, Bertho JM, et al. Synopsis of partial-body radiation diagnostic biomarkers and medical management of radiation injury workshop. *Radiat Res.* 2010;173(2):245–253.

34. Bertho JM, Demarquay C, Frick J, et al. Level of Flt3-ligand in plasma: a possible new bio-indicator for radiation-induced aplasia. *Int J Radiat Biol.* 2001;77(6):703–712.

35. Blakely WF, Miller AC, Grace MB, et al. Radiation biodosimetry: applications for spaceflight. *Adv Space Res.* 2003;31(6):1487–1493.

36. Blakely WF, Miller AC, Grace MB, McLeland CB, Muderhwa JM, Prasanna PGS. Dose assessment based on molecular biomarkers. In: *Radiation Safety Aspects of Homeland Security and Emergency Response, Proceedings of the 36th Midyear Topical Meeting; 2003.* McLean, VA: Health Physics Society; 229–234. Abstract. http://hps.org/meetings/midyear/abstract434.html. Accessed February 1, 2012.

37. Becciolini A, Giannardi G, Cionini L, Porciani S, Fallai C, Pirtoli L. Plasma amylase activity as a biochemical indicator of radiation injury to salivary glands. *Acta Radiol Oncol*. 1984;23:9–14.

38. Leslie MD, Dische S. Changes in serum and salivary amylase during radiotherapy for head and neck cancer: a comparison of conventional fractionated radiotherapy with CHART. *Radiother Oncol*. 1992;24(1):27–31.

39. Hofmann R, Schreiber GA, Willich N, Westhaus R, Bögi KW. Increased serum amylase in patients as a probable bioindicator for radiation exposure. *Strahlenther Onkol*. 1990;166(10):688–695.

40. Becciolini A, Porciani S, Lanini A, Balzi M, Faroani P. Proposal for biochemical dosimeter for prolonged space flights. *Phys Med*. 2001;17(Suppl 1):185–186.

41. Akashi M, Hirama T, Tanosaki S, et al. Initial symptoms of acute radiation syndrome in the JCO criticality accident in Tokai-mura. *J Radiat Res (Tokyo)*. 2001;42(Suppl):S157–S166.

42. Kashima HK, Kirkham WR, Andrews JR. Post-irradiation sialadenitis: a study of clinical features, histopathologic changes and serum enzyme variations following irradiation of human salivary glands. *AJR Am J Roentgenol*. 1965;94:271–291.

43. Becciolini A, Porciani S, Lanini A, Benucci A, Castagnoli A, Pupi A. Serum amylase and tissue polypeptide antigen as biochemical indicators of salivary gland injury during iodine-131 therapy. *Eur J Nucl Med*. 1994;21(10):1121–1125.

44. Chen IW, Kereiakes JG, Silberstein EB, Aron BS, Saenger EL. Radiation-induced change in serum and urinary amylase levels in man. *Radiat Res*. 1973;54:141–151.

45. Becciolini A, Porciani S, Lanini A. Marker determination for response monitoring: radiotherapy and disappearance curves. *Int J Biol Markers*. 1994;9(1):38–42.

46. Hennequin C, Cosset JM, Cailleux PE, et al. Blood amylase: a biological marker in irradiation accidents? Preliminary results obtained at the Gustave-Roussy Institut (GRI) and a literature review [in French]. *Bull Cancer*. 1989;76(6):617–624.

47. Dubray B, Girinski T, Thames HD, et al. Post-irradiation hyperamylasemia as a biological dosimetry. *Radiother Oncol*. 1992;24(1):21–26.

48. Dainiak N. Hematologic consequences of exposure to ionizing radiation. *Exp Hematol*. 2002;30:513–528.

49. Koenig KL, Goans RE, Hatchett RJ, et al. Medical treatment of radiological casualties: current concepts. *Ann Emerg Med*. 2005;45(6):643–652.

50. Voisin P, Barquinero F, Blakely B, et al. Towards a standardization of biological dosimetry by cytogenetics. *Cell Mol Biol*. 2002;48(5):501–504.

51. Blakely WF, Carr Z, Chu MC, et al. WHO 1st consultation on the development of a global biodosimetry laboratories network for radiation emergencies (BioDoseNet). *Radiat Res*. 2009;171(1):127–139.

**ATTACHMENT 1: ARMED FORCES RADIOBIOLOGY RESEARCH INSTITUTE
ADULT/PEDIATRIC FIELD MEDICAL RECORD**

AFRRI Adult/Pediatric Field Medical Record
Adapted from DD Form 1380, U.S. Field Medical Card

1. Name (last, first)	Rank/Grade ☐ Male ☐ Female
SSN — Specialty code	Religion
2. Unit — Force	Nationality
☐ A ☐ AF ☐ N ☐ MC ☐ Civilian	

☐ BC ☐ NBI	☐ Disease	☐ Psych
3. Injury — Adult — Child		☐ Airway
Front — Back — Front — Back		☐ Head
		☐ Wound
		☐ Neck/back injury
		☐ Burn
		☐ Amputation
		☐ Stress
		☐ Other (specify)

4. Level of consciousness

☐ Alert	☐ Pain response
☐ Verbal response	☐ Unresponsive

5. Pulse	Time	**6.** Tourniquet ☐ No ☐ Yes	Time
7. Morphine ☐ No ☐ Yes	Dose — Time	**8.** IV	Time

9. Treatment/observations/current medication/allergies/NBC (antidote)

10. Disposition	☐ Returned to duty ☐ Evacuated ☐ Deceased	Time
11. Provider/unit		Date (YYMMDD)

12. Reassessment

Date (YYMMDD)		Time of arrival	
Time			
BP			
Pulse			
Resp			

Date/time	**13.** Clinical comments/diagnosis
	14. Orders/antibiotics (specify)/tetanus/IV fluids

15. Provider	Date (YYMMDD)

16. Disposition	☐ Returned to duty ☐ Evacuated ☐ Deceased	Time
17. Religious services	☐ Baptism ☐ Anointing ☐ Confession — ☐ Prayer ☐ Communion ☐ Other	Chaplain

AFRRI Form 330
April 2004

ATTACHMENT 2: ARMED FORCES RADIOBIOLOGY RESEARCH INSTITUTE BIODOSIMETRY WORKSHEET

Armed Forces Radiobiology Research Institute
Biodosimetry Worksheet
(Medical Record of Radiation Dose, Contamination, and Acute Radiation Sickness Response)

Reporting Authority (person(s) creating this page of the report)

Last name: _____ First name: _____ Country of origin: _____

Unit: _____ Phone: _____ Fax: _____ Email: _____

Location: _____ Date (yymmdd): _____ Time: _____

Casualty

Last name: _____ First name: _____ Rank: _____

Country of origin: _____ Parent unit: _____ Parent unit location: _____

Parent unit phone: _____ Unit e-mail: _____ Unit fax: _____ Casualty location: _____

History of presenting injury (conventional and/or radiation): _____

History of previous radiation exposure: _____

Past medical history (general): _____

Medical countermeasures (e.g., antiemetics, transfusion), specify: _____

Administered (where, when, route): _____

Exposure conditions

Date of exposure (yymmdd): _____ Exposure location: _____ Time of exposure: _____

Weather conditions (at time of exposure): _____

Exposure results
Describe incident: _____

External exposure overview

Body exposure: ○ Total ○ Partial ○ Uncertain

Shielding confounder: ○ Yes ○ No

Contamination overview

External contamination: ○ Yes ○ No

Internal contamination: ○ Yes ○ No

Contaminated wound: ○ Yes ○ No

If wound(s) are radiation contaminated, please provide details here: _____

Biodosimetric assays overview	Sampling date, time yymmdd (time)	Estimated time post-exposure (h)	Dose (Gy)	Reference radiation quality and dose rate (Gy/min)
Time onset of vomiting:				
Lymphocyte counts or depletion kinetics:				
Urine bioassay:				
Cytogenetic biodosimetry:				
Other:				

ARS response category overview (maximum grading 0-4; see pages 4 through 6 for guidance)

N: _____ C: _____ G: _____ H: _____ = RC: _____ days after radiation exposure: _____

AFRRI Form 331 (12/2007)   **Patient's service number:** _____   PRINT   Page 1 of 6

Contamination: Dose Assessment (person(s) creating this page of the report)

Last name: _____   First name: _____   Unit: _____

Phone: _____   Fax: _____   E-mail: _____   Country: _____

Date dose assessed (yymmdd): _____   Time dose assessed: _____   Place: _____

Contamination: external/internal

Substance trademark (if applilcable): _____   Solid: ◯ Yes ◯ No

Particulate (P): ◯ Yes ◯ No   Gaseous (G): ◯ Yes ◯ No

Liquid (L): ◯ Yes ◯ No   Aerosol (L/G): ◯ Yes ◯ No

Radionuclide(s): _____   Aerosol (P/G): ◯ Yes ◯ No

Activity (Bq): _____   Chemical compound(s): _____

Comments:

Contamination distribution

Adult   **Child**

Route of intake (in case of internal contamination)

Inhalation: ◯ Yes ◯ No   Ingestion: ◯ Yes ◯ No   Other: ◯ Yes ◯ No

Cutaneous: ◯ Yes ◯ No   Injection: ◯ Yes ◯ No   If yes, specify: _____

Contamination assessment

Contamination measurement: _____   Detection device: _____

Counts per minute: _____   Estimated activity: _____

Decontamination measures: _____   Residual contamination: _____

Measures taken to prevent uptake: _____

Measures taken to increase excretion: _____

Measures taken to minimize re-absorption: _____

AFRRI Form 331 (12/2007)   **Patient's service number:** _____   [PRINT]   Page 2 of 6

External Exposure: Dose Assessment (person(s) creating this page of the report)

Last name: _____ First name: _____ Unit: _____

Phone: _____ Fax: _____ E-mail: _____ Country of origin: _____

Date dose assessed (yymmdd): _____ Time dose assessed: _____ Place: _____

Nature of exposure: radiation source

Alpha (α): ○ Yes ○ No   Beta (β): ○ Yes ○ No   Neutron (n): ○ Yes ○ No

Gamma (γ): ○ Yes ○ No   X-ray (x): ○ Yes ○ No   Mixed (n/γ): ○ Yes ○ No

Dose rate (at distance measured from): _____   Distance to source: _____

Activity of source (if known): _____   Duration of exposure: _____

Confounding factors used in dose reconstruction (e.g., shielding): ○ Yes ○ No

Type of dosimeter (if applicable): _____   Body location of dosimeter: _____

Facility where dosimeter was read: _____   Dosimeter reading: _____

Biological dosimetry type and facility where performed (if applicable): _____

Dose distribution

Comments:

Adult   Child

Blood chemistry analysis	First	Second	Third	Fourth
Data collected (yymmdd):				
Time collected:				
Data analyzed (yymmdd):				
Time analyzed:				
Serum amylase (U/L): (reference value: 21-160 U/L)				
Serum C-reactive protein (mg/L): (reference value: ~1 mg/L)				
Other:				

AFRRI Form 331 (12/2007)   **Patient's service number:** _____   PRINT   Page 3 of 6

ARS Responses Assessment: (person(s) creating this page of the report)

Last name: _____ First name: _____ Unit: _____ Country of origin: _____

Phone: _____ Fax: _____ E-mail: _____ Place: _____

Signs and Symptoms

Date assessed (yymmdd): _____

Time assessed: _____

Neurovascular system — Degree of severity 1 (mild) to 4 (severe); none=0; see page 6 for degrees of severity

Nausea: _____

Vomiting: _____

Headache: _____

Anorexia: _____

Fever: _____

Hypotension: _____

Tachycardia: _____

Neurological deficits: _____

Cognitive deficits: _____

Fatigue/weakness: _____

Maximum grading N: _____

Cutaneous system — Degree of severity 1 (mild) to 4 (severe); none=0; see page 6 for degrees of severity

Erythema: _____

Pruritis (itching): _____

Edema: _____

Bullae (blisters): _____

Desquamation: _____

Ulcer or necrosis: _____

Hair loss: _____

Onycholysis: _____

Maximum grading C: _____

Gastrointestinal system — Degree of severity 1 (mild) to 4 (severe); none=0; see page 6 for degrees of severity

Diarrhea: Frequency: _____

Consistency: _____

Melena (bloody stools): _____

Abdominal cramps or pain: _____

Maximum grading G: _____

Hematopoietic system — Blood cell counts and degree of severity (see page 6 for degrees of severity)

(C=cell count; D=ARS degree)

	C	D	C	D	C	D	C	D	C	D	C	D	C	D
Lymphocytes ($\times 10^9$)/liter:														
Granulocytes ($\times 10^9$)/liter:														
Neutrophils ($\times 10^9$)/liter:														
Platelets ($\times 10^9$)/liter:														
Blood loss:														
Infection:														

Maximum grading H:

Response category (RC) =

Days after exposure:

AFRRI Form 331 (12/2007)   **Patient's service number:** _____   [PRINT]   Page 4 of 6

ARS Responses Assessment (continued from page 4)

Date format: yymmdd (time)	Onset (date/time)	Duration (hours)
Nausea:		
Vomiting:		
Headache:		
Anorexia:		
Fever:		
Hypotension:		
Tachycardia:		
Neurological deficits:		
Cognitive deficits:		
Fatigue/weakness:		
Maximum grading N:		
Erythema:		
Pruritis (itching):		
Edema:		
Bullae (blisters):		
Desquamation:		
Ulcer or necrosis:		
Hair loss:		
Onycholysis:		
Maximum grading C:		
Diarrhea: Frequency:		
Consistency:		
Melena (bloody stools):		
Cramps or pain:		
Maximum grading G:		
Lymphopenia:		
Granulopenia:		
Neutropenia:		
Thrombopenia:		
Blood loss:		
Infection:		
Maximum grading H:		

Comments:

Adapted from:

1. NATO Standardization Agreement (STANAG 2474). Determination and Recording of Ionizing Radiation Exposure for Medical Purposes. Appendix 1, 2003.
2. Fliedner TM, Friesecke I, Beyrer K, eds. Medical Management of Radiation Accidents: Manual on the Acute Radiation Syndrome. Oxford: British Institute of Radiology; 2001. p. 1-66.
3. Gorin N-C, Fliedner TM, Gourmelon P, et al. Consensus conference on European preparedness for haematological and other medical management of mass radiation accidents. Ann Hematol. 2006;85(10):671-679.
4. Radiation Event Medical Management (REMM). Guidance on Diagnosis & Treatment for Health Care Providers. Accessed 24 Oct 2007, from http://www.remm.nlm.gov/ars.htm.
5. Waselenko JK, MacVittie TJ, Blakely WF, et al. Medical management of the acute radiation syndrome: recommendations of the Strategic National Stockpile Radiation Working Group. Ann Int Med. 2004;140:1037-1051.

AFRRI Form 331 (12/2007)   Patient's service number: _____   PRINT   Page 5 of 6

124

APPENDIX

Grading System for Response of Neurovascular, Gastrointestinal, Cutaneous, and Hematopoietic Systems

Symptom	Degree 1	Degree 2	Degree 3	Degree 4
Neurovascular system				
Nausea:	Mild	Moderate	Intense	Excruciating
Vomiting:	Occasional (one per d)	Intermittent (2–5 times per d)	Persistent (6–10 times per d)	Refractory (> 10 times per d)
Headache:	Minimal	Moderate	Intense	Excruciating
Anorexia:	Able to eat & drink	Intake decreased	Intake minimal	Parenteral nutrition
Fever:	< 38°C	38–40°C	> 40°C for < 24 h	> 40°C for > 24 h
Hypotension:	Heart rate >100 beats/ m; blood pressure > 100/70 mm Hg	Blood pressure < 100/70 mm Hg	Blood pressure < 90/60 mm Hg; transient	Blood pressure < 80/? mm Hg; persistent
Neurological deficits:	Barely detectable	Easily detectable	Prominent	Life-threatening, loss of consciousness
Cognitive deficits:	Minor loss	Moderate loss	Major impairment	Complete impairment
Fatigue/weakness:	Able to work	Interferes with work or normal activity	Needs assistance for self care	Prevents daily activities
Cutaneous system				
Erythema:	Minimal, transient	Moderate (< 10% body surface area)	Marked (10–40% body surface area)	Severe (> 40% body surface area)
Pruritis (itching):	Sensation of itching	Slight and inter-mitten pain	Moderate and persistent pain	Severe and persistent pain
Edema:	Persistent, asymptomatic	Symptomatic, tension	Secondary dysfunction	Total dysfunction
Blistering:	Rare, sterile fluid	Rare, hemorrhage	Bullae, sterile fluid	Bullae, hemorrhage
Desquamation:	Absent	Patchy dry	Patchy moist	Confluent moist
Ulcer or necrosis:	Epidermal only	Dermal	Subcutaneous	Muscle/bone involvement
Hair loss:	Thinning, not striking	Patch, visible	Complete, reversible	Complete, irreversible
Onycholysis:	Absent	Partial	Partial	Complete
Gastrointestinal system				
Diarrhea:				
Frequency, stools/d:	2–3	4–6	7–9	≥ 10; refractory diarrhea
Consistency:	Bulky	Loose	Very loose	Watery
Melena (bloody stools):	Occult	Intermittent	Persistent	Persistent; large amount
Abdominal cramps/pain:	Minimal	Moderate	Intense	Excruciating
Hematopoietic system				
Lymphocyte changes: (reference value, $1.4–3.5 \times 10^9$ cells/L)	1–2d: ≥ 1.5	1–2d: 1–1.5	1–2d: 0.5–1	1–2d: < 0.5
	3–7d: ≥ 1	3–7d: 0.5–1	3–7d: 0.1–0.5	3–7d: < 0.1
Granulocyte changes: (reference value, $4–9 \times 10^9$ cells/L)	1–2d: ≥ 2	1–2d: 4–6; mild	1–2d: 6–10; moderate	1–2d: > 10; marked
	3–7d: ≥ 2	3–7d: > 2	3–7d: > 5	3–7d: > 5
Thrombocyte (platelets) changes: (reference value, $140–400 \times 10^9$ cells/L)	1–2d: ≥ 100	1–2d: 50–100	1–2d: 50–100	1–2d: 50–100
	3–7d: ≥ 100	3–7d: 50–100	3–7d: 20–50	3–7d: < 20
Blood loss:	Petechiae, easy bruising, normal hemoglobin level	Mild blood loss with < 10% decrease in hemoglobin level	Gross blood loss with 10%–20% decrease in hemoglobin level	Spontaneous bleeding or blood loss with > 20% decrease in hemoglobin level
Infection:	Local, no antibiotic therapy required	Local; only local antibiotic therapy required	Systemic; p.o. antibiotic treatment sufficient	Sepsis; i.v. antibiotics necessary

Chapter 7

BEHAVIORAL AND NEURO-PHYSIOLOGICAL CONSEQUENCES OF RADIATION EXPOSURE

ANDRE OBENAUS, PhD*; G. ANDREW MICKLEY, PhD[†]; VICTOR BOGO, MA[‡]; BRUCE R. WEST, MS[§]; AND JACOB RABER, PhD[Y]

*Departments of Pediatrics, Radiation Medicine, Radiology, and Biophysics and Bioengineering, Loma Linda University, 11175 Campus Street, CSP A-1120, Loma Linda, California 92354
[†]Lieutenant Colonel, United States Air Force; Armed Forces Radiobiology Research Institute, Bethesda, Maryland 20814
[‡]Armed Forces Radiobiology Research Institute, Bethesda, Maryland 20814
[§]Major, United States Army; Human Response Officer, Radiation Policy Division, Defense Nuclear Agency, 6801 Telegraph Road, Alexandria, Virginia 22310
[Y]Departments of Behavioral Neuroscience and Neurology, Division of Neuroscience, Oregon National Primate Research Center, Oregon Health & Science University, Department of Behavioral Neuroscience, Oregon Health & Science University, 3181 Southwest Sam Jackson Park Road, L470, Portland, Oregon 97239

INTRODUCTION

Understanding the behavioral and neurophysiological consequences of radiation exposure are of great importance. Although this chapter in the previously published *Textbook of Military Medicine* covered this topic in great detail, this chapter expands and updates the current understanding of radiation effects, specifically describing new clinical and research advancements in behavioral and relevant noninvasive imaging modalities.

The use of nuclear weapons in military conflicts will significantly challenge the ability of the armed forces to function; the thermal and overpressure stresses of conventional weapons are significantly intensified during a nuclear battle, and military personnel will have to contend with the hazards of exposure to ionizing radiation, which will be the main producer of casualties for nuclear weapons of 50 kt or less. Present projections of nuclear combat operations suggest that between one half and three quarters of the infantry personnel targeted by a tactical nuclear weapon would receive an initial radiation dose of 1.5 to 30.0 Gy.[1] This acute dose of ionizing radiation could dramatically affect a soldier's ability to complete combat tasks successfully, and in turn may ultimately affect the outcome of the armed conflict. In addition to these more acute effects, the long-term effects of ionizing radiation on soldier performance need to be considered.

Information about the consequences of ionizing radiation may be derived from the following: (*a*) the nuclear detonations over Hiroshima and Nagasaki, (*b*) clinical irradiations, (*c*) nuclear accidents, and (*d*) laboratory animal research (Figures 7-1 and 7-2). The Hiroshima and Nagasaki data are of limited value because there was no scientific assessment of behavior and the reports were anecdotal, often conflicting, and not easily tied to specific radiation doses. Clinical irradiations are also of questionable value because precise measures of behavior are not usually recorded, and patients are behaviorally compromised by their illnesses or the chemical therapy being used. Nuclear accidents have been few and behavioral information that has been obtained from these (ie, Chernobyl) is not consistent. In addition, factors that may affect behavioral disruption after irradiation in the context of a battlefield include (but are not limited to) the physical well-being of the subject (ie, sick or healthy, tired or rested), the presence or absence of physical shielding or pharmacological radioprotectants, and the exposure or nonexposure of the subject to radiation alone or to radiation and other stresses of the nuclear battlefield (such as blast, heat, or flash). Therefore, although information on human radiation exposure is normally preferred, the paucity of data forces significant reliance on animal research.

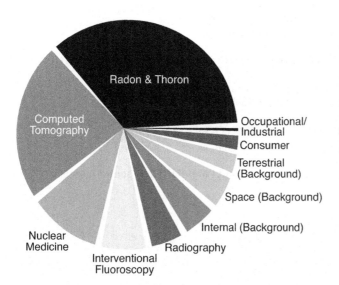
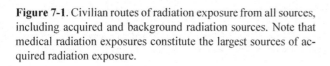

Figure 7-1. Civilian routes of radiation exposure from all sources, including acquired and background radiation sources. Note that medical radiation exposures constitute the largest sources of acquired radiation exposure.

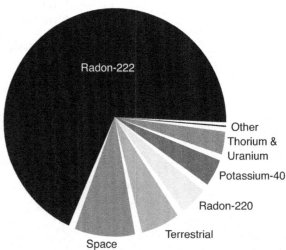

Figure 7-2. Distribution of ubiquitous background radiation.

HUMAN RETROSPECTIVE CASE STUDIES

Humans have been exposed to radiation from environmental and industrial sources, clinical therapy, accidents, wartime detonations at Hiroshima and Nagasaki, and even inadvertently during experiments in research laboratories. Many of these exposures contribute little information about the behavioral effects of ionizing radiation because, in most cases, behavioral data were not collected. Many of the data that were gathered are difficult to evaluate because there is no information about the radiation dose received, the level of baseline performance, or other circumstances. But the data are congruent with animal model findings and also suggest new hypotheses for testing.

Linear-No-Threshold Dose Response

An underlying tenant of radiobiology, particularly when addressing human risk factors, is the concept of a linear-no-threshold dose response. Because low doses are thought to result primarily in the induction of cancer, extrapolation methods are used to assess potential risk after radiation exposure. The linear-no-threshold dose response has demonstrated excellent concordance with epidemiological studies from survivors of Nagaski and Hiroshima, with a clear linear relationship between dose and cancer incidence.[2] The linear-no-threshold model for radioprotection has been recently reviewed and suggests that this model is still the most effective method for describing the risks of cancer.[3] While much research supporting the linear-no-threshold model has been derived from genomic instability[4] and radiation bystander-effects studies,[5] the experimental variables between studies do not allow for firm conclusions. More work is required to better understand the relationship between dose, dose rate, and time from the exposure to disease initiation (currently, cancer). While immune responses and sickness behavior (a consequence of cancer-inducing or other properties of irradiation) will affect behavior, it seems that there is a threshold for the effects of irradiation on behavior and cognition, although it is not yet precisely known what this threshold would be.

Radiation Accidents

Two radiation accidents are particularly instructive because both exposures occurred in the early days of fissionable radiation material production for nuclear weapons and involved radiation doses large enough to produce an early transient incapacitation (ETI). Despite safety precautions to ensure that the plutonium-rich holding tanks did not contain enough fissionable material to permit a critical reaction, such an accidental event took place in 1958 at the Los Alamos Scientific Laboratory,[6] where a worker received an average (and fatal) total-body dose of 45 Gy and an upper-abdominal dose estimated at 120 Gy of mixed neutron-gamma radiation. During the accident, the worker either fell or was knocked to the floor. For a short period, he was apparently dazed and turned his plutonium-mixing apparatus off and on again. He was able to run to another room but soon became ataxic and disoriented. He was incapacitated and drifted in and out of consciousness for over a half hour before he was rushed to a local hospital. Before his death 35 hours after irradiation, the worker regained consciousness and a degree of coherence. From approximately 2 to 30 hours after the accident, he showed significant behavioral recovery and at some points actually experienced euphoria, although his clinical signs were grave.[6]

The 1964 case of an employee at a uranium-235 recovery plant closely paralleled that of the Los Alamos worker. This accident took place in Providence, Rhode Island, when the worker was trying to extract fissionable material from uranium scraps. A criticality occurred and the worker was thrown backward and stunned for a period of time. He received a head dose of 140 Gy and an average body dose of 120 Gy. Unlike the Los Alamos worker, however, the worker did not lose consciousness. After a period of disorientation and confusion, he stood up and ran from the building to an emergency shack; a distance of over 200 yards, but his awareness of his surroundings during this early period has been questioned. Ambulance transport lasted almost 2 hours, during which time behavior was not observed. When the worker arrived at Rhode Island Hospital, he had transient difficulty enunciating words. Significant behavioral recovery occurred from 8 to 10 hours after the accident. During this period, the worker was alert, cooperative, and talked of future activities in a euphoric manner, inconsistent with his terminal diagnosis. In the hours before his death at 49 hours after the accident, the worker's condition deteriorated significantly.[7]

These human sequelae are comparable to animal research suggesting that supralethal radiation produces early performance decrements (EPDs). Both of the accident victims experienced behavioral deficits to some degree quickly after exposure, but they were transient. The behavioral recovery phase was similar in both patients, as were their final behavioral actions prior to death. The data agree with general conclusions reached in a review of several radiation accidents, in which a remission of early symptoms occurred before the onset of the manifest illness phase was recorded.[8] Compared to these high-dose accidents, lower radiation doses or partial-body exposures may produce milder but more persistent behavioral changes that are characterized by weakness and fatigability. An accident victim exposed to ionizing radiation from an unshielded klystron tube received as much as 10 Gy to portions of his upper torso and experienced fatigue that lasted for more than 210 days after exposure.[9]

The 1986 Chernobyl nuclear reactor accident also produced behavioral deficits in individuals attempting to perform their duties in high-radiation environments. A Soviet firefighter who fought the blaze of the burning reactor core suffered performance deficits and eventually had to withdraw because of his exposure to radiation.[10] Similarly, a Soviet physician who had received significant radiation exposures while treating patients could not continue to perform his duties.[11] Both eventually recovered from their behaviorally depressed states. These accident data add to the growing literature suggesting that sublethal doses of radiation can induce human performance decrements.

In the more than 20 years since the Chernobyl incident, significant data have emerged regarding cancer incidence connected to the accident.[12] The most prominent cancer types from the affected population have been thyroid and leukemia cancers, but bladder, kidney, and breast cancers have also been reported. It is important to note that only thyroid cancers (particularly in children and adolescent populations) have been shown to have a clear relationship to Chernobyl radiation exposure. Worgol et al also reported cataractogenesis as an outcome of Chernobyl radiation exposure, particularly in reactor liquidators.[13] In fact, a recent review suggests that a dose of 0.5 Gy may be sufficient to induce cataract formation, and may have a doubling dose of around 2 Gy.[14] Other data that are emerging include increased incidence of trisomy 21[15,16] and schizophrenia,[17] and potentially accelerated aging (ie, Alzheimer disease).[18] Reports from Chernobyl and other radiation accidents hint at an association between radiation exposure and cardiovascular disease,[19] but more research is required. It is important to remind the reader that while putative associations between radiation exposure and a host of disease states have been suggested, there is only clear epidemiological evidence for a link between radiation exposure and cancer.[20,21] More research is needed to definitively ascribe increased onset of disease with radiation exposure, particularly in those related to low-dose exposures.[22]

There has been scant work on the behavioral effects of radiation exposure in human populations. Large-scale epidemiological studies on the behavioral effects of radiation exposure are needed. While the Chernobyl accident provided a wealth of data on cancer incidence,[23] behavioral and psychological data collection was only started 7 years after the accident.[24] These behavioral studies focused on three areas: (1) morbidity surveys based on population statistics, (2) cognitive impairment in children, and (3) mental health studies of cleanup workers.[25] Bromet and colleagues reported significant adverse psychological effects in radiation-exposed populations, particularly in depression and anxiety with somatic symptoms.[26] The associated risk factors were being female, having young children (although no psychological effects were found in these children[27]), financial difficulties, and the perception that the Chernobyl accident had an adverse effect on one's health.

Concern about the mental and cognitive performance of children in the affected areas around Chernobyl was expressed given the higher incidence of thyroid tumors in this population.[28] A number of studies have shown no significant link between cognitive performance in children who were exposed to radiation at a young age or in utero.[29–31] Finally, numerous cognitive studies of cleanup workers at Chernobyl were assessed, but the results have not been independently verified. As noted, Loganovksy and Loganovskaja reported an increased incidence of schizophrenia,[32] but this linkage was not definitive. Polyukhov et al reported accelerated aging (radiation progeriod syndrome) based on psychological and cardiovascular testing.[33] Although suggestive, the associations between cognitive performance decrements and radiation exposure in humans are tenuous at this time, particularly at low doses.

Clinical Irradiations

Numerous studies have been undertaken to assess human performance after clinical irradiations. The Halsted test battery for frontal-lobe functional deficits was used in four patients exposed to 0.12 to 1.90 Gy of mixed neutron-gamma radiations.[34] Test scores at days 1 and 4 and 1 year after exposure were within the normal ranges. Patients with advanced neoplastic disease received whole-body irradiation with 0.15 to 2.0 Gy given as a single dose, or in 2 to 5 fractions separated by intervals of up to 1 hour.[35] These subjects were pretrained and served as their own controls in performing tests designed to assess hand-eye coordination. Tests were performed immediately after exposure and at later intervals, but at no time did a performance decrement exist that could be ascribed to these relatively low radiation doses. However, because the behavioral design of these experiments was secondary to medical treatment, the results are inconclusive. The paucity of radiobiological data on human behavior and the need to predict military performance after ionizing radiation exposure has led to an extensive Defense Threat Reduction Agency (DTRA; formerly the Defense Nuclear Agency) program on the estimation of human radiation effects.[36]

Clinical datasets, particularly from radiotherapy, can provide some understanding of radiation effects on the brain. Treatment of childhood tumors has demonstrated significant late cognitive abnormalities and complications of endocrine dysfunction in long-term survivors.[37] An important caveat is that the type, size, and location of the tumor can effect these complications. Radiotherapy is more closely associated with endocrine dysfunction than cognitive changes[37,38]; however, numerous studies have demonstrated differences in intelligence quotient scores in children treated with radiation for posterior fossa tumors.[39] In adults with low-grade gliomas, there have been some reports of neurocognitive decrements.[40] A cross-sectional study (195 patients) noted that patients who received fractional doses less than 2 Gy did not have adverse cognition, but higher fractional doses than 2 Gy were more likely to result in disability. A recent review confirms this viewpoint.[41] Cofactors such as epilepsy (and use of antiepileptic drugs) correlated more strongly with cognitive deficits than did radiotherapy. In a recent follow-up study of head and neck cancer, patients' tumor localization was a highly significant covariant for cognitive deficits.[38] Such studies underline the difficulty in assessing radiation risks from human radiotherapy studies. An original study by Taphoorn[40] was recently extended to follow up with patients after radiotherapy, with a mean of 12 years after treatment (range 6–28 years).[42] The radiotherapy patients (regardless of fractionated dose) all demonstrated significant declines in attentional and executive functioning and information speed processing. Thus, while early postradiotherapy decrements were not conclusive, long-term, neurocognitive declines are an important factor to consider after radiation exposures.

There are a number of studies that suggest cognitive decrements after radiotherapy even when the treatment site is distant from central nervous system (CNS) structures (Figure 7-3). Cognitive impairments after breast cancer treatment,[43] cervical cancer,[44] and testicular cancer[45] (however, a recent report disputes the testicular cancer results[46]) have all been described, but more study is required to determine the effects of radiation on behavior. In summary, there are no good studies evaluating radiation effects and behavioral out-

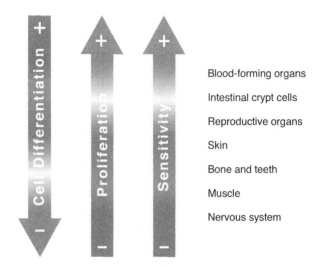

Figure 7-3. Relative tissue sensitivity. This figure illustrates the concept that highly proliferative organs (eg, blood-forming organs) have increased radiosensitivity, while those regions that are highly differentiated (eg, brain) have the lowest radiosensitivity.

comes. Although radiotherapy studies provide hints at some significant decrements in cognition, further study is needed.

Predicting Radiation-Induced Changes in Military Performance

In 1984, the Defense Nuclear Agency (currently the DTRA) published a study predicting certain effect distributions for combat personnel exposed to ionizing radiation. For every soldier who receives a radiation dose of greater than 30 Gy (a supralethal and behaviorally incapacitating dose), another will receive a lethal (4.5 Gy) dose that may alter behavior. Two more soldiers will receive doses that are sublethal but greater than the present maximum (0.5 Gy) allowed for troop safety.[47] Given this wide range of expected doses and the ambiguity of the expected outcomes for human behavior, the DTRA has established methods for estimating the behavioral effects of acute radiation doses (0.75–45.0 Gy) on combat troops.

To predict human radiation-induced performance deficits, the DTRA used a survey method, first identifying the physical symptoms expected after various radiation doses, then determining the soldiers' estimates of their own changes in performance while experiencing these symptoms. While the provided examples are somewhat dated, they illustrate the point. Briefly, this involved (*a*) an extensive review of the literature on human radiation (including radiation therapy patients, Japanese atomic bomb victims, and radiation accident victims) to identify the symptoms that might be expected after the radiation doses of interest; (*b*) the compilation of symptom complexes that reflect various combinations of the expected radiogenic symptoms, including gastrointestinal distress, fatigability, weakness, hypotension, infection, bleeding, fever, fluid loss, and electrolyte imbalance[48]; (*c*) the development of accurate descriptions of the severity of each symptom category at each postirradiation time of interest; (*d*) an analysis of tasks performed by five different crews, including a field artillery gun (155-mm self-propelled Howitzer) crew; a manual-operations, field artillery, fire-direction crew; a tank (M60A3) crew; a Chinook helicopter (CH 47) crew; and an antitank guided missile crew in a TOW (tube-launched, optically-tracked, wire command data link, guided missile) armed vehicle; (*e*) the development of questionnaires that require experienced crewmembers (noncommissioned or warrant officers) to predict task degradation during particular symptom complexes; and (*f*) the evaluation of monkey performance data from a visual discrimination (physically undemanding) task or a wheel-running (physically demanding) task.[49] The animal data was analyzed in the absence of sufficient human data to estimate the rapid behavioral decrements that follow large (10–45 Gy) radiation doses.

For each crew position, sophisticated statistical techniques made it possible to construct minute-by-minute performance estimates and also smoothed the summary curves as a function of radiation dose and time. The analysis involved grouping the results from individual crewmembers into two categories: physically demanding tasks and physically undemanding tasks. Helicopter tasks were also assessed separately. The degree of performance deficit for each of the five crew positions was described in terms of the following categories: (*a*) combat effective (performance capability 75%–100% of normal), (*b*) degraded (performance capability 25%–75% of normal), and (*c*) combat ineffective (performance capability 0–25% of normal).

This scheme was then used to summarize the expected changes in the performance of combatants after various doses of radiation exposure.[36] In general, the data indicate that the capabilities of crew members performing tasks of a similar demand are similarly degraded. The capabilities of crewmembers performing physically demanding tasks were degraded more than the capabilities of members performing physically undemanding tasks. This latter observation agrees with the data from animal studies on physical effort after irradiation. For example, if crewmembers performing a physically demanding task were exposed to 10 Gy (Figure 7-4), they would be combat effective for only a little over 1 hour. This period would be followed by an

extended time (roughly 1 month) of degraded performance before they became combat ineffective prior to death. The outlook for performance (but not ultimate prognosis) is a little better for a person performing a physically undemanding task after a 10 Gy irradiation. This soldier would remain combat effective for 1.7 hours after exposure. Following this initial period of coping, a transient performance degradation of 2.8 days would ensue before a short recovery and then a gradual decline, ending in death at 1 month after irradiation.

To obtain an independent confirmation of performance degradations predicted for radiation sickness by

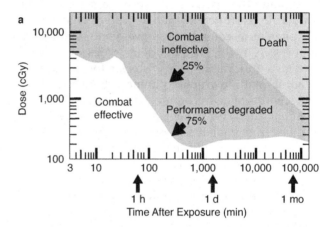

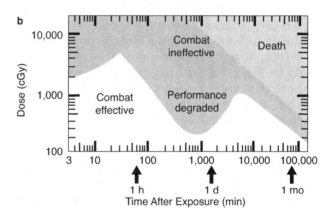

Figure 7-4. Behavioral responses following radiation exposure. Combat effective: 75%–100% normal capacity; degraded: 25%–75% normal capacity; combat ineffective: 0–25% normal capacity. **(a)** Expected behavioral response to radiation exposure for persons performing a physically demanding task (1 Gy = 100 cGy = 100 rad). **(b)** Expected behavioral response to radiation exposure for persons performing a physically undemanding task.

Data source: Anno GW, Brode HL, Washton-Brown R. *Initial Human Response to Radiation.* Washington, DC: Defense Nuclear Agency; 1982. DNA-TR-81-237.

this study, results were compared (where possible) to actual performance decrements measured in members of the US Coast Guard.[50,51] The decrements occurred during motion-sickness episodes with symptoms similar to those of radiation sickness. This comparison revealed that the estimates of radiogenic performance decrements made by responders to the questionnaire were similar to the actual radiation-induced declines in short-term task performance that were measured during motion sickness.

Although these are the best estimates of human radiation-induced behavioral deficits that are currently available, their limitations are recognized. These predictions apply to the physiological effects of a one-time whole-body irradiation. The data do not predict the behavioral effects of protracted radiation exposures that would occur with fallout, nor do they attempt to account for degradation from the psychological effects that are unique to nuclear combat.

For the military, an abrupt inability to perform (ETI) is a potentially devastating behavioral consequence of radiation exposure.[52] An idealized individual ETI profile is shown in Figure 7-5. Prior to irradiation, performance is at maximum efficiency, but 5 to 10 minutes after exposure to a large, rapidly delivered dose of ionizing radiation, performance falls rapidly to near zero, followed by partial or total recovery 10 to 15 minutes later. Delayed ETIs may also occur at about 45 minutes and 4 hours after the initial irradiation.

Radiation-Induced Brain Damage Based on Clinical Studies

Radiogenic damage to the brain, in the forms of altered performance and neuropathology, may occur after an exposure of less than 15 Gy and is a well-accepted finding at higher doses. A review of many standard radiobiology textbooks reveals the common belief that the adult nervous system is relatively resistant to damage from ionizing radiation exposure.[53] These conclusions have been derived, in part, from early clinical reports suggesting that radiation exposures, given to produce some degree of tumor control, had no immediate observable morphological effects on the nervous system.[54] However, this view eroded when it was demonstrated that the latency period for the appearance of radiation damage in the nervous system is simply longer than in other organ systems.[55] Subsequent interest in the pathogenesis of delayed radiation necrosis in clinical medicine has produced a significant body of literature. Recent studies of radiation-induced brain damage in human patients have used computed tomography to confirm CNS abnormalities that are not associated with the tumor under treatment but occur

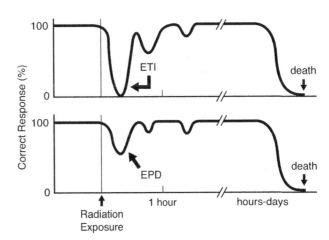

Figure 7-5. Idealized performance time-course profiles for an acute, radiation-induced behavioral decrement. Soon after a sufficiently large dose of radiation, several animal species exhibit early transient incapacitation (upper panel) or early performance decrements (lower panel). Smaller transient deficits may occur around 45 minutes and 4 hours later. Early transient incapacitation has been reported at doses as low as 3 Gy, while early performance decrements require larger doses of 100–300 Gy.
EPD: early performance decrement
ETI: early transient incapacitation
Data sources: (1) Bruner A. Immediate dose rate effects of 60Co on performance and blood pressure in monkeys. *Radiat Res.* 1977;70:378–390. (2) Pitchford T. *Beagle Incapacitation and Survival Time After Pulsed Mixed Gamma Neutron Irradiation.* Bethesda, MD: Armed Forces Radiobiology Research Institute; 1968.

because of the radiotherapy.[56]

General (although not universal) agreement exists that there is a threshold dose below which no late radiation-induced morphological sequelae occur in the CNS. In humans, the "safe" dose has been a topic of considerable debate. Depending on the radiation field size, the threshold for CNS damage has been estimated to be 30 to 40 Gy if the radiation is given in fractions,[57] although spinal cord damage may occur with fractionated doses as low as 25 Gy.[58] The difference between a safe and a pathogenic radiation dose to the brain may be as small as 4.3 Gy.[59]

It is clear that the technique used to assess neuropathology can profoundly influence its detection. In an inspection of neutron-irradiated brain tissue stained with silver to detect degenerating neural elements, punctate brain lesions were found within 4 days after exposure to 2 to 8 Gy protons and electrons.[60] The degeneration was linear through this dose range and the cellular profile suggested that beta astrocytes were the primary targets. At higher doses (20–100 Gy), the findings suggested a saturation effect. The lesions were not detectable using standard hematoxylin and eosin stains. These effects are similar to a multiinfarction syndrome in which the effects of small infarctions accumulate and may become symptomatic. This pathology was observed at a dose of radiation previously believed to be completely safe, suggesting that the brain is radiosensitive.

In an organ like the brain, different topographical regions may vary in their susceptibility to ionizing radiation. The most sensitive area is the brainstem.[61] The brain cortex may be less sensitive than the subcortical structures,[62] such as the hypothalamus,[63] the optic chiasm, and the dorsal medulla.[64] Although radiation lesions tend to occur more frequently in brain white matter,[65–67] the radiosensitivity of white matter also appears to vary from region to region.[62]

In this regard, researchers have produced measures of the functional sensitivity of some brain areas and the insensitivity of others.[68,69] The activation of behaviors through electrical stimulation of the lateral hypothalamus (but not the septal nucleus or substantia nigra) is still possible after 100 Gy.[70,71] However, years after clinical irradiations, dysfunction of the hypothalamus remains prominent even without evidence of hypothalamic necrosis.[72] Local subcortical changes may exist in the reticular formation and account for radiation-induced hyperexcitability of the brain.[73,74] Similarly, postirradiation spike discharges are more likely to be seen in hippocampal electroencephalographs than in the cortical electroencephalographs.[75] The idea of selective neurosensitivity is further supported by experiments in which electrical recordings were made from individual nerve fibers after irradiation.[76] These data reveal a hierarchy of radiosensitivity in which gamma nerve fibers are more sensitive than beta fibers, and alpha nerve fibers are the least sensitive.

A recent series of papers described the use of magnetic resonance imaging (MRI) and magnetic resonance spectroscopy to monitor radiation damage in the CNS.[77,78] Noninvasive imaging modalities allow temporal and spatial assessment of tissue alterations. Adult rodents were assessed over the course of 1 to 18 months after a single exposure of 1 to 4 Gy iron-56 (a component of cosmic radiation). Although no visual abnormalities were reported from anatomical MRI, the authors reported that quantifiable MRI and magnetic resonance spectroscopy results allowed identification of biophysical changes in all memory-related regions of interest prior to evident histological damage. As early as 1 month after brain-only radiation exposure, they reported no neuronal loss, but damage to the nonneuronal cells was indicated by decreased quantitative measures of brain water mobility (diffusion-weighted imaging) and increased edema (T2-weighted imaging;

Figure 7-6). These findings were supported by immunohistochemical data, suggesting that apparent diffusion coefficients, computed from diffusion-weighted imaging, are one of the most sensitive MRI biomarkers to monitor early disturbances within brain tissue after radiation exposure. Evaluation of the dynamic nature of radiation effects within the brain showed that up to 18 months after a single exposure to radiation, MRI can demonstrate temporal changes that correspond to evolving glial cell changes.[79] These studies demonstrate that quantification of noninvasive imaging modalities can delineate short- and long-term radiation effects. While many imaging studies are animal investigations, these reports could be readily translated to the clinical setting if needed.

Latent Central Nervous System Radiation

The phenomenon of latent CNS radiation damage with doses above threshold has been well documented.[53,80,81] The long latent period has led to considerable speculation on the likely pathogenesis of late radiation lesions: (*a*) radiation may act primarily on the vascular system, with necrosis secondary to edema and ischemia, and (*b*) radiation may have a primary effect on cells of the neural parenchyma, with vascular lesions exerting a minor influence.[54]

The first evidence in support of a vascular hypothesis was obtained when human brains that had been exposed to X-rays were examined.[55] It was suggested that delayed damage of capillary endothelial cells may occur, leading to a breakdown of the blood-brain barrier (Figure 7-7). Mao and colleagues[82,83] demonstrated a time- and dose-dependent loss of the vasculature following gamma and proton radiation exposure in rodents. Significant decrements in vessel growth were found[83] and could be observed as long as 12 months after a single 8- or 28-Gy exposure.[84] The microvascular loss within the eye could be prevented by treatment with a metalloporphyrin antioxidant mimetic.[84] Together, these findings strongly suggest that radiation exposure results in long-term alterations in vascular function.

Further evidence for vascular dysfunction has shown that radiation-induced blood-brain-barrier breakdown results in vasogenic edema, elevated blood pressure leading to impaired circulation of cerebral spinal fluid, and eventually neuronal and myelin degeneration.[85,86] The finding that hypertension accelerates the appearance of vascular lesions in the brain after irradiation with 10 to 30 Gy also supports a hypothesis of vascular pathogenesis.[87] The occlusive effects of radiation on arterial walls may cause a transient cerebral ischemia.[88]

Figure 7-6. Quantitative analysis of magnetic resonance imaging data reveals alterations 1 month after brain-only radiation exposure. (**a**) No visual anatomical changes were observed in rats on either imaging for edema (T2-weighted imaging), in water mobility (diffusion-weighted imaging), or enhanced blood-brain barrier leak. (**b**) However, quanti-

fication of water content (edema) within the hippocampus and entorhinal cortex (data not shown) revealed increased tissue edema. (**c**) Decreased water mobility (quantitative diffusion-weighted imaging, the apparent diffusion coefficient) revealed restricted water mobility in the irradiated brains compared to control. The decrements in water mobility are reflective of the differential neuropathology in microstructure evolving with radiation dose.

*: $P < 0.05$; **: $P < .01$ vs 0 Gy: ##: $P < 0.01$ vs 2 Gy; &: $P < 0.05$; &&: $P < 0.01$ vs 4 Gy; ADC: apparent diffusion coefficient; BBB: blood-brain barrier; T2: T2-weighted imaging

Data source: Huang L, Smith A, Cummings P, Kendall EJ, Obenaus A. Neuroimaging assessment of memory-related brain structures in a rat model of acute space-like radiation. *J Magn Reson Imaging.* 2009;29:785–792.

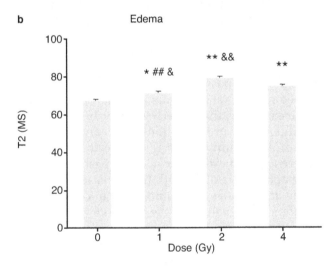

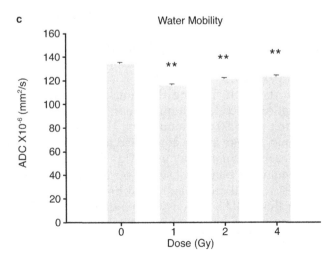

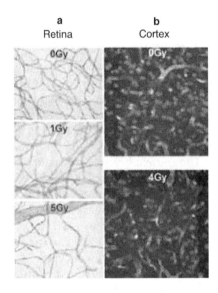

Figure 7-7. Vascular alterations following radiation exposure. (**a**) Rat retinal vascular morphological changes at 12 months following iron-56 irradiation of 0, 1, and 5 Gy of the rodent eye. Significant endothelial cells and vessel loss at 1 and 5 Gy was observed late after a single radiation exposure. (**b**) Cranial irradiation evoked morphological microvessel changes in the rat brain cortex at 12 months following iron-56 irradiation. In an unirradiated, age-matched control, the microvessels were normal, of uniform size with smooth contours. However, 12 months following 4-Gy radiation exposure, the microvessels within the cortex were torturous with nonuniform contours (see also Archambeau JO, Mao XW, McMillan PJ, et al. Dose response of rat retinal microvessels to proton dose schedules used clinically: a pilot study. *Int J Radiat Oncol Biol Phys.* 2000;48:1155–1166; Mao XW, Crapo JD, Mekonnen T, et al. Radioprotective effect of a metalloporphyrin compound in rat eye model. *Curr Eye Res.* 2009;34:62–72).

Slides courtesy of Dr V Mao, Loma Linda University, Loma Linda, CA.

ANIMAL STUDIES

Animals, such as mice, share many features with humans at the anatomical, cellular, biochemical, and molecular levels. They also share brain functions, such as anxiety, hunger, circadian rhythm, aggression, memory, sexual behavior, and other emotional responses with humans; therefore, many studies use animal models to approximate human behavioral responses following irradiation and to develop therapeutic interventions for radiation-induced CNS impairments. In laboratory animals, single doses of radiation up to 10 Gy did not produce any late morphological changes in the brain or spinal cord.[62,89] However, necrotic lesions were seen in the forebrain white matter from doses of 15 Gy.[85,90]

In a series of reports, Kiani and colleagues demonstrated that there are significant alterations in the vasculature of the hamster cremaster muscle following a single dose of radiation.[91–93] Both vascular density (capillaries) and blood flow were reduced at 3 to 30 days after irradiation[92] and these effects remained evident for as long as 6 months after a single 10-Gy dose.[91] Mao and colleagues reported similar decrements in the retinal vasculature after components of space irradiation, such as proton and iron-56 irradiations.[82,83] Perfusion and oxygenation deficits in the mouse brain were reported recently after a single 20-Gy exposure.[94] Kiani and colleagues demonstrated that the numbers of anatomical and perfused vessels were decreased up to 30 days after radiation.[94] In conjunction with these findings, they also reported that there was an increase in the distance to the nearest perfused vessel (irradiated approximately 45 μm at 3 days postirradiation, controls approximately 20 μm).[94] Although there was some return toward control intervessel distances, they never completely returned to control values.

A supportive finding for this apparent decrement in perfused vessel distance was the discovery that local tissues had a 200% increase in tissue hypoxia levels at 3 days postirradiation.[94] Although these very elevated levels of tissue hypoxia slowly declined over the next 120 days, they never reached control levels. Oxygenation pattern modeling also showed significant differences in irradiated tissues compared to age-matched controls.[93] No studies have examined the role of tissue hypoxia after brain radiation.

The hippocampus, like all regions of the brain, is dependent upon an intact and functioning vasculature to deliver oxygen and nutrients. Radiation has short-term (less than 1 month) and long-term (greater than 1 month) effects on brain function. In rodent studies, long-term effects can evolve over 1,

3, or even 12 months following irradiation. Cognitive effects are defined as effects on learning and memory. As behavioral changes can influence performance on cognitive tests, potential effects of irradiation on noncognitive behavioral measures need to be carefully considered in the interpretation of the cognitive effects. For example, potential alterations in measures of anxiety, sensorimotor function, motivation, social hierarchy, and vision can affect performance on tests of spatial learning and memory. Behavioral and cognitive performance are also influenced by genetic and environmental factors; therefore, they need to be carefully considered when assessing effects of irradiation on the brain. Thus, even after a comparable radiation exposure, the genetic makeup of an individual might critically modulate the impact of the irradiation on brain function. As was noted in the introduction, the effects of irradiation on brain function are also sex-dependent and different in female and male C57Bl6/J WT mice.[95] Female and male C57Bl6/J mice express different forms of genetic risk factors for age-related cognitive decline and show differences in developing cognitive impairments following challenges such as traumatic brain injury and cardiac bypass surgery.[96] Various studies have pooled behavioral data from male and female mice to increase statistical power. However, because of the sex differences in irradiation effects and increased variations within female mice due to individual differences in the estrous cycle, it is best not to pool male and female data. With the increase of women in the armed forces, it is important to consider sex differences in evaluating the potential effects of irradiation on brain function.

In addition to sex, age can also influence susceptibility to changes in brain function after irradiation exposure. Some impairments might become detectable or more profound in aged animals following irradiation earlier in life, and animals of different ages are likely to show different susceptibilities to altered radiation-induced changes in brain function following a specific time interval.

Efforts in elucidating the mouse genome have dramatically accelerated human-mouse comparative research. Over 90% of mouse and human genes are syntenic. Employing an automated alignment of rat, mouse, and human genomes, it was shown that 87% of human and mouse-rat sequences are aligned, and that 97% of all alignments with human sequences larger than 100 kb agree with an independent 3-way synteny map.[97] Finally, nearly 99% of human genes have mouse equivalents.[98–114]

Radiation Dose

A variety of radiation parameters, including dose, can significantly influence EPDs (see Figure 7-5). Low doses of radiation can sometimes produce behavioral changes, such as locomotor activation,[69] that contrast with the locomotor depression observed after high doses.[71] Beyond a certain threshold, more radiation tends to produce increasingly depressed measures of performance.[104,115,116] The radiation dose-response curves for measures of behavior in some ways parallel the curves observed for a number of end points, such as emesis and lethality.[117]

Radiation Dose Rate

Another radiation factor that can influence behavior is exposure dose rate.[118] Fractionated (or split) doses have been used to model the cumulative effects of radiation or to model radiation exposure over an extended period of time. As such, these studies may be useful in describing the impact on behavior after radiation exposure. Most studies report that a single dose results in more effective disruption of behavior than to split doses.[113,119–127]

Radiation in Space

As military operations move to space, new radiation hazards will challenge humans' abilities to carry out missions.[128,129] The behavioral effects of ionizing radiation (such as from protons and high-Z particles) in space are being actively explored.[130,131] A unique feature of the space radiation environment is the presence of high-energy charged particles, including protons, which comprise approximately 90% of the cosmic rays and fully ionized atomic nuclei, such as iron-56. These radiations may pose a significant hazard to space flight crews not only during military missions but also at later times when slow-developing, adverse effects might become more apparent. The hazards associated with the space environment will likely impact many organs and systems, and in the CNS, exposure to such radiation may directly affect structure and function within the brain (eg, behavioral performance), but also may change the tissue sensitivity to secondary insults such as trauma, stroke, or degenerative disease.

The effects of space irradiation on behavior and cognition might be more profound than that of earth irradiation for a few reasons. First, the energy of the irradiation is much higher in space than on Earth. In addition, there are other environmental stresses in space that might affect performance and interact with the effects of irradiation, such as the lack of circadian variations in light encountered on Earth, weightlessness, and being confined to a relatively small space for prolonged periods of time.

Similar to the sex-dependency of effects of cesium-137C irradiation described above, the effects of space irradiation on cognitive performance might also be sex dependent. When female and male mice were exposed to iron-56 irradiation at a dose of 1, 2, or 3 Gy and fear conditioning was assessed, male mice showed enhanced cognitive performance, while female mice showed reduced cognitive performance, as compared to sex-matched, sham-irradiated mice.

Irradiation and Sensory and Perceptual Changes

Sensory and perceptual processes are distinct, yet interrelated. The sensory process involves stimuli that impinge on the senses, such as vision, audition, olfaction, gustation, and skin sensation.[132] The perceptual process involves the translation of these stimuli by the brain into appropriate overt or covert interpretation or action. Ionizing radiation can be sensed and perceived, and radiation-induced sensory activation can in fact occur at extremely low levels.[133] For instance, the olfactory response threshold to radiation is less than 10 mrad, and the visual system is sensitive to radiation levels below 0.5 mrad. Ionizing radiation is as efficient as light in producing retinal activity, as assessed by the electroretinogram. The visibility of ionizing radiation was reported shortly after the discovery of X-rays and is now firmly established.[114]

Vision

Although the visual system can detect a low radiation dose, large doses are required to produce pathological changes in the retina. This is especially true for the rods, which are involved in black and white vision.[134] Necrosis of rods has been reported after irradiation doses of 150 to 200 Gy in rats and rabbits, and after 600 Gy in monkeys. Cone (color vision) ganglion cells are even more resistant to radiation. At these high radiation doses, cataracts occur.[135–139]

Although pathological changes in the visual system occur only at high doses, visual function is affected at lower doses. Rats trained to a brightness discrimination task are not able to differentiate between shades of gray after 3.6 Gy or to make sensitivity changes after exposure to 6 Gy of whole-body X-rays.[114] In mice, low-rate, whole-body irradiation adversely affected brightness discrimination tested 3 to 5 months after exposure. Humans experienced temporary decrements in scotopic visual sensitivity 1 day after being exposed to 0.3 to 1.0 Gy of X-radiation.[140] Long-term

(20–36 days) changes in dark adaptation are reported in patients exposed to 4 to 62 Gy of X-rays.[141]

With regard to visual acuity, only long-term deficits were reported in monkeys at 1 to 3 years after whole-body exposure to 3 to 60 Gy of radiation.[114,142] However, the potential effects of irradiation on attention may have caused some of these effects.[143]

Audition and Vestibular Function

Few adverse auditory changes have been noted after radiation exposure. Two grays of X-ray irradiation to the head produced no changes in cochlear microphonics in rats examined up to 90 days after exposure.[138,144,145]

The physiological substrate of hearing deficits might involve changes in the mouse ear, reported following 20 to 30 Gy of whole-body X-rays, which included cellular necrosis in the organ of Corti and in the epithelial cells of the ear canals.[114] Rats exposed to a whole-body dose of 1 to 30 Gy of gamma or X-radiation showed damage in the cochlea but not in the cristae of the vestibular inner ear or the middle ear. Human patients who received 40 to 50 Gy of therapeutic gamma radiation developed inflammation of the middle ear but only a temporary loss of auditory sensitivity and temporary tinnitus.[146,147]

Vestibular function may be more radiosensitive than audition. Depression in vestibular function may exist at doses close to the LD_{50}, and symptoms of vestibular disruption may last longer at higher than at lower doses.[148,149]

Other Senses

Olfactory and gustatory changes have been reported in patients exposed to therapeutic radiation.[150] There are altered taste perceptions in patients exposed to 36 Gy of X-rays, with a metallic taste being the most common report. Transient changes in taste and olfactory sensitivity are also reported in radiotherapy patients and in rats.[114]

Radiation may affect the skin senses, but it is often difficult to distinguish the direct receptor changes due to secondary changes arising from effects on the vascular system.[135] Radiation-induced changes in pain perception may be species dependent; gamma photons produce a dose-dependent analgesia in mice,[151] but gamma or X-rays may not alter the analgesic effects of morphine or the anesthetic effects of halothane in rats except under certain conditions.[152,153]

In summary, whole-body radiation doses below LD_{50} do not appear to produce permanent sensory changes. However, there may be transient alterations at doses of 1 to 5 Gy. High levels of radiation can cause longer-lasting sensory impairments and impair perceptual function.

Effects of Irradiation on Naturalistic Behaviors

Naturalistic behaviors (spontaneous locomotion, anxiety, social interaction, consumption behaviors, taste aversion, and emesis) are often evaluated in the study of radiation effect may affect performance on cognitive tests.[75,103,107,114,127,129,134,135,143,145,154–196]

Effects of Irradiation on Cognitive Performance

Regarding the effects of radiation on cognitive function, it is especially important to distinguish short- and long-term effects on brain function. Brain function can be altered at the time of or shortly after irradiation. Obviously, potential alterations in cognitive function during or shortly after irradiation on the battlefield can be detrimental for executing the aims of a specific operation or effort. In addition to these relatively short effects, there may also be long-term effects that need to be considered. In the extreme, potential effects of irradiation earlier in life might alter one's susceptibility to develop age-related cognitive decline and neurodegenerative diseases like Alzheimer's disease.

In human studies, environmental factors such as diet, sleep cycle, and stress levels are much more difficult to control for. For instance, a few cases of acute retrograde amnesia were reported by individuals who survived the bombing of Hiroshima.[197] Five years after the attack, deficits in memory and intellectual capacity were noted in individuals experiencing radiation sickness.[18] These data are consistent with other human studies reporting memory deficits in patients who had undergone therapeutic irradiations.[198] Radiation-induced brain injury is a limiting factor during therapeutic irradiation of the brain.[199] Overt tissue injury generally occurs only after relatively high doses. However, there is a strong likelihood of developing adverse reactions in terms of cognitive decline after relatively lower doses,[200] but in humans, the memory impairments may have been strongly influenced by other environmental stressors of war or associated with the armed forces.

Cognitive changes following irradiation have a diverse character and, in humans and animals, often include hippocampus-dependent functions involving learning and memory and spatial-information processing.[201–203] The susceptibility to developing selective hippocampus-dependent cognitive impairments remains elusive. One possibility is that these radiation effects involve alterations in the ability to generate new neurons throughout life and loss of mature neurons in the dentate gyrus,[203–205] alterations in receptor subunits involved in learning and memory,[206] and measures of neuronal signaling as assessed using in-vivo and in-vitro electrophysiology,[207] genetic risk factors,[96] and changes in oxidative stress.[203,208,209]

Early Effects

Early radiation effects are particularly pertinent to the armed forces because its members deal with the potential immediate effects of irradiation on cognitive performance during critical missions. Delayed reaction time was noted in an animal response task fallout study. Delayed reaction times were noted in each study group.[210,211] It is important to consider that fatigue and weakness, more often seen following irradiation above a threshold than as a dose-response effect, will likely affect cognitive performance and contribute to cognitive impairments.

Early Transient Incapacitation and Other Early Performance Decrements

In various animal models, ETI is a strikingly short, intense phenomenon. A less severe variant of ETI is EPD, in which performance is reduced rather than totally suppressed (see Figure 7-5). Initially, it was presumed that ETI and EPD would occur only at supralethal radiation doses and that, after behavioral recovery, death would occur in hours or days. However, high doses may not be necessary to produce these effects,[115,118] particularly when performing a more difficult task requiring both visual discrimination and memory.[118] Thus, relatively low doses of radiation may cause rapid, transient disruptions in performance.[210–218]

The issues of task demands and task complexity influencing the effective radiation level are common in the investigation of ETI. For instance, the dose of radiation required to disrupt performance was com-pared for three tasks: the visual discrimination task (with a 5-second response time), a physical activity task, and an equilibrium-maintenance task.[115,116,219] The data suggest that a range of performance decrements result from radiation exposure, with visual function least affected and physical activity most affected. Recovery time and behavioral effectiveness after radiation exposure have obvious implications for military missions.[115,129]

Late Effects

Retrograde amnesia is a short-term memory loss or an inability to recall recent events following trauma or a novel event.[133] The mechanisms of radiogenic amnesia are unclear but might involve sensory disruption, primarily of the visual system.[220–224] Classical conditioning research data indicate that radiation exposure can alter learning and memory and do not merely reflect nonassociative factors.[225]

It should be emphasized that the effects of irradiation on cognitive function are complex. Decreased, unaltered, and increased performance has been reported. This complexity might depend on the age of animals at the time of irradiation; the cognitive testing paradigm; the genetic makeup and sex of the animals; potential environmental conditions present prior, during, or after the irradiation; the dose of irradiation used; the interval between irradiation and cognitive testing; and the cognitive test and test design used (Figure 7-8).[96,114,145,202,203,209,226–234]

Although some of the behavioral radiobiology literature suggests that learning and performance are relatively radioresistant, most studies have reported postirradiation changes. For instance, maze-learning behavior was reduced after X-ray exposure up to 10 Gy.[158] More challenging tasks might be more radiosensitive than easier ones. Indeed, rats were found to have a temporary reduction in their ability to reorganize previously learned material after exposure to 4 Gy of gamma radiation (Figure 7-9).[159]

NEUROPHYSIOLOGICAL CHANGES IN THE HIPPOCAMPUS FOLLOWING RADIATION

There are a number of methods for assessing CNS-induced functional changes within the brains of humans and experimental animals. Some approaches, such as electroencephalography, are truly noninvasive, whereas others—like in-vivo depth electrodes (extracellular recordings)—are not. Electrophysiological recordings from excised tissues are also used. These excised tissues can come from a host of brain regions, but the most common is the hippocampus, an important structure for spatial learning and memory, passive avoidance, and some forms of object recognition. Human tissues are also available, primarily as neurosurgical resections during the course of amelioration of disease, such as epilepsy or tumors.[59,115,142,143,159,162,229,235–243]

Radiation Exposure of the Central Nervous System

The deleterious effects of radiation are not limited to mitotically active cell types, such as neuronal precursors in the CNS,[203] but also alter nondividing cells,

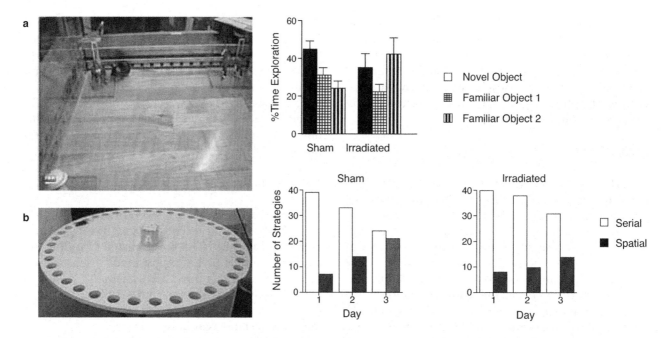

Figure 7-8. Effects of cesium-137 irradiation on hippocampus-independent, novel object recognition and hippocampus-dependent search strategies in spatial learning and memory in the Barnes maze. (**a**) Mice were habituated to an open field without any objects over 3 days. On the fourth day, the mice were trained in three trials containing three objects kept in the same location (left panel). In the novel object recognition trial, one object was replaced with a novel one. While sham-irradiated mice spent significantly more time exploring the novel object than the two familiar ones, mice irradiated with cesium-137 at a dose of 10 Gy and tested 3 months later did not (*$P < 0.05$ vs both familiar objects; Villasana and Raber, unpublished observations). (**b**) In the Barnes maze, mice were tested to locate a hidden escape tunnel over 3 days. As the mice learned the task, they switched from using serial searches (searching consecutive holes in either direction until the escape tunnel was located) to spatial searches (directly searching the hole containing the escape tunnel or the adjacent holes). However, with training, the percentage of spatial searches was higher and the percentage of serial searches lower in sham-irradiated mice than mice irradiated with cesium-137 at a dose of 10 Gy and tested 3 months later.
Data source: Raber J, Rola R, LeFevour A, et al. Radiation–induced cognitive impairments associated with changes in hippocampal neurogenesis. *Radiat Res.* 2004;162:39–47.

such as CNS neurons. Currently, little information is available on the effects of radiation on CNS function using electrophysiological techniques. An array of studies in the last 20 years has examined functional and electrophysiological alterations within the CNS following radiation exposure, but many of these have been surveys. Few electrophysiological studies examine the dose response of CNS injury to radiation.[199]

The hippocampi of humans and experimental animals are often the most studied because this brain region is similar in laminar structure, cellular composition, and function. Excised tissues provide a variety of electrophysiological, extracellular, intracellular, and, more recently, patch clamp recordings, which allow the study of cellular ion channels, each unique in the type of functional data they provide. As noted previously, there are numerous electrophysiological studies examining epileptic and tumor tissues from humans, but no studies involving radiation exposure. In animal studies, electrophysiological field excitatory postsynaptic potential recordings can be evaluated on

the basis of the physiological question posed (Figure 7-10).

Table 7-1 briefly summarizes some of the types of information that can be gleaned from electrophysiological recordings. Synaptic excitability can be evaluated by constructing input–output curves at incrementally increasing stimulation intensities. Paired-pulse facilitation (PPF) is often used to test changes in presynaptic glutamate release. PPF is evoked by paired-pulse stimulation, in which a second electrophysiological response is elicited at interpulse intervals ranging from 20 to 200 milliseconds using 30% to 50% of maximal response derived from the input–output tests. Typically, the second response is facilitated and PPF is calculated as a ratio of the second/first electrophysiological response. The function of feedback-inhibitory interneurons can be assessed by paired-pulse inhibition. Similar to PPF, two stimuli are applied at 10- to 200-millisecond interpulse intervals and the second response is typically reduced because of feedback inhibition of the primary hippocampal neurons. Long-

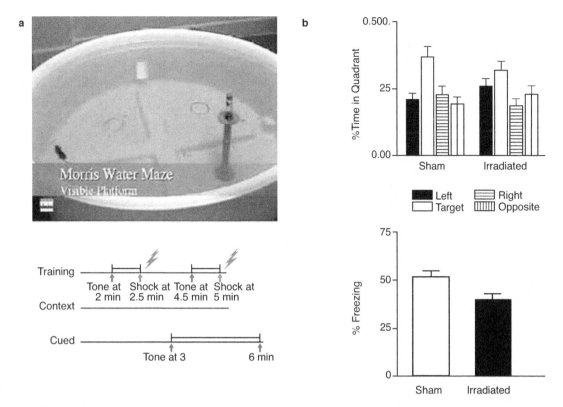

Figure 7-9. Effects of cesium-137 irradiation on hippocampus-dependent spatial memory retention in the water maze probe trial and hippocampus-dependent contextual fear conditioning. **(a)** In the water maze, 2-month-old C57Bl6/J male mice were trained to locate a visible platform in 12 trials over 2 days (left panel shows the water maze with the clearly visible platform). The mice were trained to locate visible platforms in four different locations. Subsequently, they were trained to locate a hidden platform in 12 trials over 2 days. One day after the last hidden-training trial, the mice were tested in a probe trial (no platform). While sham-irradiated mice spent more time searching the quadrant of the pool where the hidden platform was previously located, mice irradiated with cesium-137 at a dose of 10 Gy and cognitively tested 3 months later did not ($P < 0.05$ vs any other quadrant).[1] **(b)** Two-month-old C57Bl6/J male mice were trained in a fear conditioning paradigm. As indicated in the left panel, mice received two tone-shock pairings. The next day, hippocampus-dependent fear conditioning was assessed in the same environment in which the mice were trained. No tone or shock was administered. Sham-irradiated mice showed significantly more freezing (immobility measure) than mice irradiated with cesium-137 at a dose of 10 Gy ($P < 0.05$ vs sham-irradiated mice).

(1) Raber J, Rola R, LeFevour A, et al. Radiation-induced cognitive impairments are associated with changes in indicators of hippocampal

term potentiation (see Figure 7-10) is used to test cellular plasticity and can be evoked by high-frequency stimulation of hippocampal pathways, which leads to potentiated responses (> 200% increases). Intracellular and patch clamp recordings are used to assess the fundamental characteristics of neurons under investigation, including action potential amplitudes and duration and the ability of the cell to maintain its resting membrane potential. While numerous other cellular electrophysiological tests exist, the few cited here demonstrate the wealth of neurophysiological function that can be obtained in these studies.

Pellmar and colleagues have reported the most comprehensive data using in-vitro hippocampal slices to model acute radiation-induced injury. Two models were developed, one employing peroxide application[244] and another that exposes slices directly to gamma irradiation.[245] Direct exposure of hippocampal slices to gamma rays resulted in a dose- and dose-rate-dependent decrease of evoked activity. While lower doses resulted in synaptic impairment, high doses resulted in postsynaptic efficacy decrements, and decreased action potential generation (ie, decreased neuronal output). The observed postsynaptic damage was not sensitive to dose rate. In conclusion, these studies demonstrate that radiation can alter the integrated functional activity of hippocampal neurons.[245] Depleted uranium exposure is also thought to result in neurotoxicity.[246] Further study is required to determine the effects of depleted uranium on CNS

TABLE 7-1

MAJOR NEUROPHYSIOLOGICAL OUTPUTS FROM ELECTROPHYSIOLOGY

Parameter	Definition
Extracellular	
Input-output relation-ship	Presynaptic vs postsynaptic excitability, synaptic efficacy
Paired-pulse facilita-tion	Short-term plasticity, presynaptic glutamate release
Long-term potentiation	Long-term plasticity and cellular model of learning and memory
Paired-pulse inhibition	Assess feedback inhibitiory neurons (GABAergic)
Intracellular	
Resting membrane potential	Resting membrane potential of the cell
Input resistance	Input resistance of the cell
Action potential amplitude	Size of the action potential
Action potential duration	Duration of the action potential

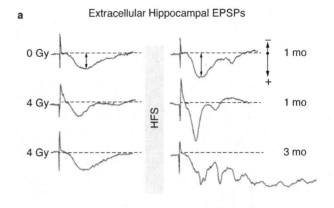

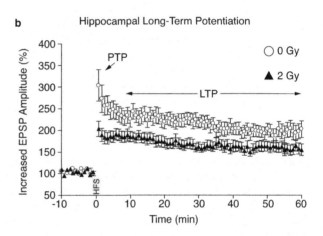

function. Radiotherapy treatment reports can yield some insight into altered physiology, but most are not directly applicable.[245,247–252]

Space Radiation Exposure of the Central Nervous System

More recently, the effects of heavy ion radiation on the CNS, specifically the CA1 region of the hippocampus, have been described. Extracellular in-vitro recordings were obtained following brain-only exposure to iron-56, a component of space radiation, which demonstrated a number of changes that were dose and time sensitive. First, synaptic efficacy was increased after radiation exposure but appears to be more prominent earlier (1 month) after irradiation rather than later (12 months). No enhancement was found within the CA1 using PPF at any of the time points investigated. Long-term potentiation, an established model of learning and memory in hippocampal slices, is altered after radiation exposure at 1 month after radiation exposure. These decrements in long-term potentiation become more pronounced over the 12-month observation period, consistent with and suggesting progressive deterioration of the synaptic circuitry within the hippocampus. These findings were

Figure 7-10. Neurophysiological alterations following radiation exposure within the CA1 region of the hippocampus. **(a)** Cranial radiation (iron-56, 600 MeV) resulted in hyperexcitibility within the CA1 of the hippocampus. High-frequency stimulation was used to simulate learning and memory (long-term potentiation), as evidenced by increased amplitude of the extracellular excitatory postsynaptic potentials (double-headed arrows). Evidence for altered hippocampal circuitry, in the form of increased excitability, was observed at 3 months following a single radiation exposure, which then returned to "normal" at later time points (> 6 months). **(b)** Decrements in learning and memory using a model system (long-term potentiation) have been observed following iron-56 irradiation. These decrements were also observed immediately after high-frequency stimulation and were manifested as an immediate decrease in the extracellular excitatory postsynaptic potential amplitude in the posttetanic potentiation phase and was followed by a sustained decrease in the output of the hippocampus (ie, decreased learning and memory).
EPSP: excitatory postsynaptic potential
HFS: high-frequency stimulation
LTP: long-term potentiation
PTP: posttetanic potentiation
Data source: Obenaus A, Vlkolinsky R, Loma Linda University, Loma Linda, CA.

not dose dependent. However, at every time point, the 2-Gy dose appeared to be more deleterious, a finding that has been previously reported.[251] One of the more interesting observations was that at early time points (1 and 3 months), there was increased hyperexcitability within the CA1 region of the hippocampus after radiation exposure. Multiple population spikes appeared to be more pronounced at higher doses, particularly in the 4-Gy animals (see Figure 7-10). These findings are in agreement with the earlier studies by Pellmar et al[253,254] that demonstrate altered excitability following radiation exposure. In addition, while many of the studies use different radiation types and qualities, the fact that similar decrements in neurophysiological function have been reported suggests the possibility that common cellular pathways are altered.

To investigate the underlying physiological mechanisms responsible for these observed changes, a series of experiments using patch clamp recordings were used to determine if the intrinsic properties of the pyramidal cell neurons were altered. No changes were found in the input resistance, resting membrane potential, action potential amplitude, or duration of the evoked pyramidal cells at any of the postirradiation time points that were investigated (3, 6, and 12 months). This would suggest that many of the electrophysiological changes in the hippocampus after iron-56 irradiation are likely due to synaptic and cellular reorganization with no changes in the intrinsic neuronal properties. Pharmacological isolation methods to remove the excitatory drive within the hippocampus allow investigation of the miniature inhibitory postsynaptic potentials that are GABAergic (γ-aminobutyric-acid-producing). A dose-dependent decrease in the miniature inhibitory postsynaptic potentials consistent with decreased inhibitory tone 18 months after radiation was observed. This decrease in inhibitory tone, particularly its dose dependence, is consistent and mechanistically plausible to account for the increased hyperexcitability after radiation exposure.

Recent work was reported that evaluated the functional effects of radiation on neuroinflammation. Using a peripheral immunological stressor, lipopolysaccharide, the response of the immune system was evaluated in animals that received brain-only radiation.[251,252] These results suggested altered processing of peripheral immune signals by the irradiated CNS. While the exact cellular and molecular radiation targets remain unknown, it has been hypothesized that space radiation may impact the functional properties of neurons and thus lead to an imbalance in neuronal network activity. Such an imbalance could potentially lead to neurological manifestations that may impact

intellectual performance and behavioral patterns (ie, learning and memory) during long-term space missions.

There is a dearth of in-vivo, adult radiation exposure research using electrophysiological methods, but several studies have used brainstem recordings to demonstrate an increased latency and length of auditory waves after 2-Gy whole-body irradiation. Follow-up microscopy revealed changes only in the cells within the brainstem auditory nuclei.[255] Reder et al[250] reported time- and dose-dependant changes in the receptive field of the lateral geniculate nucleus following proton radiation, but found no cellular necrosis or vascular damage; however, the afferents to the nucleus were disrupted.

Other model systems have been used to study the effects of radiation exposures.[248] Electrophysiological assessment of cerebellar neurons in culture following laser radiation detected damage to mitochondria and cellular membranes and increased membrane conductance to some ion species.[256]

Long-term changes within the CNS following irraditaion are reminiscent of those associated with senescence. For example, Carlson et al suggested that the increased metabolic rate in irradiated animals may accelerate aging.[257] Later, using brain-only irradiation with argon and iron particles at a dose of 0.5 Gy, Philpott et al observed a progressive decline in motor performance and morphological changes in synaptic density in the hippocampus of C57Bl/6 mice.[131,258] Iron-56 radiation was also shown to impair spatial learning and reference memory where the deficits were related to synaptic neurotransmitter release.[259] Many of these functional changes have also been reported during normal aging.[260]

To further investigate if radiation mimics or alters the temporal evolution of aging, experiments were conducted using mice that exhibited accelerated aging and age-related behavioral abnormalities.[207,251] Amyloid precursor protein transgenic mice (APP23) showed significant deficits in synaptic transmission and electrophysiological correlates of learning and memory. A 2-year temporal study evaluating the CA1 region of the hippocampus found that radiation accelerated the onset of age-related electrophysiological decrements. In APP mice without radiation exposure, decrements in learning and memory were observed at greater than 14 months of age, but in radiation-exposed mice these same deficits were observed as early as 9 months of age. At 6 months of age, the radiation-treated animals also showed a transient reduction in inhibition that then later appeared to recover. Radiation did not significantly affect overall survival of APP23 mice. It was concluded that irradiation of the brain may accelerate Alzheimer's-disease–related neurological deficits.[251]

Radiation-Induced Hyperexcitability

Increased evoked hippocampal synaptic activity at 1 month after 0- to 4-Gy iron-56 ions,[252] and increased evoked and spontaneous hyperexcitablity after either proton or iron-56 radiation exposure have been found (see Figure 7-10). These alterations are reminiscent of seizure disorders.[261] Intracellular (patch clamp) recordings evaluating functional changes within individual neurons in the face of altered networks were used to show that intrinsic neuronal membrane properties, such as input resistance, membrane time constant, action potential thresholds and duration, and spike frequency adaptation were not significantly altered at 1 to 3 months after brain-only radiation exposure.[262] These data suggest that the increased excitability observed in the extracellular recordings was likely the result of increased excitatory or decreased inhibitory neurotransmission, mediated in part by alterations in inhibitory neurotransmitter receptors.[263,264] More

recently, an interesting report demonstrated that high radiosurgical doses of photon radiation decreased the frequency of observed and electroencephalography-defined seizures in a rat model of epilepsy.[265] There were no changes in brain tissue at 20, 40, or 60 Gy and only moderate changes at 100 Gy, and the report further suggests that radiosurgical approaches to epilepsy treatment are warranted. Finally, age-related changes in a variety of measures also showed that older rats have increased inflammatory responses compared to younger rats after whole-body irradiation.[266] Younger rats have a sustained decrease in neurogenesis compared to older rats.

Interaction of Irradiation With Other Environmental Factors

Nuclear war would produce few "pure" radiation injuries. It is more likely that victims will experience burns, wounds, and perhaps trauma from chemical agents and environmental stresses combined with the damage from ionizing radiation (Figure 7-11). The physiological effects and treatment of irradia-

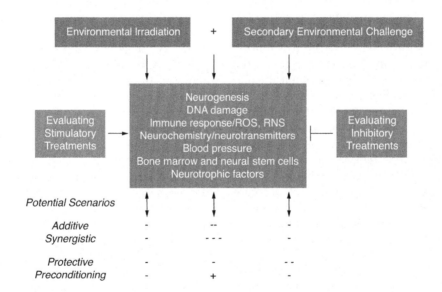

Figure 7-11. Schema of potential effects of combined injury on brain function. When the brain is challenged not only with irradiation but with a secondary environmental insult as well, the resulting effects on brain function are complex and hard to predict without experimental evidence. For example, the two insults might have additive or synergistic effects on brain function. However, it is also possible that the first insult serves as a preconditioning challenge and actually relatively protects the brain against the second challenge or even reverses the direction of the effects of the irradiation on brain function. Along the same lines, individuals with higher levels of antioxidant mechanisms prior to cranial irradiation might react differently to radiation effects on cognition than individuals with lower levels of antioxidant mechanisms. Based on these complex interactions, treatments targeting mechanisms potentially contributing to altered cognitive function following irradiation should also be evaluated following combined injuries.
-: detrimental effect on brain function
+: beneficial effect on brain function
DNA: deoxyribonucleic acid; RNS: reactive nitrogen species; ROS: reactive oxygen species

tion with other environmental factors has received significant attention.[267,268] Less clear are the behavioral and cognitive consequences from combined traumas that include irradiation. In one study, mice were exposed to 3 Gy of neutron-gamma radiation, and some were then exposed to sublethal trauma (wound or burn).[269] Radiation exposure alone caused reduced measures of locomotion. While the wound injury increased the harmful effects of radiation, the burn injury did not.

In a study of the combined effects of radiation (7 Gy) and an anticholinesterase agent (physostigmine, 0.1 mg/kg, which was used in recent military missions and was postulated to have contributed to Gulf War Syndrome), rats were evaluated on a behavioral test battery that included measuring their balance on a rotating rod and recording several components of their locomotor activity.[270,271] Forty-five minutes after irradiation, a radiation-only group had a 30% deficit in performance, while a physostigmine-only group had

a 40% deficit. A combined-treatment group showed a 60% performance deficit on the rotating rod task. All measures of performance indicated that the effect of combined ionizing radiation and physostigmine was much greater than the effect of either insult alone.[272] Environmental and combat stresses may also combine with radiation injuries to increase behavioral decrements.[165,273–276]

Other environmental stresses can alter the effectiveness of radiation on behavior or lethality. For instance, daily exhaustive exercise, continuous exposure to cold (6°C), or continuous exposure to high altitude (15,000 feet) considerably reduced the time to death and the incidence of death after irradiation.[114,277]

These data suggest that the behavioral effects of radiation may interact with other environmental stresses. Therefore, any estimates of battlefield performance decrements that do not include these factors might under- or overestimate the behavioral and cognitive changes actually observed in a military conflict.

MECHANISMS AND POSSIBLE INTERVENTIONS

Although various organ systems may contribute to radiation-induced lethargy and reduced responsiveness, the nervous system's central role in behavior makes it the presumed primary mediator of radiation-induced behavioral changes (see Figure 7-11).[278–280] Although radiation-induced behavioral changes are well established, it is unclear which specific changes in the brain mediate these changes. Sufficiently large radiation doses cause permanent brain lesions, demyelination, and necrosis, which in turn produce chronic behavioral deficits. In addition, short-lived behavioral changes may be mediated by transient vascular changes that induce edema or ischemia in the brain. Alternatively, behavioral changes might be mediated by significant alterations in brain function due to changes in neurochemistry and neurophysiology.

Radiogenic Pathology of the Nervous System

The anatomical specificity of radiation-induced brain injury may in part explain the ability of a particular dose of ionizing radiation to disrupt one type of behavior but not another.[116] Classically conditioned reflexes seem more radioresistant than motor coordination, and ionizing radiation might mainly affect the functions of the subcortical brainstem.[68,281–284]

Evidence for the direct action of radiation on the parenchymal cells of the nervous system (rather than the indirect effects through the vascular bed) was first provided when brain tissue in irradiated human pa-

tients was examined.[285] None of the brain lesions could be attributed to vascular damage because they were (*a*) predominantly in white matter and not codistributed with blood vessels, (*b*) not morphologically typical of ischemic necrosis, and (*c*) often found in the absence of any vascular effects.[286–290] Thus, direct neuronal and/or glial mechanisms caused at least some of the observed brain injury in the irradiated subjects.

In the brain, hypertension accelerates the onset of radiation-induced vascular damage but not white-matter lesions.[87] Thus, vascular damage is distinct from pathogenesis of white-matter lesions, and ischemia and edema are likely not important in white-matter pathogenesis. Selective necrosis of white matter might be due to slow reproductive loss of glia or their precursors. Certain types of glial cells are particularly sensitive to radiation effects.[291,292] The earliest sign of white-matter damage is widening of the nodes of Ranvier and segmental demyelination as early as 2 weeks after an irradiation dose of 5 to 60 Gy.[293] Clinical evidence also supports radiation-induced demyelination. After radiotherapy for head and neck cancers, several patients experienced sensations like electric shock (referenced to sensory levels below the neck).[294] These symptoms gradually abated and disappeared after 2 to 36 weeks. This transient radiation myelopathy could be a result of temporary demyelination of sensory neurons. Mitotic activity in the subependymal plate (important in glial production) did not recover after radiation doses capable of producing necrosis, but did recover after doses that did not produce necrosis, supporting the concept that glial cells are primary targets for radiation-induced brain injury.[295]

Both vascular and glial changes may be important in the development of late radiation-induced brain damage.[54] The preponderance of one type of cell damage over another depends on the radiation dose used. Vascular effects occur at lower doses of irradiation but after a longer latent period than effects mediated through damage to glia.[54] Thus, while radiation-induced brain injury is well accepted after high doses (greater than 15 Gy), increasing evidence supports radiation-induced brain injury at lower doses. The mechanisms underlying this brain injury have not been adequately explored.

In addition to axonal demyelination, other direct neuronal damage may occur in irradiated adult animals. Although mitotic neurons of the prenatal and neonatal brain are extremely sensitive to radiation, the neurons of more mature animals are relatively resistant and less likely to result in cell death.[114,150,296] However, as early as 1962, neurogenesis was proposed to take place in the adult brain as well.[297] Adult and juvenile neurogenesis was found to be especially prominent in the granule cell populations of the hippocampus and the olfactory bulb. Neurogenesis in other brain regions has been reported but is still controversial. This might be partially due to a detection limit at low levels of neurogenesis. The newly formed cells have the ultrastructural characteristics of neurons,[298] and the number of granule cells in the hippocampus increases in adult rodents.[299,300] In mice, neurogenesis quickly reduces after birth and levels of neurogenesis are relatively low at 6 months of age. Neurogenesis was also reported in the hippocampal subgranular cell layer of adult rabbits and shown to be quite radiosensitive (4.0–4.5 Gy).[301,302] Thus, certain populations of proliferating neurons in the adult brain can be damaged or destroyed by relatively low doses of ionizing radiation. These findings have been confirmed in nonhuman primates and humans and collectively suggest that certain neuronal populations in the adult brain are radiosensitive due to their mitotic state.[303] It should be pointed out, however, that there is no simple relationship between neurogenesis and cognitive function, and the exact role of reduced neurogenesis in radiation-induced cognitive changes is still unclear.

In addition to alterations in neurogenesis, there are subtle dendritic alterations following X-irradiation in the cerebral cortex of the monkey. They include decreased dendritic intersections, branchings, and length, as well as reduced packing density of neuronal elements.[304] Consistent with these findings, altered levels of the dendritic marker microtubule-associated protein 2 were reported in the mouse hippocampus and cortex.

Cellular Models

In addition to animal models, cellular models are also being used to assess the potential effects of irradiation on brain function. Cellular models are particularly useful for mechanistic questions and to determine the direct and indirect effects of irradiation on a particular cell type (see Figures 7-3 and 7-11). In general, irradiation produces DNA (deoxyribonucleic acid) and other cellular lesions that cause a severe stress response.[305] The cellular response includes activation of injury pathways, such as those involved in DNA repair, cell-cycle checkpoints, and apoptosis.[305] In turn, these pathways might involve reactive oxygen species (ROS) or reactive nitrogen species, impaired mitochondrial function, cell survival, and cell death pathways.[306] The effects of irradiation can be studied in homogeneous cultures (for example, those consisting of cells such as progenitor cells, which are particularly sensitive to irradiation or in mixed cultures). Mixed cultures can contain different sources of cell lines. Alternatively, these effects can be studied in primary 2- or 3-dimensional cultures, or "brain balls." For example, the role of ROS irradiation effects is being studied in cellular models. ROS affects the basal redox state of cells[307] and proliferation and differentiation of glial precursors, and may also contribute to the enhanced susceptibility of neural precursors to effects of irradiation.[308] In addition to ROS, reactive nitrogen species might be involved as well. While nitric oxide (NO) can inhibit the apoptotic pathway through cyclic-guanosine-monophosphate-dependent mechanisms and caspase inhibition, NO can have proapoptotic effects via mitochondria, DNA damage, and inhibition of proteasome.[305] In the developing brain, ionizing radiation induces an early increase of neuronal NO synthase activity and a further augmentation in the NO steady-state concentration.[309] Consistent with in-vivo data supporting the involvement of apoptosis in radiation-induced cell death in the developing brain,[310] radiation-induced cell death of neural precursor cells in vitro was shown to be caspase-3-dependent.[311] The advantage of in-vitro systems is that relatively simple, more mechanistic questions can be addressed. For example, a cellular model system showed more apoptosis in irradiated cells after inhibition of NO synthase, indicating NO was protective in the early irradiation response.

A combination of cellular models and whole-animal models are particularly useful when studying the effects of brain irradiation and in developing potential therapeutic strategies. For example, in a 2007 study, it was shown that brain irradiation enhances the survival of implanted neural progenitor cells in normal and tumor-bearing brains.[312] Recently, it was shown that implantating cells in nonirradiated brains has detrimental effects on hippocampus-dependent object recognition, while implantating cells in an irradiated brain enhances object recognition.[313] Together, these data emphasize that the microenvironment in irradiated and nonirradiated brains might be such that opposite therapeutic effects are encountered. Similar paradoxical effects are seen with inhibitors of oxidative stress.[314]

Alterations in Nervous System Function and Potential Therapeutic Targets

With the exception of immature neurons, the adult brain is relatively resistant to radiation-induced cell death; however, the mature brain is quite sensitive to functional changes in neurophysiology and neurochemistry. These functional changes, following low or intermediate doses of ionizing radiation (less than 15 Gy), might contribute to the radiation-induced behavioral changes.[315,316]

Neurochemistry

Sodium. One of the best-studied neurochemical changes following irradiation is ionic flow across the semipermeable neuronal membrane. The flow of sodium ions is believed to be involved in the control of neuronal excitability[317] and can be disrupted after either a very high or very low dose of radiation. A study using the radioactive isotope sodium-24 compared the sodium intake across the membrane of the squid giant axon before and after exposure to X-rays.[318] There was a significant increase in sodium intake during the initial hyperactive period following a dose of 500 Gy. Similar results were reported using frog sciatic nerves irradiated with 1,500 to 2,000 Gy of alpha particles, although a simultaneous decrease in the rate of sodium extrusion also occurred.[319] Peripheral nerves may be less radiosensitive than neurons in the CNS. The artificially stimulated uptake of sodium into brain synaptosomes was significantly reduced by an ionizing radiation exposure (high-energy electrons) of 0.1 to 1,000 Gy.[320] This effect was later confirmed using 1 to 100 Gy of gamma radiation.[321]

Dopamine and norepinephrine. The brain has been described as a radiosensitive biochemical system[315] and many changes in brain neurochemistry have been observed after irradiation. One to two days after an exposure to 3 Gy of X-radiation, neurosecretory granules in the hypophysial-hypothalamic system showed a transient increase in number over the controls.[322] Brain monoamines have been reported to leak from the neuronal terminals of rats irradiated with 40 Gy of X-rays, as well.[323] These changes may correlate with alterations of neurotransmitter systems following irradiation.

Catecholamine functioning appears to be damaged following exposure to intermediate or high doses of ionizing radiation. After 100 Gy, there is a transient disruption in dopamine functioning (similar in some ways to dopamine-receptor blockade).[324] Similarly, a 30-Gy radiation exposure increases the ability of the dopamine receptor blocker haloperidol to produce cataleptic behavior.[325] Radiation-induced effects on dopamine have been correlated in time with ETI, suggesting that changes in this neurotransmitter system may play a role in behavioral disruptions. However, other neuromodulators (such as prostaglandins) also seem to influence dopaminergic systems and might contribute to radiation-induced behavioral changes.[325] On the day of exposure to 6.6 Gy of gamma radiation, there was a transient reduction in the norepinephrine content within the monkey hypothalamus; the norepinephrine levels returned to normal 3 days later.[326] Although similar effects have been reported in one study,[327] another study found no change in noradrenaline content after 8.5 Gy of X-rays.[328] Monoamine oxidase, an enzyme that breaks down catecholamines, was significantly reduced by a supralethal, 200-Gy dose of mixed neutron-gamma radiation. This enzymatic change occurred within 4 minutes of exposure and lasted for at least 3 hours. In contrast, a very marked increase in monoamine oxidase activity was observed when animals received the same dose of radiation rich in gamma rays.[329]

5-hydroxytryptamine. Similar to norepipnehrine, there is contradiction about the effects of irradiation on 5 hydroxytryptamine (5 HT). While a radiogenic stimulation of 5 HT release following approximately 10 Gy was reported in one study, other studies observed a decrease or no change in 5-HT levels.[328,330,331]

Acetylcholine. A variety of measures involving the neurotransmitter acetylcholine (ACH) are altered by exposure to ionizing radiation. ACH synthesis rapidly increases in the hypothalamus of the rat after less than 0.02 Gy of beta radiation, but is inhibited at only slightly higher radiation doses.[315] A dose of 4 Gy of cobalt-60 gamma radiation produces a long-term increase in the rate of ACH synthesis in dogs.[332] Also, high-affinity choline uptake (a correlate of ACH turnover and release) slowly increases to 24% above control levels 15 minutes after irradiation with 100 Gy.[324] Choline uptake is back to normal by 30 minutes after exposure. Massive doses of gamma or X-rays (up to

600 Gy) are required to alter brain acetylcholinesterase activity,[333] whereas much smaller doses depress plasma acetylcholinesterase by 30%.[334]

Cyclic adenosine monophosphate. Cyclic nucleotides, such as cyclic adenosine monophosphate (cAMP), act as second messengers in synaptic transmission. After irradiation at a dose of 50 Gy, concentrations of cAMP are reduced in rats[335] and monkeys.[336] The transient nature of these changes also suggests their possible role in EPDs.

Histamine. The massive release of histamine after exposure to a large dose of ionizing radiation has been proposed as a mediator of radiogenic hypotension and EPDs.[337] Exposure to large doses of ionizing radiation results in postirradiation hypotension in monkeys,[118,338,339] with arterial blood pressure decreasing to less than 50% of normal.[340] Postirradiation hypotension also produces a decrease in cerebral blood flow immediately after a single dose of either 25 or 100 Gy of cobalt-60 gamma radiation.[118,123,341–343] This hypotension may be responsible for ETI after a supralethal dose of ionizing radiation.[118,341,343] In support of this hypothesis, the antihistamine chlorpheniramine maleate is effective in reducing performance decrements and postirradiation hypotension in monkeys.[340,344,345] However, other studies do not support a close association between blood pressure and behavioral changes.[118,346,347] Thus, changes in blood pressure may not be sufficient to explain behavioral and cognitive changes. Changes in blood pressure might also be pertinent to the potential therapeutic effects of antiinflammatory compounds that have antihypertensive effects as well (see "Inflammation" below).

Histamine is a very active biogenic amine and putative neurotransmitter located in neurons and mast cells throughout the body, especially around blood vessels.[348] Attempts to alter the development of behavioral deficits by treating animals with antihistamines before exposure have been encouraging.[95,96,340,349,350] Diphenhydramine (a histamine H1 receptor antagonist) inhibits radiation-induced cardiovascular dysfunction.[351] Because these histamine blockers produce only partial relief from radiation effects, the histamine hypothesis explains only a portion of the behavioral and physiological deficits observed after radiation exposure.[352]

Opioids. Cross-tolerance between endorphins and morphine has been demonstrated for a variety of behavioral and physiological measures.[71,114,193,353–361] Given the similarity of radiation and opiate-induced symptoms, endorphins might be involved in some aspects of radiogenic behavioral changes. For example, ionizing radiation produces dose-dependent analgesia in mice, and this can be reversed by the opiate antagonist naloxone.[151] Morphine-induced analgesia

in rats was enhanced 24 hours after neutron (but not gamma) irradiation, so combined delayed effects of endogenous and exogenous analgesics may be radiation specific.[152] Ionizing radiation exposure can also attenuate naloxone-precipitated abstinence syndrome in morphine-dependent rats.[362]

Further supporting a role for endorphins in radiation-induced behavioral changes, mice exhibit a similar stereotypic locomotor hyperactivity following morphine injection and after receiving 10 to 15 Gy of cobalt-60 gamma radiation.[106] This effect of irradiation is reversed by administering naloxone or by pre-exposing the mice to chronically stressful situations (a procedure that produces endorphin tolerance).[363–368] In addition, naloxone given immediately before exposure to 100 Gy of high-energy electrons attenuates ETI in rats.[366] Conversely, rats either undergo no change[187] or are more sensitive to radiation effects after chronic treatment with naloxone on a schedule that increases the number of endorphin receptors.[369] Similar to histamine, the manipulation of opioid systems cannot fully account for postirradiation performance deficits. Thus, multiple neurotransmitter systems might be involved in radiation-induced brain injury.

Inflammation

Following irradiation, neurogenesis is inversely correlated with the activation of microglia, and the antiinflammatory drug indomethacin partially restores radiation-induced decreases in neurogenesis.[370] Antiinflammatory drugs might antagonize radiation-induced cognitive injury as well. For example, the angiotensin-converting enzyme inhibitor ramipril[371] and angiotensin II type I receptor blocker L-158809[372] prevent or ameliorate fractionated, whole-brain, irradiation-induced cognitive impairments in rats. Angiotensin-converting enzyme converts angiotensin I to angiotensin II, a vasopressor that binds to the angiotenin II type 1 and type 2 receptors. While binding to type I receptors causes vasoconstrictive effects, binding to type II receptors produces vasodilating effects. Angiotensin II is proinflammatory, but angiotensin-converting enzyme inhibitors are used to reduce blood pressure as well. Because hypotension following irradiation might relate to early cognitive radiation-induced injury, as described earlier, different therapeutic approaches might be required to treat early radiation-induced cognitive injury.

ROS inhibitors are also tested for their ability to antagonize radiation-induced cognitive injury. However, the complex dual role of ROS in learning and memory—from being required for memory and long-term potentiation, but detrimental following chronically highly elevated levels—should be kept in mind. The beneficial effects of high ROS levels preirradiation in regard to cognitive changes following irradiation (as seen in mice lacking EC-SOD [extracellular superoxide dismutase]) underlines the need to consider ROS levels prior to irradiation as well. It could be argued that in most instances, ROS levels will be elevated in military personnel during combat missions.

Bone Marrow and Neural Stem Cells

Bone-marrow transplants have been used to challenge radiation-induced damage to the blood-forming systems (see Figure 7-3). This treatment might provide some behavioral benefits as well.[373] Measures of activity and lethality were recorded in rats that were irradiated with 6.5 Gy of X-rays. Twenty percent of the nontreated rats died, whereas 86% of the marrow-treated group survived. The initial decreases in spontaneous locomotor activity were less severe in the marrow-treated rats. Instead of showing a second drop in activity 10 days after irradiation, the treated rats showed near-normal activity for the entire 35 days of testing.[155] A similar outcome for behavior was observed in rats exposed to 7.5 Gy of whole-body X-rays, except for shielded, marrow-containing bones.[373] Consistent with these findings, implantation of bone-marrow stromal cells in the brains of neonatal mice enhanced object recognition 6 months later.[374] Similar beneficial effects might be seen when bone-marrow stromal cells or neural stem cells are given following irradiation. Although bone marrow or neural stem cell transplantation may be impractical in military situations, shielding may enable stem cells to survive. In addition, there is evidence that these cells serve as vehicles of neurotrophic factors, such as brain-derived neurotrophic factor. If this turns out to be the case, administration of one or a mixture of these neurotrophic factors might be sufficient to produce similar effects with regard to regenerating the injured brain and enhancing cognitive performance.

Antiemetics

The prodromal phase of radiation sickness, occurring hours to days after radiation exposure, includes nausea, vomiting, diarrhea, and abdominal cramp-ing.[187] The prodromal phase is distinct from acute radiation sickness in that the absorptive, secretory, and anatomic changes associated with radiation damage are not easily identifiable.[375] It is during the prodromal phase of radiation sickness that gastrointestinal motility changes[376,377] and motor activity in the gut contributes to some of the effects of radiation.[378,379] Although considerable research on antiemetics has been done, its focus has been mainly limited to drugs effective in radiation therapy.[181,380,381] In this regard, various antiinflammatory drugs (such as dexamethasone and steroids) have been useful in managing patients' emesis.[382,383] However, therapy makes few task demands on the recipients; in the military, antiemetics that are effective against radiation-induced vomiting must also not disrupt behavioral performance. That requirement significantly reduces the number of potentially useful antiemetics. For example, metoclopramide, dazopride, and zacopride (5-HT3 receptor blockers) were tested for antiemetic effects in monkeys exposed to 8 Gy of gamma radiation.[380] While all three drugs are effective antiemetics, only zacopride has no readily observable behavioral effects; metoclopramide disrupts motor performance and dazopride produces drowsiness.[180,311,384–388]

Shielding

In addition to pharmacological radioprotection, the immediate effects of radiation may be mitigated by shielding (placing material between the radiation source and the subject). Studies have focused on either head shielding (body exposed) or body shielding (head exposed). Head shielding offered significant protection from ETI. However, equivocal study results raise questions about the exclusive role of the brain in the production of radiation-induced performance deficits. As with radiation-induced taste aversion, postirradiation behaviors may be influenced by peripheral mechanisms that have not been fully explored.[179,389–393] These peripheral mechanisms might involve neuroimmune interactions as well. Together, these results suggest the need to determine the effects of therapeutics on various organs and outcome measures following whole-body irradiation. This will require a multidisciplinary approach and specific funding opportunities, like center grants, to engage such a broad approach.

SUMMARY

The success or failure of military operations is often measured in terms of missions completed or tasks performed. Exposure to ionizing radiation can significantly impede this success. In the case of low-to-intermediate doses of radiation (up to 10 Gy), performance changes may be slow to develop, may be relatively long lasting, and will usually abate before the onset of chronic radiation effects, such as cancers.

After large doses, the behavioral effects are often rapid (within minutes), and they usually abate before the onset of the debilitating chronic radiation sickness. These rapid effects can also occur after intermediate doses. But all tasks are not equally radiosensitive; tasks involving complex, demanding requirements are more easily disrupted than simple tasks, with the exception of certain naturalistic behaviors that are also radiosensitive. Radiation parameters such as dose, dose rate, fractionation, and quality can all influence the observed degree of performance changes. For example, electron radiation can produce more behavioral deficits than other radiation types, such as neutron radiation. In addition, combined injuries will probably be prevalent in future nuclear conflicts. Trauma interacts with radiation exposure in a complex fashion to modulate the direction and magnitude of the cognitive changes. The time interval and sequence of the two insults might be critical in how cognitive function is affected.

Possible sensory and neurophysiological mediators of radiation-induced behavioral changes have been identified. Long changes in performance may be mediated in part by radiogenic brain damage from ischemia, edema, direct damage to the parenchymal tissues themselves (such as dendrites and glia), or more subtle changes, such as alterations in a specific neurotransmitter or second messenger system. Various levels of neurotransmitters (such as acetylcholine, dopamine, and histamine), putative neurotransmitters (such as endorphins), and other neurochemicals (such as ROS) undergo significant changes after radiation exposure. Like the modifications of morphology and electrophysiology, many of these neurochemical changes may also be capable of mediating the performance decrements observed after ionizing radiation exposure.

More transient cerebrovascular changes after radiation exposure may also produce short-lived behavioral deficits. Postirradiation alterations in brain metabolism and the disruption of the normal electrophysiology of the axon and synapse may have important roles in certain performance changes. A wide range of neurochemical alterations following irradiation, such as the reduced ability of synaptic sodium channels to respond to stimulation, have been characterized. The radiosensitivity of the brain is revealed by the fact that alterations in the basic substrate of neural excitation are observed at doses of less than 1 Gy.

The literature on radiation-induced cognitive injury in animals is extensive. Limited human data are derived from radiation accidents or therapeutic studies, and correlate with the animal studies' findings. Based on all data now available, the Human Response Program of the DTRA has estimated the expected performance changes in irradiated soldiers. These projections depend on factors such as radiation dose, time after exposure, and task difficulty. Although complex, human and laboratory animal data should permit the description, prediction, and (eventually) amelioration of the behavioral effects of ionizing radiation exposure. However, many of the pharmacological compounds that protect animals from the lethality of ionizing radiation are associated with adverse behavioral changes. Increased efforts are warranted to further explore the potential for using behaviorally compatible antiemetics that have beneficial effects on multiple organ systems and outcome measures. Further research investigating selective physical shielding and cognitive injury following irradiation will facilitate development of post-radiation guidelines for preservation of physical and behavioral performance.

Acknowledgement

This work was partly supported by NASA grants NNJ08ZSA001N, NNX12AB54G, NSCOR NNJ08ZSA003N, and DoD grant W81XWH-09-1-0426.

REFERENCES

1. Young R, Auton D. The Defense Nuclear Agency Intermediate Dose Program. In: Proceedings of the Psychology in the Department of Defense, Ninth Symposium. Colorado Springs, CO: US Air Force Academy; 1984.

2. United Nations Scientific Committee on the Effects of Atomic Radiation. *Effects of Ionizing Radiation: Report to the General Assembly, With Scientific Annexes.* Vol 1. New York, NY: United Nations; 2008.

3. Martin C, Sutton D, West C, Wright E. The radiobiology/radiation protection interface in healthcare. *J Radiol Prot.* 2009;29:A1–A20.

4. Morgan WF. Non-targeted and delayed effects of exposure to ionizing radiation: I. Radiation-induced genomic instability and bystander effects in vitro. *Radiat Res*. 2003;159:567–580.

5. Hall E. The bystander effect. *Health Phys*. 2003;85:31–35.

6. Shipman T, Lushbaugh C, Peterson D, et al. Acute radiation death resulting from an accidental nuclear critical excursion. *J Occup Med*. 1961;3:146–192.

7. Karas J, Stanbury J. Fatal radiation syndrome from an accidental nuclear excursion. *N Engl J Med*. 1965;272:755–761.

8. Wald N, Thoma GE Jr. Radiation accidents: medical aspects of neutron and gamma ray exposures. *ORNL*. 1961;PtB:1–177.

9. Howland J. *The Lockport Incident: Accidental Exposure of Humans to Large Doses of X-Irradiation. Diagnosis and Treatment of Acute Radiation Injury*. Geneva, Switzerland: World Health Organization; 1961: 11–26.

10. Telyatnikov L. The top story of 1987. Paper presented at the Great American Firehouse Exposition and Muster; Baltimore, MD; 1987. Online Computer Library Catalogue number 18595371.

11. Young RW. Chernobyl in retrospect. 1988;39(1-3):27–32.

12. Cardis E, Howe G, Ron E, et al. Cancer consequences of the Chernobyl accident: 20 years on. *J Radiol Prot*. 2006;26:127–140.

13. Worgul BV, Kundiyev YI, Sergiyenko NM, et al. Cataracts among Chernobyl clean-up workers: implications regarding permissible eye exposures. *Radiat Res*. 2007;167:233–243.

14. Ainsbury EA, Bouffler SD, Dörr W, et al. Radiation cataractogenesis: a review of recent studies. *Radiat Res*. 2009;172:1–9.

15. Little J. The Chernobyl accident, congenital anomalies and other reproductive outcomes. *Paediatr Perinat Epidemiol*. 1993;7:121–151.

16. Verger P. Down syndrome and ionizing radiation. *Health Phys*. 1997;73:882–893.

17. Loganovsky KN, Volovik SV, Manton KG, Bazyka DA, Flor-Henry P. Whether ionizing radiation is a risk factor for schizophrenia spectrum disorders? *World J Biol Psychiatry*. 2005;6:212–230.

18. Manton KG, Volovik S, Kulminski A. ROS effects on neurodegeneration in Alzheimer's disease and related disorders: on environmental stresses of ionizing radiation. *Curr Alzheimer Res*. 2004;1:277–293.

19. Trivedi A, Hannan MA. Radiation and cardiovascular diseases. *J Environ Pathol Toxicol Oncol*. 2004;23:99–106.

20. Balonov M. Third annual Warren K. Sinclair keynote address: retrospective analysis of impacts of the Chernobyl accident. *Health Phys*. 2007;93:383–409.

21. Modan B. Cancer and leukemia risks after low level radiation—controversy, facts and future. *Med Oncol Tumor Pharmacother*. 1987;4:151–161.

22. Shore R. Low-dose radiation epidemiology studies: status and issues. *Health Phys*. 2009;97:481–486.

23. Ron E. Thyroid cancer incidence among people living in areas contaminated by radiation from the Chernobyl accident. *Health Phys*. 2007;93:502–511.

24. Rahu M. Health effects of the Chernobyl accident: fears, rumours and the truth. *Eur J Cancer*. 2003;39:295–299.

25. Bromet E, Havenaar J. Psychological and perceived health effects of the Chernobyl disaster: a 20-year review. *Health Phys*. 2007;93:516–521.

26. Bromet E, Gluzman S, Schwartz J, Goldgaber D. Somatic symptoms in women 11 years after the Chornobyl accident: prevalence and risk factors. *Environ Health Perspect*. 2002;110(Suppl 4):625–629.

27. Bromet E, Goldgaber D, Carlson G et al. Children's well-being 11 years after the Chernobyl catastrophe. *Arch Gen Psychiatry*. 2000;57:563–571.

28. Jargin S. Thyroid carcinoma in children and adolescents resulting from the Chernobyl accident: possible causes of the incidence increase overestimation. *Cesk Patol*. 2009;45:50–52.

29. Litcher L, Bromet E, Carlson G, et al. School and neuropsychological performance of evacuated children in Kyiv 11 years after the Chornobyl disaster. *J Child Psychol Psychiatry*. 2000;41:291–299.

30. Bar Joseph N, Reisfeld D, Tirosh E, Silman Z, Rennert G. Neurobehavioral and cognitive performances of children exposed to low-dose radiation in the Chernobyl accident: The Israeli Chernobyl Health Effects Study. *Am J Epidemiol*. 2004;160:453–459.

31. Health Consequences of the Chernobyl Accident. Results of the IPHECA Pilot Project and Related National Programmes. Geneva, Switzerland: World Health Organization; 1995.

32. Loganovsky K, Loganovskaja T. Schizophrenia spectrum disorders in persons exposed to ionizing radiation as a result of the Chernobyl accident. *Schizophr Bull*. 2000;26:751–773.

33. Polyukhov A, Kobsar I, Grebelnik V, Voitenko V. The accelerated occurrence of age-related changes of organism in Chernobyl workers: a radiation-induced progeroid syndrome? *Exp Gerontol*. 2000;35:105–115.

34. Hasterlik R, Marinelli L. Physical dosimetry and clinical observations on four human beings involved in an accidental critical assembly excursion. *Proceedings of the International Conference on Peaceful Uses of Atomic Energy*. Vol 11. Geneva, Switzerland: International Atomic Energy Commission; 1956.

35. Payne R. Effects of ionizing radiation exposure on human psychomotor skills. *US Armed Forces Med J*. 1959;10:1009–1021.

36. Anno GH, Wilson DB, Dore MA. *Nuclear Weapon Effect Research at PSR—1983: Acute Radiation Effects on Individual Crewmember Performance*. Washington, DC: Defense Nuclear Agency; 1985. Technical Report TR-85-52; NTIS AD-A166-282-4-XAB.

37. Anderson N. Late complications in childhood central nervous system tumour survivors. *Curr Opin Neurol*. 2003;16:677–683.

38. Alicikus ZA, Akman F, Ataman OU, et al. Importance of patient, tumour and treatment related factors on quality of life in head and neck cancer patients after definitive treatment. *Eur Arch Otorhinolaryngol*. 2009;266:1461–1468.

39. Grill J, Kieffer V, Kalifa C. Measuring the neuro-cognitive side-effects of irradiation in children with brain tumors. *Pediatr Blood Cancer*. 2004;42:452–456.

40. Taphoorn M. Neurocognitive sequelae in the treatment of low-grade gliomas. *Semin Oncol*. 2003;30:45–48.

41. Calabrese P, Schlegel U. Neurotoxicity of treatment. *Recent Results Cancer Res*. 2009;171:165–174.

42. Douw L, Klein M, Fagel SS, et al. Cognitive and radiological effects of radiotherapy in patients with low-grade glioma: long-term follow-up. *Lancet Neurol*. 2009;8:810–818.

43. Quesnel C, Savard J, Ivers H. Cognitive impairments associated with breast cancer treatments: results from a longitudinal study. *Breast Cancer Res Treat*. 2009;116:113–123.

44. Greimel E, Winter R, Kapp K, Haas J. Quality of life and sexual functioning after cervical cancer treatment: a long-term follow-up study. *Psychooncology*. 2009;18:476–482.

45. Schagen S, Boogerd W, Muller M, et al. Cognitive complaints and cognitive impairment following BEP chemotherapy in patients with testicular cancer. *Acta Oncol*. 2008;47:63–70.

46. Pedersen AD, Rossen P, Mehlsen MY, Pedersen CG, Zachariae R, von der Maase H. Long-term cognitive function following chemotherapy in patients with testicular cancer. *J Int Neuropsychol Soc*. 2009;15:296–301.

47.   Young R, Myers P. The human response to nuclear radiation. *Med Bull.* 1986;43:20–23.

48.   Baum SJ, Anno GH, Young RW, Withers HR. Nuclear weapon effect research at PSR—1983. In: *Symptomatology of Acute Radiation Effects in Humans After Exposure to Doses of 75 to 4500 Rads (cGy) Free-in-Air.* Vol 10. Washington, DC: Defense Nuclear Agency; 1985. Technical Report TR-85-50; NTIS AD-A166-280-8-XAB.

49.   Franz CG, Young RW, Mitchell WE. *Behavioral Studies Following Ionizing Radiation Exposures: A Data Base.* Bethesda, MD: Armed Forces Radiobiology Research Institute; 1981. Technical Report TR81-4; NTIS AD-A115-825-2.

50.   Anno GH, Young RW, Bloom RM, Mercier JR. Dose response relationships for acute ionizing-radiation lethality. *Health Phys.* 2003;84:565–575.

51.   Anno GH, Baum SJ, Withers HR, Young RW. Symptomatology of acute radiation effects in humans after exposure to doses of 0.5–30 Gy. *Health Phys.* 1989;56:821–838.

52.   Seigneur LJ, Brennan JT. *Incapacitation in the Monkey (Macaca Mulatta) Following Exposure to a Pulse of Reactor Radiation.* Bethesda, MD: Armed Forces Radiobiology Research Institute; 1966. Scientific Report SR66-2.

53.   Cassaret G. *Radiation Histopathology.* Vol 2. Boca Raton, FL: CRC Press; 1980.

54.   Hopewell J. Late radiation damage to the central nervous system: a radiobiological interpretation. *Neuropathol Appl Neurobiol.* 1979;5:329–343.

55.   Lyman R, Kupalov R, Scholz W, et al. Effects of roentgen rays on the central nervous system. Results of large doses on the brains of adult dogs. *AMA Arch Neurol Psychiat.* 1933;29:56–87.

56.   Hohwieler M, Lo T, Silverman M, Freiberg S. Brain necrosis after radiotherapy for primary intracerebral tumor. *Neurosurgery.* 1986;18:67–74.

57.   Pallis C, Louis S, Morgan R. Brain myelopathy. *Brain.* 1961;84:460–479.

58.   Dynes JB, Smedal MI. Radiation myelitis. *Am J Roentgenol Radium Ther Nucl Med.* 1960;83:78–87.

59.   Marks J, Wong J. The risk of cerebral radionecrosis in relation to dose, time and fractionation. A follow-up study. *Prog Exp Tumor Res.* 1985;29:210–218.

60.   Switzer RC III, Bogo V, Mickley GA. Histologic effects of high energy electron and proton irradiation of rat brain detected with a silver-degeneration stain. *Adv Space Res.* 1994;14(10):443–451.

61.   Arnold A, Bailey P, Harvey R. Intolerance of primate brain stem and hypothalamus to conventional high energy radiations. *Neurology.* 1954;4:575–585.

62.   Lindgren M. On tolerance of brain tissue and sensitivity of brain tumors to irradiation. *Acta Radiol Suppl.* 1958;170:5–75.

63.   Yoshii Y, Maki Y, Tsunemoto H, Koike S, Kasuga T. The effect of acute total-head X irradiation on C3H/He mice. *Radiat Res.* 1981;86:152–170.

64.   Ross JA, Levitt SR, Holst EA, Clemente CD. Neurological and electroencephalographic effects of X irradiation of the head in monkeys. *AMA Arch Neurol Psychiat.* 1954;71:238–249.

65.   Ibrahim MZ, Haymaker W, Miquel J, Riopelle AJ. Effects of radiation on the hypothalamus in monkeys. *Arch Psychiatr Nervenkr.* 1967;210:1–15.

66.   Roizin L, Akai K, Carsten A, et al. Post X ray myelinopathy (pathogenicm mechanisms). In: Yonawa T, ed. *International Symposium on the Aetiology and Pathogenesis of Demyelinating Diseases.* Neiho Sha: Japan Press Co; 1976: 29–57.

67.   van der Kogel A. Radiation induced damage in the central nervous system: an interpretation of target cell responses. *Br J Cancer Suppl.* 1986;7:207–217.

68. Abdullin GZ. *Study of Comparative Radiosensitivity of Different Parts of Brain in Terms of Altered Function.* Washington, DC: Office of the Secretary/Department of Commerce; 1962. Atomic Energy Commission TR-5141.

69. Hunt EL, Kimeldorf D. Behavioral arousal and neural activation as radiosensitive reactions. *Radiat Res.* 1964;21:91–110.

70. Christensen H, Flesher A, Haley T. Changes in brain self-stimulation rates after exposure to x-irradiation. *J Pharm Sci.* 1969;58:128–129.

71. Mickley G, Teitelbaum H. Persistence of lateral hypothalamic-mediated behaviors after a supralethal dose of ionizing radiation. *Aviat Space Environ Med.* 1978;49:863–873.

72. Mechanick JI, Hochberg FH, LaRocque A. Hypothalamic dysfunction following whole brain irradiation. *J Neurosurg.* 1986;65:490–494.

73. Rosenthal F, Timiras P. Changes in brain excitability after whole-body x-irradiation in the rat. *Radiat Res.* 1961;18:648–657.

74. Rosenthal F, Timiras PS. Threshold and pattern of electroshock seizures after 250 r whole-body x-irradiation in rats. *Proc Soc Exp Biol Med.* 1961;108:267–270.

75. Gangloff H. Acute effects of X irradiation on brain electrical activity in cats and rabbits. In: *Effects of Ionizing Radiation on the Nervous System Proceedings.* Vienna, Austria: International Atomic Energy Agency; 1962: 187–196.

76. Gerstner H. Effect of high-intensity x-irradiation on the A group fibers of the frog sciatic nerve. *Am J Physiol.* 1956;184:333–337.

77. Obenaus A, Huang L, Smith A, Favre CJ, Nelson G, Kendall E. Magnetic resonance imaging and spectroscopy of the rat hippocampus 1 month after exposure to 56Fe-particle radiation. *Radiat Res.* 2008;169:149–161.

78. Huang L, Smith A, Cummings P, Kendall EJ, Obenaus A. Neuroimaging assessment of memory-related brain structures in a rat model of acute space-like radiation. *J Magn Reson Imaging.* 2009;29:785–792.

79. Huang L, Smith A, Badaut J, Obenaus A. Dynamic characteristics of 56Fe-particle radiation-induced alterations in the rat brain: magnetic resonance imaging and histological assessments. *Radiat Res.* 2010;173:729–737.

80. Berg NO, Lindgren M. Time-dose relationship and morphology of delayed radiation lesions of the brain of the rabbit. 1958;167:1–118.

81. Russell DS, Wilson CW, Tansley K. Experimental radio-necrosis in the brains of rabbits. *J Neurol Neurosurg Psychiatry.* 1949;12:187–195.

82. Archambeau JO, Mao XW, McMillan PJ, et al. Dose response of rat retinal microvessels to proton dose schedules used clinically: a pilot study. *Int J Radiat Oncol Biol Phys.* 2000;48:1155–1166.

83. Mao XW. A quantitative study of the effects of ionizing radiation on endothelial cells and capillary-like network formation. *Technol Cancer Res Treat.* 2006;5:127–134.

84. Mao XW, Crapo JD, Mekonnen T, et al. Radioprotective effect of a metalloporphyrin compound in rat eye model. *Curr Eye Res.* 2009;34:62–72.

85. Caveness WF. Pathology of radiation damage to the normal brain of the monkey. *Natl Cancer Inst Monogr.* 1977;46:57–76.

86. Caveness W. Experimental observations: delayed necrosis in normal monkey brain. In: Gilbert H, Kagen A, eds. *Radiation Damage to the Nervous System.* New York, NY: Raven Press, 1980.

87. Hopewell JW, Wright EA. The nature of latent cerebral irradiation damage and its modification by hypertension. *Br J Radiol.* 1970;43:161–167.

88. Hirata Y, Matsukado Y, Mihara Y, Kochi M, Sonoda H, Fukumura A. Occlusion of the internal carotid artery after radiation therapy for the chiasmal lesion. *Acta Neurochir (Wein).* 1985;74:141–147.

89. Haymaker W, ed. Morphological changes in the nervous system following exposure to ionizing radiation. In: *Effects of Ionizing Radiation on the Nervous System Proceedings*. Vienna, Austria: International Atomic Energy Agency; 1962: 309–358.

90. Kemper TL, O'Neill R, Caveness WF. Effects of single dose supervoltage whole brain radiation in *Macaca mulatta*. *J Neuropathol Exp Neurol*. 1977;36:916–940.

91. Nguyen V, Gaber MW, Sontag MR, Kiani MF. Late effects of ionizing radiation on the microvascular networks in normal tissue. *Radiat Res*. 2000;154:531–536.

92. Roth N, Sontag M, Kiani M. Early effects of ionizing radiation on the microvascular networks in normal tissue. *Radiat Res*. 1999;151:270–277.

93. Kiani MF, Ansari R, Gaber MW. Oxygen delivery in irradiated normal tissue. *J Radiat Res (Tokyo)*. 2003;44:15–21.

94. Ansari R, Gaber MW, Wang B, Pattillo CB, Miyamoto C, Kiani MF. Anti-TNFa (TNF-alpha) treatment abrogates radiation-induced changes in vascular density and tissue oxygenation. *Radiat Res*. 2007;167:80–86.

95. Villasana L, Rosenberg J, Raber J. Sex-dependent effects of 56Fe irradiation on contextual fear conditioning in C57BL/6J mice. *Hippocampus*. 2010;20:19–23.

96. Villasana L, Acevedo S, Poage C, Raber J. Sex- and ApoE isoform-dependent effects of radiation on cognitive function. *Radiat Res*. 2006;166:883–891.

97. Brudno M, Poliakov A, Salamov A, et al. Automated whole-genome multiple alignment of rat, mouse, and human. *Genome Res*. 2004;14:685–692.

98. Tecott LH. The genes and brains of mice and men. *Am J Psychiatr*. 2003;160:646–656.

99. Mickley G. Psychological phenomena associated with nuclear warfare: potential animal models. In: Young R, ed. *Proceedings of the Defense Nuclear Agency Symposium Workshop on the Psychological Effects of Tactical Nuclear Warfare*. Washington, DC: Defense Nuclear Agency; 1987. DNA-TR-87-209; 7-1–7-35.

100. Bogo V, Franz CG, Jacobs AJ, Weiss JF, Young RW. Effects of ethiofos (WR-2721) and radiation on monkey visual discrimination performance. *Pharmacol Ther*. 1988;39:93–95.

101. Kimeldorf DJ, Jones DC, Castanera TJ. Effect of x-irradiation upon the performance of daily exhaustive exercise by the rat. *Am J Physiol*. 1953;174:331–335.

102. Hall E. *Radiobiology for the Radiologist*. Hagerstown, MD: Harper and Row; 1973.

103. Casarett A. *Radiation Biology*. Englewood Cliffs, NJ: Prentice Hall, Inc; 1968.

104. Bogo V. Effects of bremsstrahlung and electron radiation on rat motor performance. *Radiat Res*. 1984;100:313–320.

105. Casarett AP. Swim-tank measurement of radiation-induced behavioral incapacitation. *Psychol Rep*. 1973;33:731–736.

106. Mickley GA, Stevens KE, White GA, Gibbs GL. Endogenous opiates mediate radiogenic behavioral change. *Science*. 1983;220:1185–1187.

107. Davis R. The radiation syndrome. In: Schrier A, Harlow H, Stollnitz F, eds. *Behavior of Nonhuman Primates*. New York, NY: Academic Press; 1965: 495–524.

108. Bogo V. *Comparative Effects of Bremsstrahlung, Gamma, and Electron Radiation on Rat Motor Performance*. Bethesda, MD: Armed Forces Radiobiology Research Institute; 1984.

109. Bogo V, Zeman G, Dooley M. Radiation quality and rat motor performance. *Radiat Res*. 1989;118:341–352.

110. George RE, Chaput RL, Verrelli DM, Barron EL. The relative effectiveness of fission neutrons for miniature pig performance decrement. *Radiat Res*. 1971;48:332–345.

111. Thorp J. *Beagle and Miniature Pig Response to Partial Body Irradiation: Dose Relationships*. Bethesda, MD: Armed Forces Radiobiology Research Institute; 1970. TN70-5; DTIC: AD717591.

112. Curran C, Conrad D, Young R. *The Effects of 2,000 rads of Pulsed Gamma Neutron Radiation Upon the Performance of Unfettered Monkeys*. Bethesda, MD: Armed Forces Radiobiology Research Institute; 1971. SR71-3; DTIC: AD724653.

113. Hunt W. Comparative effects of exposure to high-energy electrons and gamma radiation on active avoidance behaviour. *Int J Radiat Biol Relat Stud Phys Chem Med*. 1983;44:257–260.

114. Kimeldorf D, Hunt E. *Ionizing Radiation. Neural Function and Behavior*. New York, NY: Academic Press; 1965.

115. Bogo V, Franz C, Young R. Effects of radiation on monkey discrimination performance. In: Fielden E, Fowler J, Hendry J, Scott D, eds. *Proceedings of the Eighth International Congress of Radiation Research*. Edinburgh, Scotland: International Congress of Radiation Research; 1987.

116. Franz C. Effects of mixed neutron gamma total body irradiation on physical activity performance of rhesus monkeys. *Radiat Res*. 1985;101:434–441.

117. Young R. Prediction of the Relative Toxicity of Environmental Toxins as a Function of Behavioral and Non-Behavioral End Points. Washington, DC: The Catholic University of America; 1979.

118. Bruner A. Immediate dose rate effects of 60Co on performance and blood pressure in monkeys. *Radiat Res*. 1977;70:378–390.

119. Germas J, Shelton Q. *Performance of the Monkey Following Multiple Supralethal Pulses of Radiation*. Bethesda, MD: Armed Forces Radiobiology Research Institute; 1969.

120. Young R, McFarland W. *Performance of the Monkey (Macaca mulatta) After Two 2500 rad Pulses of Mixed Gamma Neutron Radiation*. Bethesda, MD: Armed Forces Radiobiology Research Institute; 1972.

121. Mele P, Franz C, Harrison J. Effects of ionizing radiation on fix ratio escape performance in rats. *Soc Neurosci Abstr*. 1987;13(2):998.

122. Barnes DJ, Brown GC, Fractor BS. Differential effects of multiple and single irradiations upon the primate equilibrium function. Brooks Air Force Base, TX: US Air Force School of Aerospace Medicine; 1971. USAFSAM-TR-71-1.

123. Chapman PH, Young RJ. Effect of cobalt-60 gamma irradiation on blood pressure and cerebral blood flow in the Macaca mulatta. *Radiat Res*. 1968;35:78–85.

124. Chaput R, Berardo P, Barron E. *Increased Brain Radioresistance After Supralethal Irradiation*. Bethesda, MD: Armed Forces Radiobiology Research Institute; 1973.

125. Davis R, Steele J. Performance selections through radiation death in rhesus monkeys. *J Psychol*. 1963;56:119.

126. George R, Chaput R, Barron E. *The Dependence of Miniature Pig Performance Decrement Upon Gamma Ray Dose Rate*. Bethesda, MD: Armed Forces Radiobiology Research Institute; 1972.

127. Morse D, Mickley G. Dose rate and sex effects on the suppression of appetitive behavior following exposure to gamma spectrum radiation. In: *Abstracts of the 36th Annual Meeting of Radiation Research Society*. Vol 163. Philadelphia, PA: Radiation Research Society; 1988.

128. Bogo V. Radiation: behavioral implications in space. *Toxicology*. 1988;49:299–307.

129. Mickley G, Bogo V, Landauer M, Mele P. Current trends in behavioral radiobiology. In: Swenberg C, ed. *Terrestrial Space Radiation and its Biological Effects*. New York, NY: Plenum Press; 1988.

130. Hunt W, Rabin B, Joseph J, et al, eds. Effects of ion particles on behavior and brain function: initial studies. In: *Terrestrial Space Radiation and its Biological Effects*. New York, NY: Plenum Press; 1988.

131. Philpott D, Sapp W, Miquel J, et al. The effect of high energy (HZE) particle radiation (40Ar) on aging parameter of mouse hippocampus and retina. *Scan Electron Microsc*. 1985;(Pt 3):1177–1182.

132. Gleitman H. *Basic Psychology*. New York: W.W. Norton and Co; 1983.

133. Wheeler TG, Tilton BM. Duration of memory loss due to electron beam exposure. Brooks Air Force Base, TX: US Air Force School of Aerospace Medicine; 1983. USAFSAM-TR-83-33.

134. Furchtgott E. Ionizing radiations and the nervous system. In: *Biology of Brain Dysfunction*. Vol 3. New York, NY: Plenum Press; 1975: 343–379.

135. Furchtgott E. Behavioral effects of ionizing radiations. In: Furchtgott E, ed. *Pharmacology and Biophysical Agents and Behavior*. New York, NY: Academic Press; 1971: 1–64.

136. Graham ES, Farrer DN, Carsten AL, Roizin L. Decrements in the visual acuity of rhesus monkeys (Macaca mulatta) as a delayed effect of occipital cortex irradiation. *Radiat Res*. 1971;45:373–383.

137. Caveness W, Tanaka A, Hess K, Kemper TL, Tso MO, Zimmerman LE. Delayed brain swelling and functional derangement after X-irradiation of the right visual cortex in the Macaca mulatta. *Radiat Res*. 1974;57:104–120.

138. Minamisawa T, Sugiyama H, Tsuchiya T, Eto H. Effects of x-irradiation on evoked potentials from visual systems in rabbits. *J Radiat Res (Tokyo)*. 1970;11:127–133.

139. Minamisawa T, Tsuchiya T, Eto H. Changes in the averaged evoked potentials of the rabbit during and after fractionated x-irradiation. *Electroencephalogr Clin Neurophysiol*. 1972;33:591–601.

140. Kekcheyev K. Changes in the threshold of achromatic vision of man by the action of ultrashort, ultraviolet, and X rays waves. *Probl Fiziol Opt*. 1941;1:77–79.

141. Lenoir A. Adaptation und roentgenbesstrahlung. *Radio Clin*. 1944;13:264–276.

142. McDowell A, Brown W. Visual acuity performance of normal and chronic focal head irradiated monkeys. *J Genet Psychol*. 1960;93:139–144.

143. Riopelle A, ed. *Some Behavioral Effects of Ionizing Radiation on Primates*. New York, NY: Academic Press; 1962.

144. Murphy J, Harris J. Negligible effects of X irradiation of the head upon hearing in the rat. *J Aud Res*. 1961;1:117–132.

145. Jarrard LE. Effects of x-irradiation on operant behavior in the rat. *J Comp Physiol Psychol*. 1963;56:608–611.

146. Borsanyi S. The effects of radiation therapy on the ear: with particular reference to radiation otitis media. *South Med J*. 1962;55:740–743.

147. Tokimoto T, Kanagawa K. Effects of X-ray irradiation on hearing in guinea pigs. *Acta Otolaryngol*. 1985;100:266–272.

148. Moskovskaia NV. Effect of ionizing radiations on the functions of the vestibular analyzer [article in Russian]. *Vestn Otorinolaringol*. 1959;21:59–62.

149. Apanasenko Z. *Combined Effect of Double Exposure to Vibration and Chronic Irradiation on the Functional State of Vestibular Apparatus*. Washington, DC: National Aeronautics and Space Administration; 1967: 212–228.

150. Furchtgott E. Behavioral effects of ionizing radiation. *Psychol Bull*. 1963;60:157–199.

151. Teskey GC, Kavaliers M. Ionizing radiation induces opioid-mediated analgesia in male mice. *Life Sci*. 1984;35:1547–1552.

152. Burghardt W, Hunt W. The interactive effects of morphine and ionizing radiation on the latency of tail withdrawal from warm water in the rat. In: *Proceedings of the Ninth Symposium on Psychology in the Department of Defense*. Colorado Springs, CO: United States Air Force Academy; 1984: 73–76.

153. Doull J. Pharmacological responses in irradiated animals. *Radiat Res.* 1967;30:333–341.

154. Wilson RC, Vacek T, Lanier DL, Dewsbury DA. Open-field behavior in muroid rodents. *Behav Biol.* 1976;17:495–506.

155. Jones DC, Kimeldorf DJ, Rubadeau DO, Osborn GK, Castanera TJ. Effects of x-irradiation on performance of volitional activity by the adult male rat. *Am J Physiol.* 1954;177:243–250.

156. Arnold W. Behavioral effects of cranial irradiation of rats. In: Haley TJ, Snider RS, eds. *Response of the Nervous System to Ionizing Radiation.* New York, NY: Academic Press; 1962; 669–682.

157. Castanera TJ, Jones DC, Kimeldorf DJ. The effects of x irradiation on the diffuse activity performance of rats, guinea pigs and hamsters. *Br J Radiol.* 1959;32:386–389.

158. Fields PE. The effect of whole-body x-radiation upon activity drum, straightaway, and maze performances of white rats. *J Comp Physiol Psychol.* 1957;50:386–391.

159. Fields PE. The effect of whole body X radiation upon activity drum, straightaway, and maze performances of white rats. *J Genet Psychol.* 1960;97:67–76.

160. McDowell AA, Brown WL. Comparisons of running wheel activity of normal and chronic irradiated rats under varying conditions of food deprivation. *J Genet Psychol.* 1960;96:79–83.

161. Landauer M, Davis H, Dominitz J, Pierce S. Effects of acute gamma radiation exposure on locomotor activity in Swiss Webster mice. *The Toxicologist.* 1987;7:253.

162. Brown W, McDowell A. Some effects of radiation on psychologic processes in rhesus monkeys. In: Haley T, Snider R, eds. *Response of the Nervous System to Ionizing Radiation.* New York, NY: Academic Press, Inc; 1962: 729–746.

163. Leary RW, Ruch TC. Activity, manipulation drive, and strength in monkeys subjected to low-level irradiation. *J Comp Physiol Psychol.* 1955;48:336–342.

164. McDowell A, Davis R, Steele J. Application of systematic direct observational methods to analysis of the radiation syndrome in monkeys. *Percept Mot Skills.* 1956;6:117–130.

165. Mattsson JL, Yochmowitz MG. Radiation induced emesis in monkeys. *Radiat Res.* 1980;82:191–199.

166. McDowell A. The immediate effects of single dose of whole body X radiation upon the social behavior and self care of caged rhesus monkeys. *Am Psychol.* 1954;9:423.

167. Maier DM, Landauer MR. Effects of gamma radiation on aggressive behavior in male Swiss Webster mice. *Soc Neurosci Abstr.* 1987;13(2):933.

168. Vogel H Jr. The effect of X irradiation on fighting behavior in male mice. *Anat Rec.* 1950;108:547.

169. Burke R, Mattsson J, Fischer J. *Effect of Ionizing Radiation on Shock Elicited Aggression of Male Rats.* Brooks Air Force Base, TX: US Air Force School of Aerospace Medicine; 1981.

170. O'Boyle M. Suppresssion of mouse-killing in rats following irradiation. *Percept Mot Skills.* 1976;42:511–514.

171. Ader R, Hahn E. Effects of social environment on mortality to whole body x irradiation in the rat. *Psychol Rep.* 1963;13:211–215.

172. Ader R, Hahn E. Dominance and emotionality in the rat and their effects on mortality after whole-body X irradiation. *Psychol Rep.* 1963;13:617–618.

173. Maier DM, Landauer MR. Effects of acute sublethal gamma radiation exposure on aggressive behavior in male mice: a dose-response study. *Aviat Space Environ Med.* 1989;60(8):774–778.

174. Rugh R, Grupp E. X-irradiation lethality aggravated by sexual activity of male mice. *Am J Physiol.* 1960;198:1352–1354.

175. Landauer MR, Davis HD, Dominitz JA, Weiss JF. Long-term effects of the radioprotector WR 2721 on locomotor activity and body weight of mice following ionizing radiation. *Toxicology.* 1988;49:315–323.

176. Sharp J, Kelly D, Brady J. The radio attenuating effects of n decylaminoethanethiosulfuric acid in the rhesus monkey. In: Vagtborg H, ed. *Use of Nonhuman Primates in Drug Evaluation.* San Antonio, TX: Southwest Foundation for Research and Education; 1968: 338–346.

177. Davis RT. Latent changes in the food preferences of irradiated monkeys. *J Genet Psychol.* 1958;92:53–59.

178. Garcia J, Kimeldorf D, Knelling RA. A conditioned aversion to saccharin resulting from exposure to gamma radiation. *Science.* 1955;122:157–158.

179. Rabin BM, Hunt WA. Mechanisms of radiation-induced conditioned taste aversion learning. *Neurosci Biobehav Rev.* 1986;10:55–65.

180. Dubois A, Fiala N, Bogo V. Treatment of radiation induced vomiting and gastric emptying suppression with zacopride— Part 2. *Gastroenterology.* 1987;92(5):1376.

181. Young R. Mechanisms and treatment of radiation induced nausea and vomiting. In: Davis C, Lake Bakaar G, Grahame Smith G, eds. *Nausea and Vomiting: Mechanisms and Treatment.* New York, NY: Springer-Verlag; 1986: 94–109.

182. Middleton GR, Young RW. Emesis in monkeys following exposure to ionizing radiation. *Aviat Space Environ Med.* 1975;46:170–172.

183. Stapleton GE, Curtis HJ. *The Effects of Fast Neutrons on the Ability of Mice to Take Forced Exercise.* US Atomic Energy Rep. No. 9. Oak Ridge, TN: Oak Ridge National Laboratory; 1946. MDDC-696.

184. Jetter W, Lindsley O, Wohlwill F. *The Effects of X Irradiation on Physical Exercise and Behavior in the Dog; Related Hematological and Pathological Control Studies.* New York, NY: Atomic Energy Commission; 1953.

185. Jones D, Kimeldorf D, Rubadeau D, Castanera T. Relationships between volitional activity and age in the male rat. *Am J Physiol.* 1953;172:109–114.

186. Kimeldorf DJ, Jones DC. The relationship of radiation dose to lethality among exercised animals exposed to roentgen rays. *Am J Physiol.* 1951;167:626–632.

187. Bogo V. Behavioral radioprotection. *Pharmacol Ther.* 1988;39:73–78.

188. Martin BA, Michaelson SM. Exercise performance of upper-body x-irradiated dogs. *Am J Physiol.* 1966;211:457–461.

189. Smith F, Smith WW. Exercise effects on tolerance to radiation. *Am J Physiol.* 1951;165:662–666.

190. Mickley GA, Ferguson JL, Nemeth TJ, Mulvihill MA, Alderks CE. Spontaneous perseverative turning in rats with radiation-induced hippocampal damage. *Behav Neurosci.* 1989;103(4):722–730.

191. Brown W, White R. Preirradiation as a factor in the prevention of irradiation deaths in rats. *J Genet Psychol.* 1958;93:287–290.

192. Brown W, White R. A study of fatigue and mortality in irradiated rats. *Radiat Res.* 1960;13:610–616.

193. Chaput RL, Wise D. Miniature pig incapacitation and performance decrement after mixed gamma-neutron irradiation. *Aerospace Med.* 1970;41:290–293.

194. Chaput RL, Barron E. Postradiation performance of miniature pigs modified by tasks. *Radiat Res.* 1973;53:392–401.

195. Mickley GA. Behavioral and physiological changes produced by a supralethal dose of ionizing radiation: evidence for hormone-influenced sex differences in the rat. *Radiat Res.* 1980;81:48–75.

196. Wheeler T, Hardy K, Anderson L, Richards S. *Motor Performance in Irradiated Rats as a Function of Radiation Source, Dose, and Time Since Exposure*. Brooks Air Force Base, TX: US Air Force School of Aerospace Medicine; 1984; USAFSAM-TR-84-4.

197. Janis I. *Air War and Emotional Stress*. New York, NY: McGraw Hill; 1951.

198. Jammet H, Mathe G, Pendic B, et al. Study of six cases of accidental whole body irradiation [article in French]. *Rev Fr Etud Clin Biol*. 1959;4:210–225.

199. Tofilon P, Fike J. The radioresponse of the central nervous system; a dynamic process. *Radiat Res*. 2000;153:357–370.

200. Meyers CA, Brown PD. Role and relevance of neurocognitive assessment in clinical trials of patients with CNS tumors. *J Clin Oncol*. 2006;24:1305–1309.

201. Abayomi O. Pathogenesis of irradiation-induced cognitive dysfunction. *Acta Oncol*. 1996;35:659–663.

202. Raber J, Rola R, LeFevour A, et al. Radiation-induced cognitive impairments are associated with changes in indicators of hippocampal neurogenesis. *Radiat Res*. 2004;162:39–47.

203. Rola R, Raber J, Rizk A, et al. Radiation-induced impairment of hippocampal neurogenesis is associated with cognitive deficits in young mice. *Exp Neurol*. 2004;188:316–330.

204. Mizumatsu S, Monje ML, Morhardt DR, Rola R, Palmer TD, Fike JR. Extreme sensitivity of adult neurogenesis to low doses of X-irradiation. *Cancer Res*. 2003;63:4021–4027.

205. Fan Y, Liu Z, Weintein P, Liu J. Environmental enrichment enhances neurogenesis and improves functional outcome after cranial irradiation. *Eur J Neurosci*. 2007;25:38–46.

206. Shi L, Adams MM, Long A, et al. Spatial learning and memory deficits after whole-brain irradiation are associated with changes in NMDA receptor subunits in the hippocampus. *Rad Res*. 2006;166:892–899.

207. Vlkolinsky R, Titova E, Krucker T, et al. Exposure to 56Fe radiation accelerates electrophysiological alterations in the hippocampus of APP23 transgenic mice. *Radiat Res*. 2010;173:342–352.

208. Fike JR, Rola R, Limoli CL. Radiation response of neural precursor cells. *Neurosurg Clin N Am*. 2007;18:115–127, x.

209. Raber J, Villasana L, Rosenberg J, Zou Y, Huang TT, Fike JR. Irradiation enhances hippocampus-dependent cognition in mice deficient in extracellular superoxide dismuase. *Hippocampus*. 2011;21:72–80.

210. Brown G. *Behavioral and Pathological Changes Following a 1100 rad Radiation Exposure*. Ann Arbor, MI: University Microfilms International; 1984.

211. Yochmowitz MG, Brown GC. Performance in a 12-hour, 300-rad profile. *Aviat Space Environ Med*. 1977;48:241–247.

212. Barnes D, Patrick R, Yochmowitz M, et al. *Protracted Low Dose Ionizing Radiation Effects Upon Primate Performance*. Brooks Air Force Base, TX: School of Aerospace Medicine; 1977.

213. Yochmowitz MG, Brown GC, Hardy KA. Performance following a 500–675 rad neutron pulse. *Aviat Space Environ Med*. 1985;56:525–533.

214. Blondal H. Initial irradiation reaction in mice. *Nature*. 1958;182:1026–1027.

215. Pitchford T. *Beagle Incapacitation and Survival Time After Pulsed Mixed Gamma Neutron Irradiation*. Bethesda, MD: Armed Forces Radiobiology Research Institute; 1968.

216. Langham W, Kaplan S, Pickering J, et al. *The Effects of Rapid, Massive Doses of Gamma Radiation on the Behavior of Subhuman Primates*. Los Alamos, NM: Los Alamos National Laboratory; 1952.

217. Sharp J, Keller B. *A Comparison Between the Effects of Exposure to a Mixed Fission Spectrum Delivered in a Single "Pulse" and X Rays Delivered at a Slower Rate Upon Conditioned Avoidance Behavior of the Primate.* Washington, DC: Walter Reed Army Institute of Research; 1965.

218. Thorp JW, Young RW. Monkey performance after partial body irradiation. *Aerosp Med.* 1971;42:503–507.

219. Barnes D. *An Initial Investigation of the Effects of Pulsed Ionizing Radiation on the Primate Equilibrium Function.* Brooks Air Force Base, TX: US Air Force School of Aerospace Medicine; 1966. USAFSAM-TR-66-106.

220. Meyerson F. Effect of damaging doses of gamma radiation on unconditioned and conditioned respiratory reflexes. In: *Works of the Institute of Higher Nervous Activity, Pathophysiological Series.* Vol 4. Moscow, Russia: Izvestia Akademi; 1958: 25–41.

221. Hall ME, Mayer MA. Effects of alpha methyl-para-tyrosine on the recall of a passive avoidance response. *Pharmacol Biochem Behav.* 1975;3:579–582.

222. Wheeler TG, Hardy KA. Retrograde amnesia produced by electron beam exposure: causal parameters and duration of memory loss. *Radiat Res.* 1985;101:74-80.

223. Page K, Wheeler T. *Potency of Photoflash Produced Retrograde Amnesia in Rats.* Brooks Air Force Base, TX: US Air Force School of Aerospace Medicine; 1985. USAFSAM-TR-85-9.

224. Wheeler T. *Amnesia Production by Visual Stimulation.* Brooks Air Force Base, TX: US Air Force School of Aerospace Medicine; 1982. USAFSAM-TR-82-45.

225. Burt D, Ingersoll E. Behavioral and neuropathological changes in the rat following X irradiation of the frontal brain. *J Comp Physiol Psychol.* 1965;59:90–93.

226. Barnes CA, Jung MW, McNaughton BL, Korol DL, Andreasson K, Worley PF. LTP saturation and spatial learning disruption: effects of task variables and saturation levels. *J Neurosci.* 1994;14:5793–5806.

227. Benice TS, Rizk A, Kohama S, Pfankuch T, Raber J. Sex-differences in age-related cognitive decline in C57BL/6J mice associated with increased brain microtubule-associated protein 2 and synaptophysin immunoreactivity. *Neuroscience.* 2006;137:413–423.

228. Furchtgott E. Effects of total body x-irradiation on learning: an exploratory study. *J Comp Physiol Psychol.* 1951;44:197–203.

229. Arnold WJ, Blair WC. The effects of cranial x irradiation on retention of maze learning in rats. *J Comp Physiol Psychol.* 1956;49:525–528.

230. Blair WC. The effects of cranial x irradiation on maze acquisition in rats. *J Comp Physiol Psychol.* 1958;51:175–177.

231. Scarborough B, Martin J, McLaurin W. Ionizing radiation: effects of repeated low dose exposure. *Physiol Behav.* 1966;1:147–150.

232. Ordy JM, Barnes HW, Samorajski T, Curtis HJ, Wolin L, Zeman W. Pathologic and behavioral changes in mice after deuteron irradiation of the central nervous system. *Radiat Res.* 1963;18:31–45.

233. Ordy JM, Samorajski T, Zeman W, Collins RL, Curtis HJ. Long-term pathologic and behavioral changes in mice after local deuteron irradiation of the brain. *Radiat Res.* 1963;20:30–42.

234. Meier G. Irradiation, genetics, and aging: behavioral implications. In: *Effects of Ionizing Radiation on the Nervous System, Proceedings of the Symposium Held at Vienna, 5–9 June 1961.* Vienna, Austria: International Atomic Energy Agency; 1962: 187–196.

235. van Cleave C. *Irradiation and the Nervous System.* New York, NY: Rowman and Littlefield, Inc; 1963.

236. Harlow HF, Moon LE. The effects of repeated doses of total-body x irradiation on motivation and learning in rhesus monkeys. *J Comp Physiol Psychol.* 1956;49:60–65.

237. McDowell AA. Comparisons of distractibility in irradiated and nonirradiated monkeys. *J Genet Psychol*. 1958;93:63–72.

238. Ades HW, Gradsky MA, Riopelle AJ. Learned performance of monkeys after single and repeated x irradiations. *J Comp Physiol Psychol*. 1956;49:521–524.

239. McDowell AA, Brown WL. Facilitative effects of irradiation on performance of monkeys on discrimination problems with reduced stimulus cues. *J Genet Psychol*. 1958;93:73–78.

240. Kaplan S, Gentry G. *Some Effects of a Lethal Dose of X Radiation Upon Memory. A Case History Study*. Randolph Air Force Base, TX: US Air Force School of Aviation Medicine; 1954. Project No. 21-3501-0003, Report No. 2.

241. Mele PC, Franz CG, Harrison JR. Effects of sublethal ionizing radiation on schedule-controlled performance in rats. *Pharmacol Biochem Behav*. 1988;30:1007–1014.

242. Azrin NH, Dimascio A, Fuller J, Jetter W. The effect of total body x-irradiation on delayed-response performance of dogs. *J Comp Physiol Psychol*. 1956;49:600–604.

243. Brown W, Overall J, Logie L, Wicker J. Lever pressing behavior of albino rats during prolonged exposures to X irradiation. *Radiat Res*. 1960;13:617–631.

244. Myers LS Jr, Carmichael AJ, Pellmar TC. Radiation chemistry of the hippocampal brain slice. *Adv Space Res*. 1994;14:453–456.

245. Tolliver JM, Pellmar TC. Ionizing radiation alters neuronal excitability in hippocampal slices of the guinea pig. *Radiat Res*. 1987;112:555–563.

246. Pellmar TC, Keyser DO, Emery C, Hogan JB. Electrophysiological changes in hippocampal slices isolated from rats embedded with depleted uranium fragments. *Neurotoxicology*. 1999;20:785–792.

247. LeCouteur RA, Gillette EL, Powers BE, Child G, McChesney SL, Ingram JT. Peripheral neuropathies following experimental intraoperative radiation therapy (IORT). *Int J Radiat Oncol Biol Phys*. 1989;17:583–590.

248. Clatworthy AL, Noel F, Grose E, Cui M, Tofilon PJ. Ionizing radiation-induced alterations in the electrophysiological properties of Aplysia sensory neurons. *Neurosci Lett*. 1999;268:45–48.

249. Ito M, Kato M, Kawabata M. Premature bifurcation of the apical dendritic trunk of vibrissa-responding pyramidal neurones of X-irradiated rat neocortex. *J Physiol*. 1998;512(Pt 2):543–553.

250. Reder CS, Moyers MF, Lau D, Kirby MA. Studies of physiology and the morphology of the cat LGN following proton irradiation. *Int J Radiat Oncol Biol Phys*. 2000;46:1247–1257.

251. Vlkolinsky R, Krucker T, Nelson GA, Obenaus A. (56)Fe-particle radiation reduces neuronal output and attenuates lipopolysaccharide-induced inhibition of long-term potentiation in the mouse hippocampus. *Radiat Res*. 2008;169:523–530.

252. Vlkolinsky R, Krucker T, Smith AL, Lamp TC, Nelson GA, Obenaus A. Effects of lipopolysaccharide on 56Fe-particle radiation-induced impairment of synaptic plasticity in the mouse hippocampus. *Radiat Res*. 2007;168:462–470.

253. Pellmar T, Tolliver J, Neel K. Radiation-induced impairment of neuronal excitability. *Fundam Appl Toxicol*. 1988;11:577–578.

254. Pellmar TC, Schauer DA, Zeman GH. Time- and dose-dependent changes in neuronal activity produced by X radiation in brain slices. *Radiat Res*. 1990;122:209–214.

255. Anniko M, Borg E, Hultcrantz M, Webster DB. Morphological and electrophysiological study of the inner ear and the central auditory pathways following whole body fetal irradiation. *Hear Res*. 1987;26:95–104.

256. Olson JE, Schimmerling W, Gundy GC, Tobias CA. Laser microirradiation of cerebellar neurons in culture. Electrophysiological and morphological effects. *Cell Biophys*. 1981;3:349–371.

257. Carlson LD, Scheyer WJ, Jackson BH. The combined effects of ionizing radiation and low temperature on the metabolism, longevity, and soft tissues of the white rat. I. Metabolism and longevity. *Radiat Res*. 1957;7:190–197.

258. Philpott DE, Miquel J. Long term effects of low doses of 56Fe ions on the brain and retina of the mouse: ultrastructural and behavioral studies. *Adv Space Res.* 1986;6:233–242.

259. Denisova NA, Shukitt-Hale B, Rabin BM, Joseph JA. Brain signaling and behavioral responses induced by exposure to (56)Fe-particle radiation. 2002;158:725–734.

260. Pawlowski TL, Bellush LL, Wright AW, Walker JF, Colvin RA, Huentelman MJ. Hippocampal gene expression changes during age-related cognitive decline. *Brain Res.* 2009;1256:101–110.

261. Devi PU, Manocha A, Vohora D. Seizures, antiepileptics, antioxidants and oxidative stress: an insight for researchers. *Expert Opin Pharmacother.* 2008;9:3169–3177.

262. Spigelman I VR, Lopez-Valdes HE, Nelson GA, Krucker T, Obenaus A. Alterations in hippocampal electrophysiological characteristics and development of hyperexcitability after 56Fe radiation exposure. *Society of Neuroscience Annual Meeting.* 2007;362:317.

263. Murphy R L-VH, Vlkolinsky R, Obenaus A, Nelson GA, Spigelman I. Hippocampal hyperexcitability and decreased GABAergic inhibition after 56Fe radiation exposure. *Society of Neuroscience Annual Meeting.* 2008;828:823.

264. Olsen R. Absinthe and gamma-aminobutyric acid receptors. *Proc Natl Acad Sci U S A.* 2000;97:4417–4418.

265. Mori Y, Kondziolka D, Balzer J, et al. Effects of stereotactic radiosurgery on an animal model of hippocampal epilepsy. *Neurosurgery.* 2000;46:157–165; discussion 165–168.

266. Schindler MK, Forbes ME, Robbins ME, Riddle DR. Aging-dependent changes in the radiation response of the adult rat brain. *Int J Radiat Oncol Biol Phys.* 2008;70:826–834.

267. Gruber D, Walker R, Macvittie T, Conklin J. *The Pathophysiology of Combined Injury and Trauma: Management of Infectious Complications in Mass Casualty Situations.* Orlando, FL: Academic Press; 1987.

268. Walker R, Gruber D, Macvittie T, Conklin JE. *The Pathophysiology of Combined Injury and Trauma: Radiation, Burn, and Trauma.* Baltimore, MD: University Park Press; 1985.

269. Landauer MR, Ledney GD, Davis HD. Locomotor behavior in mice following exposure to fission-neutron irradiation and trauma. *Aviat Space Environ Med.* 1987;58:1205–1210.

270. Bogo V, Hill TA, Young RW. Comparison of accelerod and rotarod sensitivity in detecting ethanol- and acrylamide-induced performance decrement in rats: review of experimental considerations of rotating rod systems. *Neurotoxicology.* 1981;2:765–787.

271. Wheeler T, Cordts R. *Combined Effects of Ionizing Radiation and Anticholinesterase Exposure on Rodent Motor Performance.* Brooks Air Force Base, TX: US Air Force School of Aerospace Medicine; 1983. USAFSAM-TR-83-30.

272. Wheeler T, Cordts R. *Nonlinear Performance Interaction Upon Exposure to Anticholinesterase and Ionizing Radiation.* Brooks Air Force Base, TX: US Air Force School of Aerospace Medicine; 1984; USAFSAM-TR-84-5.

273. Antipov V, Davyov B, Verigo V, Svirezhev Y. Combined effect of flight factors. In: Calvin M, Gazenko O, eds. *Ecological and Physiological Bases of Space Biology and Medicine.* Vol. 2. Washington, DC: National Aeronautics and Space Administration; 1975: 639–667.

274. Casey HW, Cordy DR, Goldman M, Smith AH. Influence of chronic acceleration on the effects of whole body irradiation in rats. *Aerosp Med.* 1967;38:451–457.

275. Mattsson JL, Cordts RE, Deyak RR Jr. Radiation and G tolerance in rats. *Aviat Space Environ Med.* 1981;52:404–407.

276. Livshits NN, Apanasenko ZI, Kuznetsova MA, Meĭzerov ES, Zakirova RM. Effect of acceleration on the higher nervous activity of previously irradiated rats [article in Russian]. *Radiobiologiia.* 1975;15:92–99.

277. Rosi S, Ferguson R, Levy W, et al. Trauma induced alterations in cognition and expression of the behaviorally-induced immediate early gene arc are reduced by a previous exposure to 56Fe. Paper presented at: Society for Neuroscience Annual Meeting, 2009; Chicago, IL. Available at: www.dsls.usra.edu/meetings/hrp2010/pdf/Radiation/1037Fike.pdf. Accessed April 9, 2012.

278. Ingersoll EH, Carsten AL, Brownson RH. Behavioral and structural changes following x-irradiation of the forebrain in the rat. *Proc Soc Exp Biol Med.* 1967;125:382–385.

279. Arnold WJ. Maze learning and retention after X irradiation of the head. *J Comp Physiol Psychol.* 1952;45:358–361.

280. Mickley GA, Stevens KE. Stimulation of brain muscarinic acetylcholine receptors acutely reverses radiogenic hypodipsia. *Aviat Space Environ Med.* 1986;57:250–255.

281. Halpern J, Kishel SP, Park J, Tsukada Y, Johnson RJ, Ambrus JL. Radiation induced edema in primates studied with sequential brain CAT scanning and histopathology. Protective effect of sodium meclofenamate. A preliminary report. *Res Commun Chem Pathol Pharmacol.* 1984;45:463–470.

282. Winkler H. Examination of the effect of roentgen rays on hemato-encephalic barrier by means of radioactive phosphorus [article in German]. 1957;97:301–307.

283. McMahon T, Vahora S. Radiation damage to the brain: neuropsychiatric aspects. *Gen Hosp Psychiatry.* 1986;8:437–441.

284. Sheline GE, Wara WM, Smith V. Therapeutic irradiation and brain injury. *Int J Radiat Oncol Biol Phys.* 1980;6:1215–1228.

285. O'Connel J, Brunschwig A. Observations on the roentgen treatment of intracranial gliomata with special reference to the effects of irradiation upon the surrounding brain. *Brain.* 1937;60:230–258.

286. Crompton MR, Layton DD. Delayed radionecrosis of the brain following therapeutic x-irradiation of the pituitary. *Brain.* 1961;84:85–107.

287. Hopewell J, Wright E. The effects of dose and field size on late radiation damage to the rat spinal cord. *Int J Radiat Biol.* 1975;28:325–333.

288. Innes J, Carsten A. Demyelination or malacic myelopathy. *Arch Neurol.* 1961;4:190–199.

289. Pourquier H, Baker JR, Giaux G, Benirschke K. Localized roentgen-ray beam irradiation of the hypophysohypothalamic region of guinea pigs with a 2 million volt van de Graaf generator. *Am J Roentgenol Radium Ther Nucl Med.* 1958;80:840–850.

290. Zeman W. Disturbances of nucleic acid metabolism preceding delayed radionecrosis of nervous tissue. *Proc Natl Acad Sci U S A.* 1963;50:626–630.

291. Reyners H, Gianfelici de Reyners E, Maisin JR. Early cell regeneration processes after split dose X-irradiation of the cerebral cortex of the rat. *Br J Cancer Suppl.* 1986;7:218–220.

292. Reyners H, Gianfelici de Reyners E, Maisin JR. The beta astrocyte: a newly recognized radiosensitive glial cell type in the cerebral cortex. *J Neurocytol.* 1982;11:967–983.

293. Mastaglia FL, McDonald WI, Watson JV, Yogendran K. Effects of x-irradiation on the spinal cord: an experimental study of the morphological changes in central nerve fibers. *Brain.* 1976;99:101–122.

294. Jones A. Transient radiation myelopathy (with reference to Lhermitte's sign of electrical paresthesia). *Br J Radiol.* 1964;37:727–744.

295. Cavanagh JB, Hopewell JW. Mitotic activity in the subependymal plate of rats and the long-term consequences of X-irradiation. *J Neurol Sci.* 1972;15:471–482.

296. Furchtgott E. Behavioral effects of ionizing radiations. *Psychol Bull.* 1956;53:321–334.

297.   Altman J. Are new neurons formed in the brains of adult mammals? *Science*. 1962;135:1127–1128.

298.   Kaplan MS, Hinds JW. Neurogenesis in the adult rat: electron microscopic analysis of light radioautographs. *Science*. 1977;197:1092–1094.

299.   Bayer SA, Altman J. Radiation-induced interference with postnatal hippocampal cytogenesis in rats and its long term-effects on the acquisition of neurons and glia. *J Comp Neurol*. 1975;163:1–20.

300.   Bayer S. Neuron production in the hippocampus and olfactory bulb of the adult rat brain: addition or replacement. *Ann N Y Acad Sci*. 1985:457:163–172.

301.   Guéneau G, Baille V, Court L. Protracted postnatal neurogenesis and radiosensitivity in the rabbit's dentate gyrus. In: Kriegel H, Schmahl W, Gerber G, Stieve F, eds. *Radiation Risks to the Developing Nervous System*. Stuttgart, Germany: Gustav Fischer Verlag; 1986: 133–140.

302.   Guéneau G, Drouet J, Privat A, Court L. Differential radiosensitivity of neurons and neuroglia of the hippocampus in the adult rabbit. *Acta Neuropathol*. 1979;48:199–209.

303.   Rakic P. DNA synthesis and cell division in the adult primate brain. *Ann N Y Acad Sci*. 1985;457:193–211.

304.   Schade J, Caveness W. Alterations in dendritic organization. *Brain Res*. 1968;7:59–86.

305.   Dent P, Yacoub A, Contessa J, et al. Stress and radiation-induced activation of multiple intracellular signaling pathways. *Radiat Res*. 2003;159:283–300.

306.   Simonian NA, Coyle JT. Oxidative stress in neurodegenerative diseases. *Ann Rev Pharmacol Toxicol*. 1996;36:83–106.

307.   Bast A, Haenen GR, Doelman CJ. Oxidants and antioxidants: state of the art. *Am J Med*. 1991;91:2S–13S.

308.   Smith J, Ladi E, Mayer-Proschel M, Noble M. Redox state is a central modulator of the balance between self-renewal and differentiation in a dividing glial precursor cell. *Proc Natl Acad Sci U S A*. 2000;97:10032–10037.

309.   Clutton SM, Townsend KM, Walker C, Ansell JD, Wright EG. Radiation-induced genomic instability and persisting oxidative stress in primary bone marrow cultures. *Carcinogenesis*. 1996;17:1633–1639.

310.   Limoli CL, Giedzinski E, Morgan WF, Swarts SG, Jones GD, Hyun W. Persistent oxidative stress in chromosomally unstable cells. *Cancer Res*. 2003;63:3107–3111.

311.   Plumb M, Harper K, MacDonald D, Fennelly J, Lorimore S, Wright E. Ongoing Y-chromosome instability defines subclonal variants in radiation-induced leukemias in the mouse. *Int J Radiat Biol*. 1997;72:1–9.

312.   Niranjan A, Fellows W, Stauffer W, et al. Survival of transplanted neural progenitor cells enhanced by brain irradiation *J Neurosurg*. 2007;107:383–391.

313.   Acharya MM, Christie LA, Lan ML, et al. Rescue of radiation-induced cognitive impairment through cranial transplantation of human embryonic stem cells. *Proc Natl Acad Sci U S A*. 2009;106:19150–19155.

314.   Devi PU, Satyamitra M. Tracing radiation induced genomic instability in vivo in the haemopoietic cells from fetus to adult mouse. *Br J Radiol*. 2005;78:928–933.

315.   Egana E. Some effects of ionizing radiations on the metabolism of the central nervous system. *Int J Neurol*. 1962;3:631–647.

316.   Ito M, Patronas NJ, Di Chiro G, Mansi L, Kennedy C. Effect of moderate level x-radiation to brain on cerebral glucose utilization. *J Comput Assist Tomogr*. 1986;10:584–588.

317.   Catterall WA. The molecular basis of neuronal excitability. *Science*. 1984;223:653–661.

318. Rothenberg M. Studies on permeability in relation to nerve function, ionic movements across axonal membranes. *Biochim Biophys Acta.* 1950;4:96–114.

319. Gaffey C, ed. *Bioelectric Effects of High Energy Irradiation on Nerve.* New York, NY: Academic Press; 1962.

320. Wixon HN, Hunt WA. Ionizing radiation decreases veratridine-stimulated uptake of sodium in rat brain synaptosomes. *Science.* 1983;220:1073–1074.

321. Mullin MJ, Hunt WA, Harris RA. Ionizing radiation alters the properties of sodium channels in rat brain synaptosomes. *J Neurochem.* 1986;47:489–495.

322. Tanimura H. Changes of the neurosecretory granules in hypothalamo hypophysical system of rats by irradiating their heads with X rays. *Acta Anat Nippon.* 1957;32:529–533.

323. Dahlström A, Häggendal J, Rosengren B. The effect of roentgen irradiation on monoamine containing neurons of the rat brain. *Acta Radiol Ther Phys Biol.* 1973;12:191–200.

324. Hunt WA, Dalton TK, Darden JH. Transient alterations in neurotransmitter activity in the caudate nucleus of rat brain after a high dose of ionizing radiation. *Radiat Res.* 1979;80:556–562.

325. Joseph JA, Kandasamy SB, Hunt WA, Dalton TK, Steven S. Radiation-induced increases in sensitivity of cataleptic behavior to haloperidol: possible involvement of prostaglandins. *Pharmacol Biochem Behav.* 1988;29:335–341.

326. Kulinski V, Semenov L. Content of catecholamines in the tissues of macaques during the early periods after total gamma irradiation. *Radiobiologiia.* 1965;5:494–500.

327. Varagic V, Stepanovic S, Svecenski N, Hajdukovic S. The effect of X irradiation on the amount of catecholamines in heart atria and hypothalamus of the rabbit and in brain and heart of the rat. *Int J Radiat Biol.* 1967;12:113–119.

328. Johnsson JE, Owman C, Sjöberg NO. Tissue content of noradrenaline and 5-hydroxytryptamine in the rat after ionizing radiation. *Int J Radiat Biol Relat Stud Phys Chem Med.* 1970;18:311–316.

329. Catravas G, McHale C. *Activity Changes of Brain Enzymes in Rats Exposed to Different Qualities of Ionizing Radiation.* Bethesda, MD: Armed Forces Radiobiology Research Institute; 1973.

330. Prasad KN, van Woert MH. Dopamine protects mice against whole-body irradiation. *Science.* 1967;155:470–472.

331. Rixon RH, Baird KM. The therapeutic effect of serotonin on the survival of x-irradiated rats. *Radiat. Res.* 1968;33:395–402.

332. Davydov B. Acetylcholine metabolism on the thalamic region of the brain of dogs after acute radiation sickness. *Radiobiologiia.* 1961;1:550–554.

333. Sabine JC. Inactivation of cholinesterases by gamma radiation. *Am J Physiol.* 1956;187:280–282.

334. Lundin J, Clemedson CJ, Nelson A. Early effects of whole body irradiation on cholinesterase activity in guinea pigs' blood with special regard to radiation sickness. *Acta Radiol.* 1957;48:52–64.

335. Hunt WA, Dalton TK. Reduction in cyclic nucleotide levels in the brain after a high dose of ionizing radiation. *Radiat Res.* 1980;83:210–215.

336. Catravas G, Wright S, Trocha P, Takenaga J. Radiation effects on cyclic AMP, cyclic GMP, and amino acid levels in the CSF of the primate. *Radiat Res.* 1981;87:198–203.

337. Doyle TF, Strike TA. Radiation-released histamine in the rhesus monkey as modified by mast-cell depletion and antihistamine. *Experientia.* 1977;33:1047–1049.

338. Cockerham L, Pautler E, Hampton J. Postradiation blood flow in the visual cortex of primates. *The Toxicologist.* 1984;5:82.

339. Hawkins RN, Forcino CD. Postradiation cardiovascular dysfunction. *Comments on Toxicology 2*. 1988;2:243–252.

340. Doyle TF, Curran CR, Turns JE, Strike TA. The prevention of radiation-induced, early, transient incapacitation of monkeys by an antihistamine. *Proc Soc Exp Biol Med*. 1974;145:1018–1024.

341. Chapman PH, Young RJ. Effect of high energy x-irradiation of the head on cerebral blood flow and blood pressure in the Macaca mulatta. *Aerosp Med*. 1968;39:1316–1321.

342. Cockerham LG, Doyle TF, Paulter EL, Hampton JD. Disodium cromoglycate, a mast-cell stabilizer, alters postradiation regional cerebral blood flow in primates. *J Toxicol Environ Health*. 1986;18:91–101.

343. Turbyfill CL, Roudon RM, Kieffer VA. Behavior and physiology of the monkey (*Macaca mulatta*) following 2500 rads of pulse mixed gamma-neutron radiation. *Aerosp Med*. 1972;43:41–45.

344. Miletich D, Strike T. *Alteration of Postirradiation Hypotension and Incapacitation in the Monkey by Administration of Vasopressor Drugs*. Bethesda, MD: Armed Forces Radiobiology Research Institute; 1970.

345. Turns J, Doyle T, Curran C. *Norepinephrine Effects on Early Post Irradiation Performance Decrement in the Monkey*. Bethesda, MD: Armed Forces Radiobiology Research Institute; 1971.

346. McFarland WL, Levin SG. Electroencephalographic responses to 2500 rads of whole-body gamma-neutron radiation in the monkey Macaca mulatta. *Radiat Res*. 1974;58:60–73.

347. Mickley GA, Teitelbaum H, Parker GA, Vieras F, Dennison BA, Bonney CH. Radiogenic changes in the behavior and physiology of the spontaneously hypertensive rat: evidence for a dissociation between acute hypotension and incapacitation. *Aviat Space Environ Med*. 1982;53:633–638.

348. Douglas W. Histamine and 5 hydroxytryptamine (serotonin) and their antagonists. In: Goodman LS, Gilman A, eds. *Goodman and Gilman's the Pharmacological Basis of Therapeutics*. 7th ed. New York, NY: Macmillan; 1985: 605–615.

349. Doyle TF, Turns JE, Strike TA. Effect of antihistamine on early transient incapacitation of monkeys subjected to 4000 rads of mixed gamma neutron radiation. *Aerosp Med*. 1971;42:400–403.

350. Mickley GA. Antihistamine provides sex-specific radiation protection. *Aviat Space Environ Med*. 1981;52:247–250.

351. Alter W, Catravas G, Hawkins R, Lake C. Effect of ionizing radiation on physiological function in the anesthetized rat. *Radiat Res*. 1984;99:394–409.

352. Carpenter D. *Early Transient Incapacitation: A Review with Considerations of Underlying Mechanisms*. Bethesda, MD: Armed Forces Radiobiology Research Institute; 1979.

353. De Ryck M, Schallert T, Teitelbaum P. Morphine versus haloperidol catalepsy in the rat: a behavioral analysis of postural support mechanisms. *Brain Res*. 1980;201:143–172.

354. Iverson S, Iverson L. *Behavioral Pharmacology*. New York, NY: Oxford University Press; 1981.

355. Akil H, Madden J, Patrick R III, Barchas J. Stress induced increase in endogenous opioid peptides: concurrent analgesia and its reversal by naloxone. In: Kosterlitz H, ed. *Opiates and Endogenous Opiate Peptides*. Amsterdam, The Netherlands: Elsevier North Holland; 1976.

356. Grevert P, Goldstein A. Some effects of naloxone on behavior in the mouse. *Psychopharmacology (Berl)*. 1977;53:111–113.

357. Herman BH, Panksepp J. Effects of morphine and naloxone on separation distress and approach attachment: evidence for opiate mediation of social effect. *Pharmacol Biochem Behav*. 1978;9:213–220.

358. Margules D. Beta endorphin and endoloxone: hormones of the autonomic nervous system for the conservation of expenditure of bodily resources and energy in anticipation of famine or feast. *Neurosci Biobehav Rev*. 1979;3:155–162.

359. Katz R, Carroll BJ, Baldrighi G. Behavioral activation by enkephalins in mice. *Pharmacol Biochem Behav.* 1978;8:493–496.

360. Browne RG, Segal DS. Alterations in beta-endorphin-induced locomotor activity in morphine-tolerant rats. *Neuropharmacology.* 1980;19:619–621.

361. Szkely JI, Rónai AZ, Dunai-Kovács Z, Miglécz E, Bajusz S, Gráf L. Cross tolerance between morphine and beta endorphin in vivo. *Life Sci.* 1977;20:1259–1264.

362. Dafny N, Pellis NR. Evidence that opiate addiction is in part an immune response. Destruction of the immune system by irradiation-altered opiate withdrawal. *Neuropharmacology.* 1986;25:815–818.

363. Mickley GA, Sessions GR, Bogo V, Chantry KH. Evidence for endorphin-mediated cross-tolerance between chronic stress and the behavioral effects of ionizing radiation. *Life Sci.* 1983;33:749–754.

364. Mickley GA, Stevens KE, White GA, Gibbs GL. Changes in morphine self-administration after exposure to ionizing radiation: evidence for the involvement of endorphins. *Life Sci.* 1983;33:711–718.

365. Mickley GA, Stevens KE, Moore GH, Ionizing radiation alters beta-endorphin-like immunoreactivity in brain but not blood. *Pharmacol Biochem Behav.* 1983;19:979–983.

366. Alter W, Mickley G, Catravas G, et al. Role of histamine and beta-endorphin in radiation induced hypotension and acute performance decrement in the rat. In: *Proceedings of the 51st Annual Scientific Meeting of Aerospace Medical Association.* Alexandria, VA: AsMA; 1980: 225–226.

367. Danquechin Dorval E, Mueller GP, Eng RR, Durakovic A, Conklin JJ, Dubois A. Effect of ionizing radiation on gastric secretion and gastric motility in monkeys. *Gastroenterology.* 1985;89:374–380.

368. Mickley GA, Stevens KE, Burrows JM, White GA, Gibbs GL. Morphine tolerance offers protection from radiogenic performance decrements. *Radiat Res.* 1983;93:381–387.

369. Morse D, Mickley G. Interaction of the endogenous opioid system and radiation in the suppression of appetite behavior. *Abstr Soc Neurosci.* 1988;14(2):1106.

370. Monje ML, Toda H, Palmer TD. Inflammatory blockade restores adult hippocampal neurogenesis. *Science.* 2003;302:1760–1765.

371. Lee C, Payne V, Ramanan S. The ACE inhibitor, ramipril, prevents fractionated whole-brain irradiation-induced cognitive impairment. In: Proceedings from the 55th Annual Meeting of the Radiation Research Society; October 3–7, 2009; Savannah, GA. Presentation number PS1.36.

372. Robbins ME, Payne V, Tomassi E, et al. The AT1 receptor antagonist, L-158,809, prevents or ameliorates fractionated whole-brain irradiation-induced cognitive impairment. *Int J Radiat Oncol Biol Phys.* 2009;73:499–505.

373. Jones DC, Kimeldorf DJ, Castanera TJ, Rubadeau DO, Osborn GK. Effect of bone marrow therapy on the volitional activity of whole-body x-irradiated rats. *Am J Physiol.* 1957;189:21–23.

374. Peister A, Zeitouni S, Pfankuch T, Reger RL, Prockop DJ, Raber J. Novel object recognition in Apoe(-/-) mice improved by neonatal implantation of wild-type multipotential stromal cells. *Exp Neurol.* 2006;201(1):266–269.

375. Otterson M, Leming S, Moulder J, Engelsgjerd M. 5HT3 antagonist blocks contractions associated with abdominal cramping. *Gastroenterology.* 1995;108:A662.

376. Otterson M. Effects of radiation upon gastrointestinal motility. *World J Gastroenterol.* 2007;13:2684–2692.

377. Erickson BA, Otterson MF, Moulder JE, Sarna SK. Altered motility causes the early gastrointestinal toxicity of irradiation. *Int J Radiat Oncol Biol Phys.* 1994;28:905–912.

378. Otterson MF, Sarna SK, Moulder JE. Effects of fractionated doses of ionizing radiation on small intestinal motor activity. *Gastroenterology.* 1988;95:1249–1257.

379. Otterson MF, Sarna SK, Leming SC, Moulder JE, Fink JG. Effects of fractionated doses of ionizing radiation on colonic motor activity. *Am J Physiol*. 1992;263:G518–G526.

380. Dubois A. Effect of ionizing radiation on the gastrointestinal tract. *Fundam Appl Toxicol*. 1988;11:574–575.

381. Young R, ed. *Acute Radiation Syndrome*. New York, NY: Academic Press; 1987.

382. Barrett A, Barrett AJ, Powles R. Total body irradiation and marrow transplantation for acute leukemia. The Royal Marsden Hospital experience. *Pathol Biol (Paris)*. 1979;27:357–359.

383. Salazar OM, Rubin P, Keller B, Scarantino C. Systemic (half-body) radiation therapy: response and toxicity. *Int J Radiat Oncol Biol Phys*. 1978;4:937–950.

384. Dubois A, Fiala N, Boward CA, Bogo V. Prevention and treatment of the gastric symptoms of radiation sickness. *Radiat Res*. 1988;115:595–604.

385. Otterson M, Leming S, Moulder J. Central NK1 receptors mediate radiation induced emesis. *Gastroenterology*. 1997;112:A801.

386. Otterson M, Leming S, Liu X, Moulder J. The role of the NMDA receptor in radiation induced colonic motility. *Dig Dis Sci*. 1998;43:1590.

387. Otterson M, Leming S, Liu X, Moulder J. Radiation induced changes in small intestinal motility: a role for the NMDA receptor. *Gastroenterology*. 1998;114:A816.

388. Otterson M, Leming S, Callison J, Moulder J. NMDA receptor antagonists block but do not mitigate prodromal radiation sickness. In: Proceedings from the 55th Annual Meeting of the Radiation Research Society; October 3–7, 2009; Savannah, GA. Presentation number PS7.04.

389. Thorp JW, Chaput RL, Kovacic RT. Performance of miniature pigs after partial body irradiation. *Aerosp Med*. 1970;41:379–382.

390. Thorp J, Germas J. *Performance of Monkeys After Partial Body Irradiation*. Bethesda, MD: Armed Forces Radiobiology Research Institute; 1969.

391. Chapman PH, Young RJ. *Effect of Head Versus Trunk Fission-Spectrum Radiation on Learned Behavior in the Monkey*. Brooks Air Force Base, TX: School of Aerospace Medicine; 1968. Technical Report TR-68-80.

392. Chapman PH. *Behavioral and Circulatory Responses to X-Irradiation Delivered at 200 rads per Minute to Whole Body and Trunk Only*. Brooks Air Force Base, TX: School of Aerospace Medicine; 1968. Technical Report TR-68-111.

393. Chapman PH, Hurst CM. *The Effect of Head Versus Trunk X-Irradiation on Avoidance Behavior in the Rhesus Monkey*. Brooks Air Force Base, TX: School of Aerospace Medicine; 1968. Technical Report TR-68-37.

Chapter 8

PSYCHOLOGICAL ISSUES IN A RADIOLOGICAL OR NUCLEAR ATTACK

STEVEN M. BECKER, PhD*

*Professor of Community and Environmental Health, College of Health Sciences, Old Dominion University, Norfolk, Virginia 23529

INTRODUCTION

Among the most complex and challenging threats facing the United States and other nations in the 21st century is the possibility of a radiological or nuclear attack. Humankind's most powerful armaments, nuclear bombs, are the very definition of a weapon of mass destruction. They have the capacity to cause widespread and horrendous physical devastation and staggering numbers of casualties, as can be seen in photographs taken shortly after the atomic bombings of Hiroshima and Nagasaki.

Radiological weapons do not involve a nuclear detonation; rather, they either disperse radioactive materials to contaminate people (a radiological dispersal device [RDD]) or place a radiation source with the aim of intentionally exposing people (a radiation exposure device). In terms of fatalities, the consequences of a radiological attack would be many orders of magnitude smaller than a nuclear weapon detonation,[1] but in no sense does this mean that an attack involving a radiological weapon would not be serious. For example, a "dirty bomb," which combines conventional explosives and radioactive material, could kill dozens or even hundreds of people immediately (mainly from the conventional explosive), injure many, and put others at increased risk of becoming ill, depending on the location and the type and size of the attack. However, radiological weapons lack the capacity to cause the kind of massive, area-wide destruction and huge numbers of fatalities associated with an atomic bomb.

Although radiological and nuclear weapons differ in terms of how they work and impart their physical effects, what they share is the capacity to produce widespread and profound social, psychological, and behavioral impacts. These can include transient and longer-lasting individual mental health effects, as well as deep community and societal impacts.[2] Furthermore, in either a radiological or nuclear event, people's behavior (eg, whether or not populations undertake appropriate protective actions) can be one of the principal factors affecting the number of casualties. Thus, the psychological dimension of a radiological or nuclear attack needs to be a central consideration in planning, training, preparedness, and response. This chapter examines some of the potential behavioral effects and challenges posed by a radiological or nuclear attack in the contemporary context and traces out a strategy for enhancing resilience and preventing and reducing psychological impacts.

EVOLVING THREATS, NEW SCENARIOS

The psychological challenges posed by a radiological or nuclear attack (and the populations likely to be most affected) are influenced to a substantial degree by the nature of the threat and the type of scenario encountered. Thus, it is useful to begin this examination of psychological issues by considering how threats and scenarios have evolved in recent decades and how they might further change in the future. For much of the second half of the 20th century, the world faced a continuous threat of nuclear war. Cold War tensions, and sometimes even direct clashes, between the communist Eastern Bloc and the nations of the West made the risk of a highly destructive nuclear confrontation an ever-present part of daily reality. One possibility involved a tactical nuclear exchange between armies in the field, or what was sometimes referred to as a "limited nuclear war." In this scenario, shorter-range, generally smaller-yield, nuclear weapons (eg, nuclear artillery shells and landmines) would have been employed to augment conventional weapons in battlefield or theater-level military conflict. Although such nuclear combat was characterized as limited in scope, its effects would undoubtedly have been physically and psychologically devastating, both to military personnel and civilians in nearby areas. Furthermore, such a scenario would have also carried with it the risk of escalation to an even larger nuclear war.

The other danger, and the one that motivated the massive civil defense efforts of the 1950s and 1960s in the United States and Union of Soviet Socialist Republics, was the possibility of a "global" or strategic nuclear war between nations. This would have involved the use of long-range, larger-yield weapons delivered by intercontinental ballistic missiles, submarine-launched ballistic missiles, and long-range bombers. The potential impacts of such an all-out nuclear war would have been horrific, with infrastructure, command and control centers, military bases, industrial facilities, commercial centers, and perhaps entire major urban areas completely obliterated. The combined effects of blast, heat, fire, radiation, and radioactive fallout would have killed tens, perhaps hundreds, of millions of people.

During the Cold War period, consideration of the psychological issues posed by nuclear conflict focused largely on how soldiers might be affected by the limited use of nuclear weapons in the battlefield, or how civilian populations and nations as a whole might act or be affected by an all-out nuclear war.[3–8] With the fall of the Berlin Wall and the end of the Cold War, the possibility of this type of global nuclear war decreased significantly but did not disappear. Meanwhile, in recent years, a range of new threats has emerged, posing daunting challenges for emergency planners, medical and mental health professionals, the homeland security community, and the uniformed services.

Nuclear Proliferation

The list of nations possessing nuclear weapons has grown, bringing with it new perils and new possibilities for nuclear conflict. One very troubling example is North Korea, which conducted its first nuclear test in 2006 and another in 2009. The tightly controlled dictatorship, which has had very tense relations with its neighbors and the United States and regularly issues threatening statements, is also engaged in developing ballistic missiles. Both the nuclear weapons and missile programs have been the object of United Nations Security Council condemnation and targeted sanctions. Another particularly troubling example is Iran, which appears to be moving aggressively to develop nuclear weapons and delivery systems despite United Nations Security Council resolutions calling for a halt to the country's uranium enrichment activities, and despite intense diplomatic efforts and sanctions by the United Nations, the United States, the European Union, and others. Meanwhile, the list of countries seeking nuclear weapons is likely to grow longer in coming years.

Terrorism

There is now also a serious and growing possibility that nonstate actors (groups rather than nations) will obtain nuclear weapons. Among those attempting to add nuclear weapons to their arsenals are terrorist organizations. Terrorists could try to acquire or steal a weapon from a nation that possesses nuclear weapons, particularly a country experiencing serious political or social instability. Generally speaking, however, the extensive security measures surrounding nuclear armaments would make it difficult for terrorists to secure a stockpile weapon. Alternatively, terrorists could seek to create a crude nuclear bomb, known as an improvised nuclear device.[1] Despite various control efforts, proliferation of nuclear know-how and nuclear technology has continued globally. Experts disagree about precisely how difficult it would be to acquire the necessary fissile material, or exactly how long it would take to create a working, usable bomb. Whether a terrorist organization has assistance from a state sponsor or supporter could certainly affect the equation. But in no sense is the threat just a hypothetical one; rather, as nuclear researcher Matthew Bunn has warned, it is a "real and urgent danger." Terrorists are

"actively seeking nuclear weapons and the materials to make them."[9]

Undoubtedly, the best-known example of a terrorist group trying to acquire or develop a nuclear bomb is Al Qaeda. As far back as the early 1990s, the organization showed a clear interest in nuclear weapons. Since that time, Al Qaeda has had contact with nuclear scientists, attempted to acquire nuclear materials and designs, and even issued religious justifications for the use of weapons of mass destruction. The organization's top leadership has "demonstrated a sustained commitment to buy, steal or construct" a weapon of mass destruction.[10] But according to Graham Allison, director of Harvard's Belfer Center for Science and International Affairs, Al Qaeda may not be the only terrorist organization with an interest in acquiring nuclear weapons:

> If we awaken tomorrow to news of a nuclear terrorist attack, Al Qaeda will certainly be the most probable perpetrator. Unfortunately, however, the list of potential attackers does not stop there. There exists a rogues' gallery of other terrorist groups that have actively explored the nuclear options or, on current trend lines, could do so in the next few years.[11]

Furthermore, for some groups, traditional deterrence and the fear of retaliation would not be effective in stopping them from using a nuclear weapon against the United States or its allies. As Robert Gallucci has pointed out, "some of today's adversaries value their own lives less than our deaths."[12]

Impacts of an Improvised Nuclear Device

Most experts assume that a nuclear device created by a terrorist organization would be smaller and cruder than a military weapon, and that its effects would be smaller as well. Typical analyses discuss an improvised nuclear device that is 10 kilotons or smaller. That is the size, for example, considered in the Institute of Medicine's examination of medical preparedness for a nuclear event, and in the US National Planning Scenario created to help guide national, state, and local preparedness activities for a nuclear attack.[13] But even a 10-kiloton device would have immense destructive power, both in terms of physical damage and the psychological toll it would take. According to Bunn, "With enough plutonium or highly enriched uranium (HEU), a sophisticated and well-organized terrorist group could potentially make at least a crude nuclear bomb that could incinerate the heart of any major city."[9]

A RAND study of the effects of a 10-kiloton detonation in the Port of Long Beach, California, found that "within the first 72 hours, the attack would devastate a vast portion of the Los Angeles metropolitan area," including the power grid and infrastructure.[14] Some 60,000 people might be killed, 150,000 others might be exposed to hazardous radiation levels, 600,000 homes would be lost, and several million people would be displaced. Other estimates of the effects of an improvised nuclear device detonation on the US mainland are equally sobering. For example, the Nuclear/Radiological Incident Annex of the National Response Framework states that "even a small nuclear detonation in an urban area could result in over 100,000 fatalities (and many more injured). . . ."[15] Studies of detonations in the most densely populated US urban areas (eg, New York City) have indicated a potential for even higher casualty tolls. Regardless of which estimate is used, it is clear that the medical, mental health, economic, and social impacts of a nuclear attack would be shocking. Indeed, every American would be affected in some way and left to wonder whether additional attacks would occur in the future.

Radiological Weapons

Another important change in the threat environment involves the emergence of radiological weapons. Although the general idea of spraying or spreading radioactive materials to cause harm and contaminate an area is not new,[16,17] it took a combination of the widespread availability of radioactive sources, a thriving illicit trade in radioactive materials, and the emergence of modern terrorism to make radiological weapons a realistic 21st-century threat. Creating an RDD weapon, such as a dirty bomb, would require only modest financial resources and technical skills. Furthermore, only a limited geographic reach would be needed. According to Ferguson et al:

> Widespread access to radioactive sources essentially obviates the need for a multinational network. An RDD may be effectively delivered via a conventional bomb packed with radioactive material or through other dispersion modes....The relative ease of delivery of an RDD makes it a viable option for smaller groups with limited financial resources and technical know-how.[1]

The ease of creating a radiological weapon is one reason several expert assessments have concluded that a radioactive dirty bomb or other form of radiological terrorism could be close to the top of the list of likely attacks in the future.[18,19] As noted earlier, the capacity of a dirty bomb or other form of radiological terrorism to cause fatalities is limited. However, because radiological weapons can spread radioactive materials and expose people to radiation, they have the potential to sow fear, engender terror, create mass disruption, and leave enormous economic, social, and psychological impacts in their wake (Figures 8-1 and 8-2).[1]

PSYCHOLOGICAL CHALLENGES IN A COMPLEX THREAT ENVIRONMENT

In the 21st century, the terrain has shifted. Now, even as the possibility of global nuclear war has decreased but not disappeared, new dangers have emerged. The need for the nation to prepare for these challenges is reflected in the responsibilities given to the Department of Defense under the National Response Framework. Along with its traditional national defense role, the Department of Defense, when directed to do so, is now also responsible for providing support to the Department of Homeland Security and other federal, state, and local government agencies.

Today's threat environment is highly complex and includes a broad range of circumstances with varying psychological issues and implications. The following situations are among the specific possibilities that need to be taken into account in preparedness and planning.

Nuclear Attack by a Rogue Nation or a Terrorist Group on Overseas US Forces or Facilities

Such an attack could, for example, be directed against US forces engaged in combat operations or

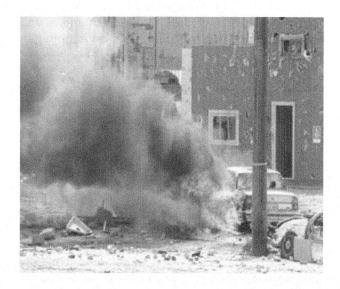

Figure 8-1. Buildings damaged and cars burning in TOPOFF (top officials) 2 "dirty bomb" national level exercise, Seattle. Reproduced from: Seattle Municipal Archives Photograph Collection. Collection Record Series 0207-01 (Fleets and Facilities Imagebank). Item number 13861.

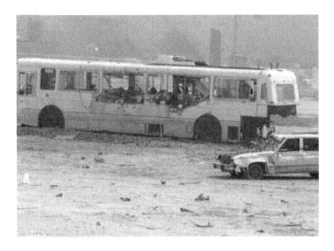

Figure 8-2. Destroyed bus after mock radiological dispersal device attack, TOPOFF (top officials) 2 exercise, Seattle. Reproduced from: Seattle Municipal Archives Photograph Collection. Collection Record Series 0207-01 (Fleets and Facilities Imagebank). Item number 138618.

peacekeeping operations, or it could be directed against an overseas base. In addition to the direct and indirect effects on military and civilian personnel in the targeted area, there would be a tremendous psychological impact on the host country, on US service members' families and communities back home, on personnel at other facilities around the world, and on the United States as a whole.

Nuclear Attack on US Forces Inside the Continental United States

A nuclear attack targeting the home base and community of a US military unit would have enormous pyschological impacts. In addition to the effects on military and civilian personnel, military families, and civilians in the targeted area, there could be substantial psychological impacts on other personnel overseas, on people working and living at or near other bases, on military communities, and on the nation as a whole.

War Between Regional Nuclear Powers

Although a conflict may not directly involve the United States, it may affect US military and civilian personnel based overseas (eg, through the spread of radioactive fallout). Such a situation would create considerable concerns about potential immediate and longer-term health effects, likely requiring substantial medical, psychological, and other follow-up programs. In addition, a continuing communication and infor-

mation effort would be needed to address the many questions, concerns, and information needs of the potentially affected military and civilian personnel, their units, and their families and communities back home.

A Series of Coordinated "Dirty Bomb" Attacks on Critical Infrastructure

A series of coordinated RDD attacks on key commercial, governmental, or military buildings inside the United States would result in direct civilian and military casualties as well as radioactive contamination left by the attacks. This, coupled with people's apprehensions about potential and perceived dangers, could lead concerned individuals to flood medical facilities, hobble administrative and business centers, and even paralyze entire sections of cities.

A Terrorist Nuclear Detonation in a US City, Followed by Deployment of US Forces

Such forces might not only have to contend with their own concerns about radiation, other dangers, and personal safety, but could also encounter almost unimaginable and gruesome sights, including widespread destruction, large numbers of corpses, and people with horrific, disfiguring burns (Figure 8-3). This point was driven home in Lifton's writings on Hiroshima,[20] in which people who had been in the city at the time of the bombing reported their reactions and experiences. "Everything I saw," commented a young university professor who had been about a mile and a half from the blast, "made a deep impression—a park nearby covered with dead bodies waiting to be cremated...very badly injured people..." and most of all, "very young girls...with their skin peeled off." For soldiers, even combat veterans, experiencing death on the battlefield is difficult enough; responding to a nuclear event and seeing widespread death and destruction on the US mainland would tax psychological resources even more. Meanwhile, there would be a tremendous psychological impact on survivors of the attack, and potential impacts on people residing anywhere near the event, the families of those deployed to render aid, and individuals across the nation.

This range of potential threats and scenarios is remarkably wide; so, too, is the array of groups that could be psychologically affected. Planning and preparedness activities related to the psychological dimensions of a radiological or nuclear attack need to take these varying possibilities into account; some of the aforementioned possibilities have received only scant attention to date in preparedness efforts.

RESPONSES AND REACTIONS TO A RADIOLOGICAL OR NUCLEAR ATTACK

Planning and preparedness efforts also need to take into account ways that people might respond or react to a situation in which radiological or nuclear weapons are used. Yet making predictions about people's psychological and behavioral responses is complicated. Despite evidence of various terrorist plots and plans, as of this writing, the world has thus far been spared a successful radiological terrorism attack. With respect to nuclear weapons, comments made by Iklé in 1958 still hold true:

> The only empirical evidence of the effect of nuclear weapons on society must come from mankind's only actual experience with nuclear bombings of cities—at Hiroshima and Nagasaki. Firsthand knowledge of man's reaction to nuclear bombs is therefore—and most fortunately—very limited (Figure 8-4).[21]

The Myth of Widespread Panic

One important finding from the two atomic bombings of Japan is that there was an absence of mass panic in the population. According to Iklé, "findings

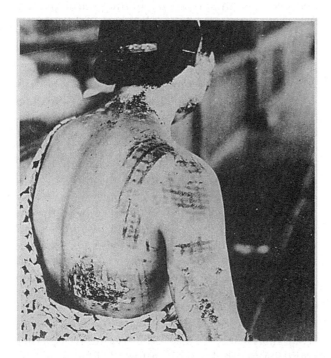

Figure 8-3. An atomic bomb survivor's skin is burned in a pattern corresponding to the dark portions of a kimono worn at the time of the explosion.
Reproduced from: National Archives and Records Administration. RG 77. Photo no. 77-MDH-6.55b (World War II Collection).

from Hiroshima, Nagasaki…and other areas of large bombings in World War II do not indicate that serious mass panic occurred at any time."[21] Indeed, contrary to what is seen in many disaster movies, the literature on disasters of all types suggests that panic is actually a relatively rare phenomenon. This does not mean that it never occurs; there have been instances involving panic, particularly when people are trapped. But on the whole, "reports from very large disasters in the past fail to show any significant mass panic among the afflicted population."[21] In general, people try to "cope with the threat and apply corrective measures using their best knowledge and capabilities."[22]

The same pattern appears to hold true in large-scale terrorist bombings. Drawing on survivor and witness accounts, Drury et al,[23] examined people's reactions and responses to the series of four coordinated bombings of the London public transportation system carried out by Islamist terrorists on July 7, 2005. The blasts, one on a bus and three on the London Underground, killed 57 people and wounded more than 700 others. The circumstances were terrifying for individuals trapped underground on bombed subway trains: "Those in the bombed underground trains were not reached by emergency services immediately, and were left in the dark, with few announcements, and with no way of knowing whether they would be rescued, or whether the rail lines were live."[23] Although it was not uncommon for people to use the word "panic" or "panicky" to describe their feelings during the event, and although many people reported experiencing fear, descriptions of people's behavior during the event tended to emphasize that they were mostly calm and that the evacuation was orderly.

Similarly, there was no evidence of mass panic during the Al Qaeda terrorist attacks on the World Trade Center in New York and the Pentagon in Washington on September 11, 2001, when hijacked commercial jets were intentionally crashed into the buildings. Accounts of people's responses suggest that behavior was generally orderly. Remarkably, more than 14,000 people were able to successfully evacuate the twin towers in New York.[24] According to Kathleen Tierney, "the rapid, orderly, and effective evacuation of the immediate impact area—a response that was initiated and largely managed by evacuees themselves, with a virtual absence of panic—saved numerous lives."[25]

Helping Behavior in Disaster

Not only was behavior following the September 11, 2001, attacks generally orderly and without mass panic; many people also engaged in helping

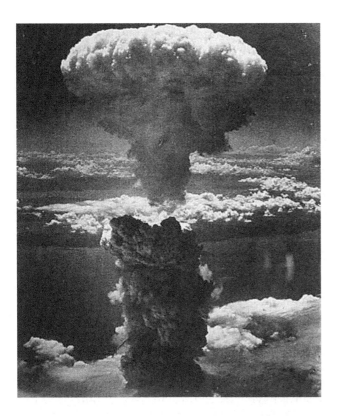

Figure 8-4. A dense column of smoke rises more than 60,000 feet into the air over the Japanese port of Nagasaki, the result of an atomic bomb dropped on August 8, 1945.
Reproduced from: National Archives and Records Administration. "Atomic Cloud Rises Over Nagasaki, Japan, 08/09/1945–08/09/1945." RG 208. Photo no. 208-N-43888 (World War II Collection).

behaviors. Tierney writes that, with the assistance of emergency workers, "occupants of the World Trade Center and people in the surrounding area helped one another to safety, even at great risk to themselves."[25] Similarly, in London, "selfish behaviors were found to be rare; mutual helping was more common."[23] These and other historical experiences suggest that in most calamities, people are less likely to experience mass panic and more likely to behave in an orderly manner and engage in prosocial helping behaviors, even in the face of danger.

Complicating Factors

When considering a large-scale radiological or nuclear attack, several factors have the potential to complicate the situation. For example, there are important limitations in extrapolating from the atomic bombings of Japan. The weapons that hit Hiroshima and Nagasaki were new, and the resulting devastation was unprecedented. People had little or no in-

formation about nuclear weapons, and they did not understand the nature or causes of the mysterious illnesses and aftereffects that occurred. Today, with the world having not only witnessed the effects of the atomic bombings in 1945 but also having experienced the Cold War, people have strong attitudes and perceptions regarding nuclear threats. In addition, they have virtually instant access to information and pictures about nuclear subjects through the Internet, social media, and the mass media. All of this has the potential to significantly affect how people understand and interpret a situation, and how they react and respond.

Perceptions, Attitudes, Fatalism

The literature on risk perception provides useful insights into how people view nuclear threats. Slovic has suggested that people assess risks on the basis of two broad dimensions: "dread risks" and "unknown risks."[26] Among the perceived characteristics of dread risks are catastrophic potential, fatal consequences, uncontrollability, inequitable distribution of risks and benefits, involuntariness, and a high risk to future generations. People's perceptions and attitudes, notes Slovic, are closely related to the dread risk factor: "the higher a hazard's score on this factor, the higher its perceived risk."[26] Nuclear weapons score higher than any other risk in terms of dread. In a study carried out by Slovic et al,[27] people were asked to rate the risk associated with 90 different activities, substances, and technologies. Nuclear weapons topped the list. Commenting on the study, Rosa and Freudenberg concluded that "nuclear risks are perceived to be the riskiest—and are the most dreaded."[28]

Complementing the risk-perception research are numerous studies of people's attitudes and expectations regarding nuclear war. Perhaps not surprisingly, in studies of the images people have of nuclear war, the dominant themes were exceedingly bleak: "physical destruction (long-term, short-term, and immediate), death, injury, weapons, politics, hell, oblivion, nothingness, pain, contamination, radiation, end of civilization, and genetic damage. Dominant emotional images included fear, terror, worry, and sadness."[29,30] A review by Fiske of more than 50 studies carried out over 4 decades found a high degree of consistency in public conceptions, attitudes, images, and perceptions of nuclear war.[31] One clear finding is that people expect a nuclear conflict to result in annihilation, and "included in that annihilation is the self."[31] In other words, people do not expect to survive. Fiske writes that, "even abstract references are clear in that respect (utter destruction, nobody left, annihilation). Moreover, when specifically asked whether they personally would expect to survive, people on average rate their chances as poor."[31]

More recent research also shows evidence of fatalism regarding radiological and nuclear terrorism, particularly among minority populations.[32,33] For example, when considering the possibility of an attack, it is not uncommon to hear comments such as "I don't think we'd have a chance" or "there is nothing you can do." In addition, studies indicate that there is some confusion about radiological and nuclear threats, and a clear pattern of low self-efficacy in the population. In surveys discussing potential terrorism threats, people say they know the least about how to protect themselves from radiological agents; only about half the population says it knows the difference between a dirty bomb and an atomic bomb; and people report lower confidence in their abilities to respond to a radiological or dirty bomb than to an earthquake or tornado, explosion or bomb, or hazardous materials accident, such as a chemical release.[34–36]

Fear of Radiation

Finally, looming large as a possible behavioral factor is the extraordinary, and perhaps unique, potential for situations involving radiation to "produce widespread fear, a profound sense of vulnerability, and a continuing sense of alarm and dread."[32] A combination of many perceived characteristics is thought to contribute to radiation's power to create apprehension and anxiety: the agent is invisible, odorless, colorless, and unable to be "apprehended by the use of the unaided senses," making it more terrifying[37,38]; it can lead to long-term contamination of an area; there are frightening historical associations and images (eg, the atomic bombs at Hiroshima and Nagasaki, the disaster at Chernobyl Nuclear Power Plant); the agent is viewed as having the potential to cause hidden and irreversible damage and as having the capacity to produce forms of illness and death that arouse particular dread (eg, cancer); it is seen as representing special dangers to young children and pregnant women; it is in many ways unfamiliar and the risks are perceived to be involuntary and even unnatural, triggering more concern than other sorts of risks[39,40]; and it is seen as posing an unbounded or open-ended threat. Because long-term health consequences may take years to develop, the danger is seen as having no end. There is a continuing sense of vulnerability and concern, and people can remain in a "permanent state of alarm and anxiety."[37]

POTENTIAL POPULATION BEHAVIORS

Population Flight

Fear is not only significant as an individual emotional reaction; as Gray and Ropeik have pointed out, it also has "powerful public health implications."[41] In situations where information is scarce, unavailable, or confusing, "fear can translate into responses that put people at risk and make managing the incident even more difficult."[42] Population flight, or spontaneous evacuation, is one important possibility. During the 1979 accident at Three Mile Island Nuclear Power Plant in Pennsylvania (Figure 8-5), for example, people received inadequate and conflicting information from authorities. Against a background of already heightened fear, a large number of people fled the area. Officials had advised pregnant women and preschool-aged children within a 5-mile radius of the reactor to leave the area. Others were told to stay indoors. Based on this advice, approximately 3,500 people should have evacuated.[43] However, for every person officially advised to evacuate, nearly 45 actually did. In all, some 150,000 people fled the area (social scientists, recognizing the trend for this sort of mass evacuation, refer to the gap between expected and actual evacuation as an "evacuation shadow").[37,44]

Chronic Stress and the Overwhelming of Healthcare Facilities

Another behavioral response that has been observed is chronic stress in unexposed people, and the overwhelming of healthcare or screening facilities by people concerned about potential health effects. The best example of this phenomenon is the 1987 radiological accident in Goiânia, Brazil,[32] when two individuals discovered a radiotherapy unit in an abandoned and partially demolished clinic. The two did not know what the machine was, but thought it may have scrap value. While trying to dismantle the unit, they ruptured the source capsule, revealing 100 g of (what was later determined to be) cesium 137. The source assembly was sold to a junkyard, and the radioactive material, which glowed blue in the dark, was spread around by curious workers and children. The incident resulted in four deaths, around 260 people and 800 acres of land showing signs of contamination, and 49 people requiring medical treatment.[45–48]

"When measured in terms of fatalities and injuries alone," Petterson observed, the event "hardly seems to be of international significance—certainly no more than any other industrial accident."[45] But because ra-

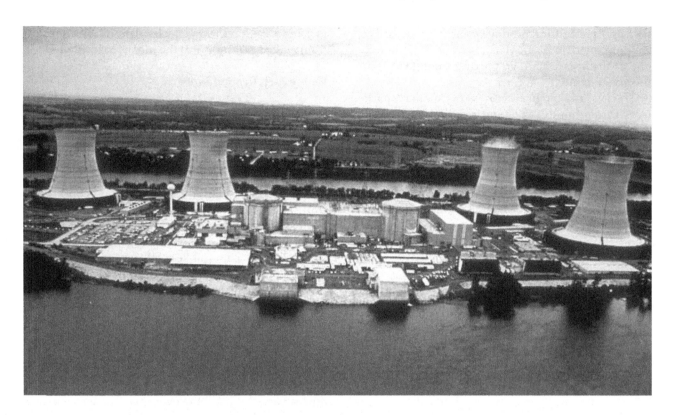

Figure 8-5. The Three Mile Island nuclear power plant near Middletown, Pennsylvania, the site of a serious accident on March 28, 1979. Inadequate, ambiguous, and conflicting information increased people's fears and likely contributed to a large spontaneous evacuation. For every person advised to leave, about 45 actually did. In all, some 150,000 people fled the area. Reproduced from: The Centers for Disease Control and Prevention Public Health Image Library. http://phil.cdc.gov/phil.

diation was involved, ripples of worry and attendant secondary impacts extended far from the epicenter of the event. Over 112,000 people, concerned about potential exposure, voluntarily sought examinations. "The fear was so intense that some people fainted in the queues, as they approached the moment of monitoring,"[49] wrote psychologist Ana Bandeira de Carvalho. Significant numbers of people also exhibited stress-induced symptoms that mimicked radiation exposure (fatigue, nausea, vomiting, diarrhea, or reddened skin).[49]

Social Stigma

A third type of fear-based behavioral response to radiation involves social stigma and discrimination against people and products from an affected area. Widespread and long-lasting stigma was powerfully evident after the atomic bombings of Hiroshima and Nagasaki. In accounts by survivors, individuals related how they were seen as tainted and as people to be avoided.[50] Survivors were seen as unacceptable as potential marriage partners. A young man breaking off his engagement with his fiancée explained: "My

father says he doesn't care who I marry as long as it isn't you. To tell the truth, my father and I both prefer not to have the blood of an atomic bomb victim in the family."[50] This stigma affected not just survivors, but succeeding generations as well. According to Mikihachiro Tatara, "knowledge that an individual comes from a Hibakusha family raises the specter that there may be 'bad blood.'… As a result, the Hibakusha Nisei [second generation] may be socially rejected out of fear that their genes will taint marriages and families."[51]

Similar reactions have also been seen after a wide variety of other situations involving radiation. Schoolchildren who were relocated from contaminated areas as a consequence of the 1986 nuclear accident at Chernobyl reported being shunned, and adolescents reportedly hid their identities as Chernobyl survivors because they feared discrimination in further education, work, and marriage.[52] After a 1999 nuclear criticality accident in Tokaimura, Japan, some residents reported that when they or their family members visited resorts, springs, or hotels in other parts of the country, they were asked not to use the public baths.[53] Products were also stigmatized after the Tokaimura accident, despite tests showing that field and agricultural products were not radioactively contaminated. In particular, it became difficult to sell one of the area's main crops, dried potatoes, under the Tokai name.[53]

The 1987 radiological accident in Goiânia "sparked fears throughout Brazil" and resulted in numerous manifestations of stigma.[54] Throughout the country, even far from the incident, "Goiânia was regarded as a place to be avoided."[32] The number of visitors to the area dropped significantly, agricultural products would not sell, and conventions planned for the city were canceled.[32,54,55] People from Goiânia faced far-reaching discrimination.[32] For example, hotels in some parts of Brazil refused Goiânia residents and some airline pilots refused to fly with them aboard, and cars with Goias license plates were stoned.[56] As a result of the discrimination, around 8,000 residents were given official certificates declaring them uncontaminated.[32]

Reactions such as flight, stress in unexposed populations, overwhelming of healthcare facilities, and stigma are not inevitable outcomes of a radiological or nuclear terrorism situation, but given the tremendous fear of radiation, they are a possibility that must be considered. Some research suggests a high propensity for population flight.[57,58] A random-digit-dial telephone survey of 800 households in the greater Washington, DC, area found that people's expressed likelihood of leaving the area immediately was higher for radiological and nuclear terrorism events than for natural disasters, technological disasters, or chemical terrorism.[57] For a radiological event, 76% indicated they were very or somewhat likely to leave immediately; for a nuclear event, the corresponding figure was 83%.[57] Households with children under 18 were the most likely to say they would leave.

The disaster literature and past disaster experiences suggest that the reaction to a radiological or nuclear attack is likely to include a great deal of calm, organized behavior, and a host of efforts to help others, even at personal risk and in the face of danger. But perceptions, concerns, and fears about radiation may also produce other kinds of behavioral responses that could inhibit helping behaviors, reduce social support, and slow recovery processes. A 2003 Department of Homeland Security report concluded, "public fear of a terrorist attack involving radioactive materials is likely to be high and could produce responses that endanger physical and mental health as well as the economic viability of affected communities."[59] Such responses are most likely when information is unavailable, inadequate, contradictory, or confusing. Thus, a crucial component of any effort to address psychological issues in a nuclear or radiological at-

tack involves having an effective communication and information strategy and the means to implement it.

Emergency Responders

It is important to note that uneasiness about radiation and radioactive materials incidents is not limited to the public; emergency responders can also be affected. A growing body of focus group, interview, and survey research has begun to provide important insights into the views, perceptions, and concerns of front-line personnel in relation to radiological and nuclear attacks. Among the groups included in such studies are police officers, firefighters, emergency medical technicians, public health professionals, physicians, nurses, and hospital personnel.

One clear and consistent finding is that responders of all types have a high level of dedication to duty and a strong commitment to professional responsibilities. Responders consistently emphasize that their work is not just about doing a job; it is also about a powerful devotion to duty, helping, and service, which would factor into the response to a radiological or nuclear attack.[32,60–62] However, many responders are concerned about radiological and nuclear incidents in ways they are not with other emergency situations. Many responders have doubts about individual and organizational readiness for responding to this "new" challenge. Although first responders appear to have a higher level of confidence than either public health workers or hospital-based healthcare providers, all responder groups express preparedness concerns. Responders also express a lower comfort level with radiation compared to many other threats, and for some this lack of familiarity translates into greater apprehension.[32,60–62]

Survey research studies have found that responders express a lower willingness to be involved in dealing with radiological and nuclear events than with most, or sometimes even all, other types of incidents.[63–68] Furthermore, the difference in willingness to respond to radiological or nuclear incidents as compared to other events is striking. A large majority (87%) of 1,711 hospital personnel surveyed in five states indicated a willingness to work in response to a fire, rescue, and collapse mass casualty incident. The figures were also high for a flood (81%), earthquake (79%), hurricane (78%), tornado (77%), ice storm (75%), and even an influenza epidemic (72%). But only 57% expressed a willingness to report for duty following a radiation event.[68] This is consistent with other surveys, where expressed willingness to report for a radiological or nuclear incident tends to hover around the 50% mark.

There is considerable uncertainty about the implications of these and other related findings.[69] Some experts have recommended that planners assume fewer first responders and health personnel will come to work after a radiation event because they will either fear contamination or will stay near home to care for their families.[70] Exactly what percentage of workers this might affect is difficult to predict because what people say in focus groups and surveys may not always mirror what occurs in an actual event; people's expressed behavioral intentions are not always good predictors of what they will actually do. In the case of emergency responders, a high level of dedication to duty could override other factors. On the other hand, there have already been real-world situations in which concerns about contamination have affected response and recovery efforts and responders' willingness to carry out certain work. This was the case after the May 2000 Cerro Grande wildfire in New Mexico, which spread to areas around the Los Alamos National Laboratory.[60] Some laboratory property was destroyed, resulting in staff evacuations and temporary closure. However, even though fires came close to critical facilities, laboratory officials declared that all major structures had been secured and no releases of radiation had occurred. In the aftermath of the fire, hundreds of professional wildland firefighters were brought in to assist with efforts to reseed burned land and rehabilitate affected areas. Approximately 100 of the firefighters asked to be released from their duties. The firefighters were concerned that they might be exposed to radioactive contaminants or other hazardous materials, despite the assurances of laboratory officials.[71–77]

In the Los Alamos event, willingness to carry out certain work was reduced by a combination of concerns about contamination and lack of trust in authorities and their assurances about safety. However, even a real-world clean-up and recovery operation is not the same thing as an unfolding radiological or nuclear attack in which people are desperate for help. In such a situation, the powerful commitment to duty and service that motivates responders would likely translate into higher levels of willingness to report than have been expressed in research studies. Responders face danger and save lives every day, and they do so with professionalism, courage, and heroism. Still, the research findings should be a red flag. They indicate that many responders have deep concerns and apprehension about situations involving radiation, and that these may dramatically increase responder

stress and make it harder for them to do their jobs. The findings also suggest that responder concerns, if left unaddressed, could result in reduced capacity for agencies to respond to a large-scale radiological or nuclear incident.[61]

Military Personnel

At the time of this writing, published, peer-reviewed "ability and willingness" studies of the type carried out with emergency responders have not been performed with military personnel. But there are indications that military personnel, like their counterparts in the emergency response community, are not always clear about radiation issues. Pastel carried out a pilot study of pretest–posttest results from military medical personnel who took the 3-day Armed Forces Radiobiology Research Institute's Medical Effects of Ionizing Radiation course. He concluded, "this pilot study suggests that the understanding of radiation and radiation exposure risks is surprisingly limited among a selected highly trained, well-educated population."[78]

Undoubtedly, there are personnel and units (eg, specialized units that have been trained to respond to a radiological or nuclear event) that are both knowledgeable and comfortable dealing with radiation issues. There are also those who live with or deal with radiation on a daily basis (eg, those serving on a nuclear-powered submarine). However, the majority of uniformed personnel likely share some of the same concerns and apprehensions that have been identified in the emergency responder community. Civilian employees assigned to military bases and other facilities may also harbor the same perceptions, attitudes, and concerns as the general public. Thus, it is possible for some of the same behavioral reactions and responses identified earlier to occur.

It is essential that appropriate training, informational materials, and emergency messages be developed and tested well in advance of a nuclear event to properly prepare the military community. Information about radiation, health effects, and related issues should be clear and credible. Input from uniformed personnel and civilian employees about potential concerns and information needs can help make communication strategies and tools more responsive and effective. It is also vital to have mechanisms in place to provide information about family and address family concerns in the event of a nuclear emergency.

SPECTRUM OF MENTAL HEALTH IMPACTS

A broad spectrum of mental health effects can result from an attack involving radiological or nuclear weapons, including the stress reactions that commonly result from all disasters (eg, natural disasters, technological disasters, terrorism).[2,53] The effects can be emotional, physical, cognitive, or interpersonal (Exhibit 8-1). Such reactions, which are highly prevalent in the emergency and early postimpact phases of a disaster, represent a normal reaction to a highly abnormal situation.[53] Disasters are:

> highly stressful, disruptive experiences. People are exposed to situations that are well outside the bounds of everyday experience, and such situations place extraordinary demands—both physical and emotional—on people. It would be remarkable, then, if individuals who experience such extreme situations did not exhibit some physiological or emotional response.[79]

Following a major disaster, large numbers of people can experience stress reactions.[79] However, human beings are often remarkably resilient, and mild or moderate stress reactions are usually transient.[53] According to Hartsough and Myers, "relief from stress and the passage of time usually lead to the reestablishment of equilibrium, but information about normal reactions, education about ways to handle them, and early attention to symptoms can speed recovery and prevent long-term problems."[80]

When considering a radiological or nuclear attack, however, the picture becomes somewhat more complicated, because exposure to invisible contaminants can produce a chronic state of alarm.[2] Even concern about the possibility of exposure can be enough to cause significant chronic stress reactions, as was demonstrated in a study by Collins and de Carvalho carried out 3 ½ years after the Goiânia radiological accident in Brazil. The study examined the behavioral responses of three groups: (1) people who had been exposed to radiation as a result of the accident, (2) people who had not been exposed but were concerned about potential exposure, and (3) a control group. The study found that people who had been exposed and people who were concerned about potential exposure showed

---

EXHIBIT 8-1

COMMON STRESS REACTIONS TO DISASTER

Emotional Effects	**Cognitive Effects**
Shock	Impaired concentration
Anger	Impaired decision-making ability
Despair	Memory impairment
Emotional numbing	Disbelief
Terror	Confusion
Guilt	Distortion
Grief or sadness	Decreased self-esteem
Irritability	Decreased self-efficacy
Helplessness	Self-blame
Loss of pleasure derived from regular activities	Intrusive thoughts and memories
Dissociation (eg, perceptual experience seems "dreamlike," tunnel vision," "spacey," or on "automatic pilot"	Worry

Physical Effects	**Interpersonal Effects**
Fatigue	Alienation
Insomnia	Social withdrawal
Sleep disturbance	Increased conflict within relationships
Hyperarousal	Vocational impairment
Somatic complaints	School impairment
Impaired immune response	
Headaches	
Gastrointestinal problems	
Decreased appetite	
Decreased libido	
Startle response	

Reproduced with permission from: Young BH, Ford JD, Ruzek JI, Friedman MJ, Gusman FD. *Disaster Mental Health Services: A Guidebook for Clinicians and Administrators.* Washington, DC: National Center for Posttraumatic Stress Disorder; 1998.

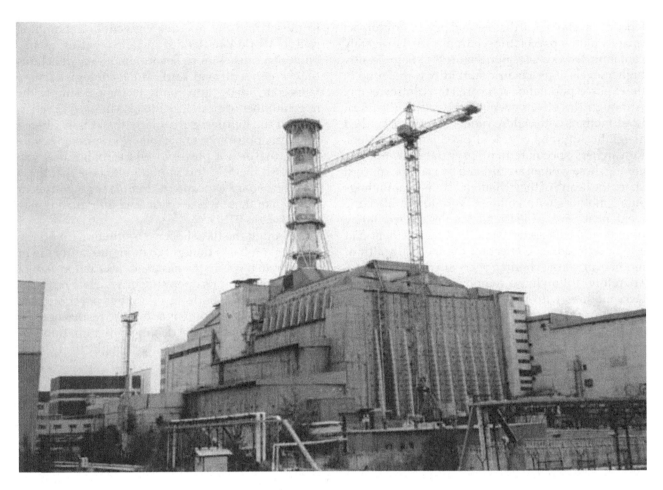

Figure 8-6. The Chernobyl Nuclear Power Plant, where an explosion and fire in the number 4 reactor caused a large release of radioactive materials and a major disaster on April 26, 1986. In the aftermath of the disaster, populations in affected areas have been gripped by a deep sense of fatalism.

similar psychological, behavioral, and cardiovascular-neuroendocrine effects.[81] This included more fear than controls, declines in performance on speed and accuracy tests, and significantly higher blood pressure. In other words, concern about potential exposure can produce stress levels similar to those caused by actual exposure to radiation. This means that psychological stresses and mental health impacts from a radiation incident can extend far beyond the immediate area of impact.[2,53]

In the aftermath of an incident involving radiation and radioactive contamination, many people are left with a continuing sense of vulnerability and a pervasive feeling of uncertainty that can last for years after the event. Whether the immediate source of danger is removed from the community or people are relocated away from the danger zone, many individuals may continue to have serious concerns about the longer-term implications of the incident.[2] Thus, although the immediate emergency may officially be over and considerable time may have passed, the incident con-

tinues to act as a powerful and persistent stressor.[82] People can become hypervigilant with respect to their own health, fearful that any symptom could be an indication of radiation-related health effects. The point is powerfully illustrated in Lifton's interviews with atomic bomb survivors. One man in his 30s who had been at Hiroshima noted, "even when I have an illness which is not at all serious—as for instance when I had very mild liver trouble—I have fears about its cause."[20] Another survivor emphasizes the constant nature of the fear, saying, "even those who look no different from the people around them live in constant fear that someday the dreaded symptoms will appear."[50]

People's concerns (and their sense of guilt) can be especially strong with relation to their children, as well. They may worry, as some Hiroshima survivors did, that their future children will inherit a radiation-related disease from them.[20] Mental health, as it relates to a survivor's children, may also be impacted after nuclear accidents. Studies carried out more than 6 years after the Chernobyl disaster found a high prevalence of psychological distress and psychiatric impact (mainly milder psychiatric syndromes) in the severely contaminated Gomel region (Figure 8-6). Significantly higher levels of psychiatric morbidity were found in the exposed population compared to a control region. Although the effects were mainly at a subclinical level, mothers with children under 18 years of age had a significantly higher risk of psychiatric disorders. Researchers speculate that "psychiatric symptoms among these women are fostered by genuine concern about the health of their children."[83,84] Similar findings about mothers with children were found after the incident at Three Mile Island. Studies carried out by Bromet and colleagues found that the accident had a long-term adverse effect on the mental health of mothers of young children years after the accident.[85] Therefore, following a radiological or nuclear attack, mothers with young children should be seen as a high-risk group warranting special services and assistance.[2,53]

More generally, chronic stress after a radiological or nuclear incident may be an important public health problem, as it can lead to conditions such as high blood pressure, cardiovascular problems, and digestive disorders. In terms of mental health, excessive worrying over a loved one on a daily basis affects one's present attitude and hopes for the future.[53] Since the Chernobyl disaster, for example, chronic stress has contributed to a deep sense of fatalism that affects significant portions of the region's population.

A smaller portion of the population is at risk for more serious and persistent mental health problems following a nuclear or radiological attack.[2] These problems can include depression, anxiety disorders, substance abuse, and posttraumatic stress disorder (PTSD). PTSD, a "prolonged post-traumatic stress response,"[86] can result in a persistent reexperiencing of a traumatic event; persistent avoidance of stimuli associated with the trauma and a numbing of general responsiveness; and persistent symptoms of increased arousal, such as irritability, outbursts of anger, or exaggerated startle response.[2,87]

Unlike the transient stress reactions that often occur after disasters, PTSD results in higher levels of impairment and dysfunction. It typically—but not always—appears in the first few months after a trauma. There can also be variations in its intensity and duration.[79] Among the most important factors associated with the PTSD development is the nature of the trauma. Individuals "exposed to life threat and perhaps, in those exposed to terror, horror, and the grotesque,"[82] which could all be factors in a nuclear attack, are at greater risk for developing PTSD. Comparing the effects of a nuclear detonation

to those from the massive conventional bombing raids of World War II, Iklé concluded that an "atomic bombing causes more severe emotional reactions than a conventional raid."[21] Psychologist Irving Janis concluded, "apparently it was not simply the large number of casualties but also the specific character of the injuries, particularly the grossly altered physical appearance of persons who suffered severe burns, that had a powerful effect upon those who witnessed them."[21] It is important to note that those with secondary exposure to trauma (eg, spouses or children of those who experienced it firsthand) may also develop PTSD.[2,79]

Although the likelihood of a situation involving nuclear combat is thought to be significantly lower today than it was in the past, such a situation cannot be ruled out. Troops operating in a nuclear environment would face both the enormous psychological stresses posed by combat and those resulting from the special challenges of dealing with radiation and radioactivity. Factors that are thought to increase the level of combat stress include surprise, lack of combat experience, poor unit cohesion, lack of preparation, prevalence of direct casualties, poor or tired leadership, and especially intense battles.[22] With respect to the radiological issues, stressors may include having to wear special protective equipment and being exposed to substantial radiation levels.[88–90]

For those in positions of command, difficult decisions about acceptable level of risk would be an additional stressor. Tradeoffs between accomplishing immediate objectives and long-term health risk may weigh heavily on commanders. More generally, concern about both immediate and future health effects would be a continuing stressor for all those operating in a nuclear environment.

Another highly stressful situation for members of the armed forces would be responding to the area affected by a nuclear detonation to render assistance to civilians. One factor would be the large numbers of bodies. According to Sullivan and Bongar, "witnessing large numbers of dead or injured people can demoralize or shock even those not directly exposed to the attack."[70] This would be dramatically amplified by seeing the bodies of dead children, including children with burns and other grotesque injuries.

The inability to help save some people would weigh heavily on personnel deployed to render assistance. Lifton cites the case of a young male social worker who was in military service at the time of the Hiroshima blast who saw a dead mother with a child still alive next to her. The social worker, who had to return to his unit, was unable to do more than provide the child with some water, which the child was too weak to drink. The image of that child, remarked the social worker, "stayed on my mind and remains as a strong impression even now."[20]

Finally, the involvement of terrorism (eg, a series of terrorist dirty bomb attacks) could also amplify psychological effects and increase the number of people severely psychologically affected for the long term, in part because of the intentionality of the act. According to Butler et al, "Many elements of terrorism are very distinct from other forms of trauma. The most obvious and salient is the element of intent—the purpose of terrorism is widespread infliction of psychological pain."[91] The possibility of additional attacks would also likely exacerbate the psychological impacts.[91]

Clearly the psychological dimension is one of the most important aspects of a radiological or nuclear incident. Reviewing 2 decades of research on the short- and long-term health, environmental, and socioeconomic consequences of the 1986 Chernobyl disaster, an international consortium of scientists concluded that the mental health impact of Chernobyl "is the largest public health problem caused by the accident to date."[92]

PREVENTING AND REDUCING THE PSYCHOLOGICAL IMPACTS OF A RADIOLOGICAL OR NUCLEAR ATTACK

Regardless of the type of nuclear threat or nuclear incident, the guiding principle in relation to psychological impacts should be prevention. According to the Institute of Medicine, "efforts must be expanded beyond treatment for individuals who are most severely affected to comprehensive prevention and health promotion."[91] This point was also emphasized by the National Council on Radiation Protection and Measurements in *Management of Terrorist Events Involving Radioactive Material*, the first comprehensive report on radiological and nuclear terrorism:

> It is far more effective to intervene early to prevent social and psychological problems from developing than it is to have to address serious problems once they have arisen. What this implies is the need to have plans, infrastructure, resources and trained personnel already in place. In other words, the social and psychosocial component cannot be an afterthought.…The cost of inadequate preparedness is greater morbidity and more long-term effects.[2]

Thus, what is needed is a comprehensive, integrated approach that enhances preparedness, fosters people's natural resilience and helping behaviors, and endeavors to prevent and reduce psychological impact. This approach includes a number of key components.

Integrating Psychological, Social, Behavioral, and Risk-Communication Issues into Response Plans

The complex psychosocial dimension must not be overlooked when preparing for a radiological or nuclear attack.[93] This not only means it is vital to make psychological issues an organic part of the planning process; it also means considering the full range of potential scenarios, including the uncomfortable and disconcerting ones identified earlier in this chapter. Furthermore, effective planning requires that the psychological component be addressed on multiple levels: individual mental health, unit-level impacts, and broader behavioral responses, such as flight and stigma. In addition, it means addressing the possibility that large numbers of concerned individuals could flood healthcare facilities. Estimates of the kinds of numbers that could be involved vary widely. Jarrett suggests that in a nuclear attack, "everyone who 'saw the flash' would be convinced" that he or she had received a significant radiation injury.[94] Sullivan and Bongar argue that:

> public health authorities should expect that for every person actually exposed…many (perhaps hundreds) more will seek medical screening. A significant percentage of nonexposed individuals seeking screening will present with psychosomatic symptoms that mimic those of victims who were actually exposed.[70]

Whatever the estimate, such an outcome should not be ignored in plans, nor should it be considered automatic or inevitable. Plans for dealing with radiological and nuclear attacks need to include robust components for reducing (via emergency messaging and public information efforts) and addressing (eg, through triage, alternate care sites, and related approaches) this challenging issue.[95–97]

Including and Practicing Psychosocial Issues in Drills and Exercises

Drills and exercises can be invaluable in improving preparedness, but, as the National Council on Radiation Protection and Measurements pointed out a number of years ago, drills and exercises are "only useful to the extent that they are similar to the conditions likely to be faced by responders."[2] Although there have undoubtedly been improvements in recent years in including psychosocial content, the vast majority of drills and exercises remain lacking in this key area. Having a small number of mock psychological casualties is useful but is not enough; rather, drills and exercises need to grapple with such challenges as population flight, stigma, chronic stress in the unaffected population, triage, the overwhelming of healthcare facilities by concerned and anxious individuals, adapting standard mental health interventions for contamination situations, counseling pregnant women about radiation effects, assisting high-risk groups (such as women with young children), and radiation risk communication for service personnel, civilian employees, decision makers and commanders, and the broader population. Furthermore, the various radiological and nuclear attack scenarios, including those identified earlier in this chapter, need to be exercised.

Individual Detection and Recording Devices

A key finding of research conducted during the 2006 London polonium incident (in which Alexander Litvinenko, a Russian émigré living in London, was poisoned with radioactive polonium-210 and subsequently died) was that people concerned about potential contamination are not satisfied with general assurances. Most people concerned about a radiation event want more than abstract explanations; they want specific, individual information about the level of exposure and the likely consequences.[98–100] Thus, it is advisable for all personnel who are expected to be in radiation areas to have individual dosimeters.[101] Having the kind of individual-level information that a personal dosimeter can provide is valuable as a radiation protection measure, a means of facilitating long-term follow-up, a way of providing specific answers to health concerns, and as a measure to help prevent psychological impacts. Blanket statements, and even group-level or unit-level radiation readings, are simply not a substitute for such individual-level data. Furthermore, not having such individual-level information is a recipe for chronic uncertainty and apprehension about potential future health effects.

Identifying Groups at Greater Risk for Psychological Effects

For all personnel affected by, or responding to, a radiological or nuclear event, the use of peer support, buddy care, psychological first aid, and the fostering of unit cohesion and similar approaches can help improve individual resilience and coping. At the same time, it is important to be aware of groups that may be at elevated risk for psychological effects and that

may require additional support and attention. As in all disaster situations, individuals with preexisting mental illness are at increased risk. So, too, are those who suffer physical injuries, lose family in the event, suffer disruption of social support, directly witness the deaths of others, or handle dead bodies.[70]

As noted, research from the incidents at Chernobyl and Three Mile Island has identified mothers with young children as being at the greatest risk of psychiatric morbidity in radiation accidents. This finding is likely to be relevant in a radiological or nuclear attack as well. In scenarios where families of service personnel are in the affected area, special attention might need to be devoted to female service members who have young children. This could be especially important given the rapidly growing role of women in the armed services, particularly the reserves (women are now estimated to make up about 25% of the Army Reserve).[102]

Special attention will also be needed for pregnant women and persons with reproductive and fertility concerns. In the aftermath of a radiological or nuclear attack, such individuals could experience extraordinary stress about potential radiation-related health impacts on the developing fetus. Some women may also feel pressure to terminate pregnancies out of fear of giving birth to a malformed child. Thus, in any radiological or nuclear attack scenario, it will be important to have accurate information and appropriate reproductive counseling available so that informed decisions can be made and emotional support can be provided.

Depending on the scenario (eg, an attack on a military base and surrounding community in the United States), many children could also be affected. In any disaster situation, children have unique vulnerabilities. They may be exposed to the same frightening sights, sounds, smells, and dangers as adults, but not have the coping skills, resources, emotional maturity, and life experience to understand and deal with what is going on around them.[103] As Danieli and Dingman have noted, children in disaster situations may experience worry, fear, nightmares, separation anxiety, and somatic complaints, as well as concern about personal safety and security.[104] Other reactions can include changes in sleep and appetite, decreases in school performance, increased sensitivity to sounds (eg, sirens), heightened startle response, and decreased interest in pleasurable activities.[104] As younger children cope, they may "engage in posttraumatic play and ask questions or talk about the event repeatedly."[104] Older children might express concerns about their safety, security, and futures, while adolescents may respond with withdrawal, substance abuse, risk-taking behaviors, or fascination with death or suicide.[104]

Healthcare professionals, service providers, parents, teachers and others will need to be aware of these potential impacts. Mental health professionals have cautioned that "extensive viewing of media coverage appears to negatively affect children of all ages."[104] Triage, radiological screening, and other processes will need to have pediatric-specific zones that can address the physical and emotional needs of children. In addition, there is a need for specialized, age-appropriate materials to answer children's questions and explain key aspects of the situation.[105]

A radiological or nuclear attack may even create a cohort of orphans, as was the case after the atomic bombings in Japan. Because of the conventional bombings that had already occurred, thousands of children had been taken out of urban areas. Their parents, however, still spent considerable time in the cities. Thus, when the atomic bombs were dropped, a large number of children suddenly became orphans.[106] If the central business district of a large US city were destroyed during a weekday by a nuclear weapon, when most children would be located at schools further from the city center, it is possible that a similar outcome could occur.

An Integrated Approach to Service Delivery

In providing services to an affected population, it is vital for the medical and psychosocial components of the response effort to be well integrated in terms of approach and personnel.[53] Authorities should ensure that those fearing they have been exposed to radiation or radioactive contaminants should be given requested medical examinations as soon as possible, and their concerns and symptoms should be taken seriously.[53] Likewise, pejorative terms such as "radiophobia" or "worried well" should be avoided when discussing people's concerns about radiation, since they could easily be seen as dismissive.[53]

In cases where people have been exposed to radiation, the best way to prevent psychological effects is to provide exposed individuals with care "that will enable them to maintain a sense of control over their health."[107] Healthcare professionals and those affected will need to collaborate in this process, matching vigilance programs to individual needs. Among other things, strategies for reducing overall risk through lifestyle change may be useful.[53]

Efforts to provide long-term assistance and compensation to affected populations should include a psychosocial component and should also take into account key lessons from current programs, such as the Radiation Exposure Screening and Education Program set up by Congress in 1990 and amended in 2000.[108]

Focus on the Crucial Role of Information and Risk Communication

If there is one factor that is crucial in a strategy for preventing social, psychological, and behavioral impacts, it is the availability of information. Sullivan and Bongar note that "inconsistent or incomplete information . . . can heighten anxiety and deplete trust."[70] Similarly, Pastel and Ritchie note that health risk communication is important for both acute and long-term risks, and that insufficient knowledge and poor public communication can increase psychological ill effects.[109] Noy concludes, "the most salient factor in a prevention program is the dissemination of knowledge."[22] There are several components in a communication strategy aimed at reducing psychological effects.

Prebriefing

Those going into a setting affected by a radiological or nuclear attack should be briefed in advance on what they are about to experience. No amount of preparation can completely mitigate the effects of seeing large numbers of dead bodies (including children), many with severe burns and mutilating injuries, but prebriefing personnel so that they know in advance what they are likely to encounter may help prepare them emotionally. Once on the scene, efforts to reduce exposure to trauma whenever possible are also helpful.

Just-in-Time Training

Just-in-time training is now an important part of preparation for a range of low-probability, high-consequence events where there is a rapid surge in workforce requirements.[110,111] Many people may need at least a minimal level of training on an urgent basis, and others who have had more extensive training in the past may require a quick refresher. The training should be highly practical, focused on essentials, and short enough to be completed soon before going into the field or otherwise responding to an event. It should also be developed and ready in advance so that it can be "on the shelf" should an event occur. Topics should include information on what to do, who does what, how to recognize dangers and protect against them, and how to assist others. Just-in-time training not only has the potential to increase operational effectiveness; it may also help familiarize personnel with key practical issues, helping manage fear and increasing a sense of efficacy.

Information About Family

Depending on the scenario, personnel could have deep concerns about the fate and well-being of family members. It is essential to develop lines of communication between families, friends, and the community to prevent unnecessary stress.[112]

Radiation Risk Communication

Those affected by, or responding to, a radiological or nuclear attack will have many concerns, questions, and fears regarding radiation and health effects. They may also have critical decisions to make regarding what actions they will take. The information they have can have a crucial impact on those decisions. For example, Sullivan and Bongar suggest that "effective preparation and official communication are critical to preventing unplanned evacuations."[70]

With respect to a radiological or nuclear attack, it is essential that people's information needs be anticipated and proactively addressed. Waiting until the time of an event to prepare messages and materials is already too late; rather, these items need to be crafted and professionally tested in advance to ensure that messages and materials are responsive and effective and that the communication resources are ready should an incident occur.[32] Materials should be scientifically accurate, clear, forthright, and credible, communicating "in a way that neither inappropriately minimizes effects nor creates unwarranted fear."[101] They should also emphasize actions that people can take to protect themselves. In addition to having messages and materials for military personnel and emergency responders, it is important that the information needs and concerns of other key audiences (eg, civilian employees on a base, families of service personnel) be anticipated and addressed.

SUMMARY

One of the most serious threats facing the United States today is the possibility of a large-scale attack involving radiological or nuclear weapons. Furthermore, the risk of an attack could grow in the coming years, due in part to factors such as the global illicit trade in radioactive materials, the proliferation of nuclear know-how and technology, and the continuing efforts of rogue nations and terrorist groups to produce or obtain radiological or nuclear weapons. Potential scenarios that need to be considered include an attack on a US city or port, the targeting of a US military base or the home community of a military unit deployed overseas, an attack on key commercial or governmental facilities in the continental United States, and the targeting of US personnel or interests overseas.

In addition to its physical effects, an attack involving radioactive materials has the capacity to produce widespread social, psychological, and behavioral impacts. These could range from transient or longer-lasting individual mental health effects to deep community impacts, such as stigma. Among those who could be affected are civilians, military personnel and their families, emergency responders, and others in the vicinity of the incident. Depending on the type of attack, psychosocial impacts could also ripple outward, touching the lives of people far from the site and across the nation. It is crucial, therefore, for social, psychological, and behavioral issues and challenges to be a central component of preparedness and response efforts.

When considering psychosocial impacts, the guiding principle at all levels—individual, community, and societal—should be prevention. This requires a comprehensive, integrated approach that enhances preparedness, ensures that assistance efforts are responsive, and fosters resilience. Specific measures include making social, psychological, and behavioral issues an organic part of response plans and the overall planning process; better incorporating psychosocial issues in training, drills, and exercises; providing realistic training and prebriefing to personnel and ensuring they have information about their families; identifying and providing additional support and attention to groups at elevated risk for psychological effects; taking people's health concerns seriously and integrating the medical and psychosocial components of the response effort; and fitting personnel expected to be in radiation areas with individual detection and recording devices. Finally, the importance of communication and information cannot be overstated as part of a strategy of prevention. Ambiguous, inconsistent, or insufficient information can greatly exacerbate psychosocial impacts and hamper recovery efforts. Thus, making people partners in the communication process and rapidly, candidly, and effectively addressing people's information needs are essential factors in the prevention or reduction of psychosocial impacts.

REFERENCES

1. Ferguson CD, Potter WC, Sands A, Spector LC, Wehling FL. *The Four Faces of Nuclear Terrorism*. New York, NY: Routledge; 2005.

2. Poston JW, Abdelnour C, Ainsworth EJ, et al. *Management of Terrorist Events Involving Radioactive Material*. Bethesda, MD: National Council on Radiation Protection and Measurements; 2001. NCRP report no. 138.

3. Vineberg R. *Human Factors in Tactical Nuclear Combat*. Alexandria, VA: Human Resources Research Office, George Washington University, under contract with the Department of the Army; 1965. Technical report 65-2.

4. Vineberg R. *Human Factors in Tactical Nuclear Combat*. Alexandria, VA: Human Resources Research Office, George Washington University, under contract with the Department of the Army; 1967. Professional paper 2-67.

5. Sessions GR. *A Summary of the Psychological Effects of Tactical Nuclear Warfare*. Colorado Springs, CO: US Air Force Academy; 1984.

6. Baker GW, Rohrer JH, eds. *Human Problems in the Utilization of Fallout Shelters*. Washington, DC: National Academy of Sciences, National Research Council; 1960. Disaster study no. 12.

7. Baker GW, Cottrell LS Jr, eds. *Behavioral Science and Civil Defense*. Washington, DC: National Academy of Sciences, National Research Council; 1962. Disaster study no. 16.

8. Smelser NJ. *Theories of Social Change and the Analysis of Nuclear Attack and Recovery*. McLean, VA: Human Sciences Research Inc; 1967.

9. Bunn M. *Securing the Bomb 2007*. Cambridge, MA: Belfer Center for Science and International Affairs, Harvard University; 2007.

10. Mowatt-Larssen R. *Al Qaeda Weapons of Mass Destruction: Hype or Reality?* Cambridge, MA: Belfer Center for Science and International Affairs, Harvard University; 2010.

11. Allison G. *Nuclear Terrorism: The Ultimate Preventable Catastrophe*. New York, NY: Times Books; 2004.

12. Gallucci RL. Averting Nuclear Catastrophe: Contemplating Extreme Responses to US Vulnerability. In: Allison G, ed. *Confronting the Specter of Nuclear Terrorism*. Vol 607. In: *The Annals of the American Academy of Political and Social Science*. Thousand Oaks, CA: Sage Publications; 2006: 51–58.

13. Committee on Medical Preparedness for a Terrorist Nuclear Event, Board on Health Sciences Policy, Institute of Medicine of the National Academies. *Assessing Medical Preparedness to Respond to a Terrorist Nuclear Event*: *Workshop Report*. Washington, DC: The National Academies Press; 2009.

14. Meade C, Molander RC. *Considering the Effects of a Catastrophic Terrorist Attack*. Santa Monica, CA: RAND Center for Terrorism Risk Management Policy; 2006. Technical report.

15. US Federal Emergency Management Agency. Nuclear/radiological incident annex of the National Response Framework (2008). http://www.fema.gov/pdf/emergency/nrf/nrf_nuclearradiologicalincidentannex.pdf. Accessed August 16, 2010.

16. Blackett PMS. *Fear, War, and the Bomb: Military and Political Consequences of Atomic Energy*. New York, NY: Whittlesey House; 1949.

17. Hirschfelder JO, Kramish A, Parker DB, Smith RC, Glasstone S, eds. *The Effects of Atomic Weapons*. New York, NY: McGraw-Hill; 1950.

18. Lugar RG. *The Lugar Survey on Proliferation Threats and Responses*. Washington, DC: US Senate Foreign Relations Committee; 2005.

19. Terrorism Survey. Frequency questionnaire, March 8–April 21, 2006, Foreign Policy and Center for American Progress. http://www.americanprogress.org/kf/terrorsurveypoll.pdf. Accessed August 16, 2010.

20. Lifton RJ. Psychological effects of the atomic bomb in Hiroshima: the theme of death. *Daedalus*. 1963;92(3):462–497.

21. Janis I. Quoted in: Iklé FC. *The Social Impact of Bomb Destruction*. Norman, OK: University of Oklahoma Press; 1958.

22. Noy S. Prevalence of psychological, somatic, and conduct casualties in war. *Mil Med*. 2001;166(S2):17–18.

23. Drury J, Cocking C, Reicher S. The nature of collective resilience: survivor reactions to the 2005 London bombings. *Int J Mass Emerg Disasters*. 2009;27(1):66–95.

24. Gershon RRM, Qureshi KA, Rubin MS, Raveis VH. Factors associated with high-rise evacuation: qualitative results from the World Trade Center Evacuation Study. *Prehosp Disaster Med*. 2007;22(3):165–173.

25. Tierney K. *Strength of a City: a Disaster Research Perspective on the World Trade Center Attack*. New York, NY: Social Science Research Council; 2002. http://essays.ssrc.org/sept11/essays/tierney.htm. Accessed August 17, 2010.

26. Slovic P. Perception of risk. In: Slovic P. *The Perception of Risk*. London, UK: Earthscan Publications Ltd; 2001: 220–231. Chap 13.

27. Slovic P, Fischoff B, Lichtenstein S. Facts and fears: understanding perceived risk. In: Slovic P. *The Perception of Risk*. London, UK: Earthscan Publications Ltd; 2001: 137–153.

28. Rosa EA, Freudenberg WR. The historical development of public reactions to nuclear power: implications for nuclear waste policy. In: Dunlap RE, Kraft ME, Rosa EA, eds. *Public Reactions to Nuclear Waste: Citizens' Views of Repository Siting*. Durham, NC: Duke University Press; 1993: 32–63.

29. Slovic P, Layman M, Flynn JH. Perceived risk, trust, and nuclear waste: lessons from Yucca Mountain. In: Dunlap RE, Kraft ME, Rosa EA, eds. *Public Reactions to Nuclear Waste: Citizens' Views of Repository Siting*. Durham, NC: Duke University Press; 1993: 64–86. Chap 3.

30. Fiske ST, Pratto F, Pavelchak MA. Citizens' images of nuclear war: content and consequences. *J Soc Issues*. 1983;39:41–65.

31. Fiske ST. Adult beliefs, feelings, and actions regarding nuclear war: evidence from surveys and experiments. In: Solomon F, Marston RQ, eds, and Institute of Medicine of the National Academies Steering Committee for the Symposium on the Medical Implications of Nuclear War. *The Medical Implications of Nuclear War*. Washington, DC: The National Academies Press; 1986: Chap 21.

32. Becker SM. Emergency communication and information issues in terrorism events involving radioactive materials. *Biosecur Bioterror*. 2004;2(3):195–207.

33. Wray RJ, Becker SM, Henderson N, et al. Communicating with the public about emerging health threats: lessons from the Pre-Event Message Development Project. *Am J Public Health*. 2008;98(12):2214–2222.

34. US Federal Emergency Management Agency. *Personal Preparedness in America: Findings From the 2009 Citizen Corps National Survey*. Washington, DC: FEMA; 2009.

35. Kano M, Wood MM, Mileti DS, Bourque LB. *Public Response to Terrorism: Findings From the National Survey of Disaster Experiences and Preparedness*. Los Angeles, CA: University of California; 2008.

36. Lasker RD. *Redefining Readiness: Terrorism Planning Through the Eyes of the Public*. New York, NY: Center for the Advancement of Collaborative Strategies in Health, The New York Academy of Medicine; 2004.

37. Erikson K. *A New Species of Trouble: The Human Experience of Modern Disasters*. New York, NY: WW Norton; 1995.

38. Salter CA. Psychological effects of nuclear and radiological warfare. *Mil Med*. 2001;166(S2):17–18.

39. Bennett P. Understanding responses to risk: some basic findings. In: Bennett P, Calman K, eds. *Risk Communication and Public Health*. Oxford, UK: Oxford University Press; 1999.

40. Stokes JW, Banderet LE. Psychological aspects of chemical defense and warfare. *Mil Psychol*. 1997;9(4):395–415.

41. Gray GM, Ropeik DP. Dealing with the dangers of fear: the role of risk communication. *Health Aff*. 2002;21(6):106–116.

42. Becker SM. Addressing the psychosocial and communication challenges posed by radiological/nuclear terrorism: key developments since NCRP report no. 138. *Health Phys*. 2005;89(5):521–530.

43. Johnson JH Jr. A model of evacuation–decision making in a nuclear reactor emergency. *Geogr Rev*. 1985;75(4):405–418.

44. Zeigler DJ, Brunn SD, Johnson JH Jr. Evacuation from a nuclear technological disaster. *Geogr Rev*. 1981;71(1):1–16.

45. Petterson JS. Perception vs. reality of radiological impact: the Goiania model. *Nucl News*. 1988;31(14):84–90.

46. De Oliveira CN, Melo DR, Liptzstein JL. Internal contamination in the Goiania Accident, Brazil, 1987. In: Gusev I, Guskova A, Mettler FA Jr, eds. *Medical Management of Radiation Accidents*. 2nd ed. Boca Raton, FL: CRC Press; 2001: 355–360. Chap 26.

47. Binns DAC. Goiania 1987: searching for radiation. In: *Goiania 10 Years Later: Proceedings of an International Conference, Goiania, Brazil, 26–31 October 1997*. Vienna, AT: International Atomic Energy Agency and Brazilian Atomic Energy Commission; 1998.

48. International Atomic Energy Agency. *The Radiological Accident in Goiania*. Vienna, AT: IAEA; 1988.

49. de Carvalho AB. Psychological aspects of a radiological accident. Paper presented at: The 9th Annual National Radiological Emergency Preparedness Conference; March 1999; Baton Rouge, LA.

50. Sekimori G, trans. *Hibakusha: Survivors of Hiroshima and Nagasaki*. Tokyo, JP: Kosei Publishing Company; 1987.

51. Tatara M. The second generation of Hibakusha, atomic bomb survivors: a psychologist's view. In: Danieli Y, ed. *International Handbook of Multigenerational Legacies of Trauma*. New York, NY: Plenum Press; 1998: 141–146.

52. *The Trace of the Black Wind: Through the Eyes of Children*. Bence M, ed. Minsk, BY: Belarusian Socio-Ecological Union; 1996.

53. Becker SM. Psychosocial effects of radiation accidents. In: Gusev I, Guskova A, Mettler FA Jr, eds. *Medical Management of Radiation Accidents*. 2nd ed. Boca Raton, FL: CRC Press; 2001: Chap 41.

54. Easterling D, Kunreuther H. The vulnerability of the convention industry to the siting of a high-level nuclear waste repository. In: Dunlap RE, Kraft ME, Rosa EA, eds. *Public Reactions to Nuclear Waste: Citizens' Views of Repository Siting*. Durham, NC: Duke University Press; 1993: 209–238.

55. Easterling D. Fear and loathing of Las Vegas: will a nuclear waste repository contaminate the imagery of nearby places. In: Flynn J, Slovic P, Kunreuther H, eds. *Risk, Media and Stigma: Understanding Public Challenges to Modern Science and Technology*. London, UK: Earthscan Publications Ltd; 2001: 133–156.

56. Kasperson RE, Kasperson JX. The social amplification and attenuation of risk. *Ann Am Acad Pol Soc Sci*. 1996;545(May):95–105.

57. Gerber BJ, Ducatman A, Fischer M, Althouse R, Scotti JR. *The Potential for an Uncontrolled Mass Evacuation of the DC Metro Area Following a Terrorist Attack: A Report of Survey Findings*. Morgantown, WV: West Virginia University; 2006.

58. Meit M, Briggs T, Kennedy A. *Urban to Rural Evacuation: Planning for Rural Population Surge*. Bethesda, MD: The Walsh Center for Rural Health Analysis, National Opinion Research Center; 2008.

59. US Department of Homeland Security and the American Nuclear Society. *The Scientific Basis for Communication About Events Involving Radiological Dispersion Devices*. Washington, DC: DHS, ANS; 2003.

60. Becker SM. Preparing for terrorism involving radioactive materials: three lessons from recent experience and research. *J Appl Secur Res*. 2009;4(1):9–20.

61. Becker SM. Risk communication and radiological/nuclear terrorism: perceptions, concerns and information needs of first responders, health department personnel, and healthcare providers. In: Johnson RH, ed. *Radiation Risk Communication: Issues and Solutions*. Madison, WI: Medical Physics Publishing; 2010: 271–280. Chap 15.

62. Becker SM, Middleton S. Improving hospital preparedness for radiological terrorism: perspectives from emergency department physicians and nurses. *Disaster Med Public Health Prep*. 2008;2(3):174–184.

63. Dimaggio C, Markenson DT, Loo G, Redlener I. The willingness of U.S. emergency medical technicians to respond to terrorist incidents. *Biosecur Bioterror*. 2005;3:331–337.

64. O'Sullivan TL, Dow D, Turner MC, et al. Disaster and emergency management: Canadian nurses' perceptions of preparedness on hospital front lines. *Prehosp Disas Med*. 2008;23(3):s11–s18.

65. Veenema TG, Walden B, Feinstein N, Williams JP. Factors affecting hospital-based nurses' willingness to respond to a radiation emergency. *Disaster Med Public Health Prep*. 2008;2(4):224–229.

66. Lanzilotti SS, Galanis D, Leoni N, Craig B. Hawaii medical professionals assessment. *Hawaii Med J*. 2002;61(8):162–173.

67. Qureshi K, Gershon RR, Sherman MF, et al. Health care workers' ability and willingness to report to duty during catastrophic disasters. *J Urban Health*. 2005;82:378–388.

68. Cone DC, Cummings BA. Hospital disaster staffing: if you call, will they come? *Am J Disaster Med*. 2006;1(1):28–36.

69. Redlener I, Garrett AL, Levin KL, Mener A. *Regional Health and Public Health Preparedness for Nuclear Terrorism: Optimizing Survival in a Low Probability/High Consequence Disaster*. New York, NY: National Center for Disaster Preparedness, Columbia University Mailman School of Public Health; 2010.

70. Sullivan GR, Bongar B. Psychological consequences of actual or threatened CBRNE terrorism. In: Bongar B, Brown LM, Beutler LE, Breckenridge JN, Zimbardo PG, eds. *Psychology of Terrorism*. New York, NY: Oxford University Press; 2007: 153–163.

71. Hill BT. *Fire Management: Lessons Learned From the Cerro Grande (Los Alamos) Fire and Actions Needed to Reduce Fire Risks*. Washington, DC: US General Accounting Office; 2000. T-RCED-00-273.

72. Becker SM. Meeting the threat of weapons of mass destruction terrorism: toward a broader conception of consequence management. *Mil Med*. 2001;166(S2):13–16.

73. Novak S. Experts debate safety issues as fire spreads to nuclear lab. *The New Mexican*. May 12, 2000: 1.

74. Davenport K. Contamination concerns. *The New Mexican*. June 12, 2000: 1.

75. Neary B. Cerro Grande fire debris worries landfill neighbors. *The New Mexican*. August 8, 2000: 1.

76. Associated Press. Firefighters worried about possible contamination. *Albuquerque Journal*. June 16, 2000: 6.

77. Local produce to be tested for radiation. *The New Mexican*. July 16, 2000: 12.

78. Pastel RH. Fear of radiation in US military medical personnel. *Mil Med*. 2001;166(S2):80–82.

79. Landesman LY, Malilay J, Bissell R, Becker SM, Roberts L, Ascher MS. Roles and responsibilities of public health in disaster preparedness and response. In: Novick Lloyd F, ed. *Public Health Administration*. New York, NY: Aspen Publishers; 2000: 646–708.

80. Hartsough DM, Myers DG. *Disaster Work and Mental Health: Prevention and Control of Stress Among Workers*. Washington, DC: Center for Mental Health Services, Substance Abuse and Mental Health Services Administration, US Public Health Service; 1985.

81. Collins DL, de Carvalho AB. Chronic stress from the Goiania 137Cs radiation accident. *Behav Med*. 1993;18:149–157.

82. Ursano RJ, Fullerton CS, McCaughey BG. Trauma and disaster. In: Ursano RJ, McCaughey BG, Fullerton CS, eds. *Individual and Community Responses to Trauma and Disaster: The Structure of Human Chaos*. Cambridge, MA: Cambridge University Press; 1994: 3–27.

83. Havenaar JM, van den Brink W, Kasyanenko AP, et al. Mental health problems in the Gomel region (Belarus): an analysis of risk factors in an area affected by the Chernobyl disaster. *Psychol Med*. 1996;26:845–855.

84. Havenaar JM, Rumyantzeva GM, van den Brink W, et al. Long-term mental health effects of the Chernobyl disaster: an epidemiologic survey of two former Soviet regions. *Am J Psychiatry*. 1997;154:1605–1607.

85. Bromet EJ, Parkinson DK, Dunn LO. Long-term mental health consequences of the accident at Three Mile Island. *Int J Ment Health*. 1990;19:48–60.

86. Young BH, Ford JD, Ruzek JI, Friedman MJ, Gusman FD. *Disaster Mental Health Services: A Guidebook for Clinicians and Administrators*. Washington, DC: National Center for Posttraumatic Stress Disorder; 1998.

87. American Psychiatric Association. *Diagnostic and Statistical Manual of Mental Disorders*. 4th ed. Washington, DC: APA; 1994.

88. Oordt MS. The psychological effects of weapons of mass destruction. In: Kennedy CH, Zillmer EA, eds. *Military Psychology: Clinical and Operational Applications*. New York, NY: The Guilford Press; 2006: 295–309.

89. Mickley GA. Psychological factors in nuclear warfare. In: Walker RI, Cerveny TJ, eds. *Medical Consequences of Nuclear Warfare*. In: Zajtchuk R, Jenkins DP, Bellamy RF, Ingram VM, eds. *Textbook of Military Medicine*. Washington, DC: Department of the Army, Office of The Surgeon General, Borden Institute; 1989: Chap 8.

90. Mickley GA, Bogo V. Radiological factors and their effects on military performance. In: Gal R, Mangelsdorff AD, eds. *Handbook of Military Psychology*. Chichester, UK: Wiley; 1991.

91. Butler AS, Panzer AM, Goldfrank LR, eds. *Preparing for the Psychological Consequences of Terrorism: A Public Health Strategy*. Washington, DC: The National Academies Press; 2003.

92. The Chernobyl Forum 2003–2005. *Chernobyl's Legacy: Health, Environmental and Socio-Economic Impacts and Recommendations to the Governments of Belarus, the Russian Federation and Ukraine*. Second revised version. Vienna, Austria: The Chernobyl Forum 2003–2005; 2006. www.iaea.org/Publications/Booklets/Chernobyl/chernobyl.pdf. Accessed August 18, 2010.

93. Baratta AJ. Psychological and social response to a nuclear terrorist event. In: Apikyan S, Diamond D, Way R, eds. *Prevention, Detection and Response to Nuclear and Radiological Threats. NATO Science for Peace and Security Series–B: Physics and Biophysics*. Dordrecht, NL: Springer; 2008: 249–257.

94. Jarrett DG. Medical aspects of ionizing radiation. *Mil Med*. 2001;166(S2):6–8.

95. Leiba A, Goldberg A, Hourvitz A, et al. Who should worry for the "worried well"? Analysis of mild casualties center drills in non-conventional scenarios. *Prehosp Disaster Med*. 2006;21(6):441–444.

96. Pilch F. *The Worried Well: Strategies for Installation Commanders*. Colorado Springs, CO: US Air Force Institute for National Security Studies, United States Air Force Academy; 2005.

97. Stone FP. *The "Worried Well" Response to CBRN Events: Analysis and Solutions*. Maxwell Air Force Base, AL: USAF Counterproliferation Center, Air University; 2007. http://handle.dtic.mil/100.2/ADA475818. Accessed August 19, 2010.

98. Rubin GJ, Page L, Morgan O, et al. Public information needs after the poisoning of Alexander Litvinenko with polonium-210 in London: cross sectional telephone survey and qualitative analysis. *BMJ*. 2007;335(7630):1143.

99. Becker SM. Communicating risk to the public after radiological incidents. *BMJ*. 2007;335(7630):1106–1107.

100. Rubin GJ. The London polonium incident: lessons for risk communication. Paper presented at: The 46th Annual Meeting of the National Council on Radiation Protection and Measurements; March 2010; Bethesda, MD.

101. Institute of Medicine Committee on Battlefield Radiation Exposure Criteria. *Potential Radiation Exposure in Military Operations: Protecting the Soldier Before, During, and After*. Mettler FA Jr, Thaul S, O'Maonaigh H, eds. Washington, DC: National Academies Press; 1999.

102. Kennedy CH, Malone RC. Integration of women into the modern military. In: Freeman SM, Moore BA, Freeman A, eds. *Living and Surviving in Harm's Way: A Psychological Treatment Handbook for Pre- and Post-Deployment of Military Personnel*. New York, NY: Routledge; 2009: 67–81.

103. Vetter RJ, Becker SM, Carbaugh E, et al. *Population Monitoring and Radionuclide Decorporation Following a Radiological or Nuclear Incident* Bethesda, MD: National Council on Radiation Protection and Measurements; 2011. NCRP report no. 166.

104. Danieli Y, Dingman RL, eds. *On the Ground After September 11: Mental Health Responses and Practical Knowledge Gained*. Binghamton, NY: The Haworth Maltreatment and Trauma Press; 2005: 1–15.

105. Gurwitch RH, Kees M, Becker SM, Schreiber M, Pfefferbaum B, Diamond D. When disaster strikes: responding to the needs of children. *Prehosp Disaster Med*. 2004;19(1):21–28.

106. The Committee for the Compilation of Materials on the Damage Caused by the Atomic Bombs in Hiroshima and Nagasaki. *The Physical, Medical, and Social Effects of the Atomic Bombings*. Ishikawa E, Swain DL, trans. New York, NY: Basic Books; 1981.

107. Vyner HM. The psychological dimensions of health care for patients exposed to radiation and other invisible environmental contaminants. *Soc Sci Med*. 1988;27(10):1097–1103.

108. Board on Radiation Effects Research, National Research Council of the National Academies. *Assessment of the Scientific Information for the Radiation Exposure Screening and Education Program*. Washington, DC: National Academies Press; 2005.

109. Pastel RH, Ritchie EC. Mitigation of psychological effects of weapons of mass destruction. In: Ritchie EC, Watson PJ, Friedman MJ, eds. *Interventions Following Mass Violence and Disasters*. New York, NY: The Guilford Press; 2006: 300–318.

110. Spitzer JD, Hupert N, Duckart J, Xiong W. Operational evaluation of high-throughput community-based mass prophylaxis using just-in-time training. *Public Health Rep*. 2007;122(5):584–591.

111. McCurley MC, Miller CW, Tucker FE, et al. Educating medical staff about responding to a radiological or nuclear emergency. *Operational Health Phys*. 2009;96(S2):S50–S54.

112. Reissman DB, Reissman SG, Flynn BW. Integrating medical, public health, and mental health assets into a national response strategy. In: Bongar B, Brown LM, Beutler LE, Breckenridge JN, Zimbardo PG, eds. *Psychology of Terrorism*. New York, NY: Oxford University Press; 2007: 434–451.

Chapter 9

LATE AND LOW-LEVEL EFFECTS OF IONIZING RADIATION

ALEXANDRA C. MILLER, PhD[*]; MERRILINE SATYAMITRA, PhD[†]; SHILPA KULKARNI, PhD[‡]; AND THOMAS WALDEN, PhD[§]

INTRODUCTION

SOMATIC CELL EFFECTS

CARCINOGENESIS: THE HUMAN DATABASE

RADIATION EFFECTS IN UTERO

GENETIC EFFECTS

TRANSGENERATIONAL EFFECTS

RADIATION-INDUCED IMMUNOSUPPRESSION

REGULATORY GUIDES FOR EXPOSURE

SUMMARY

[*] Senior Scientist, Scientific Research Department, Armed Forces Radiobiology Research Institute, 8901 Wisconsin Avenue, Building 42, Room 3122, Bethesda, Maryland 20889

[†] Staff Scientist, Scientific Research Department, Armed Forces Radiobiology Research Institute, 8901 Wisconsin Avenue, Building 42, Room 3122, Bethesda, Maryland 20889

[‡] Staff Investigator, Scientific Research Department, Armed Forces Radiobiology Research Institute, 8901 Wisconsin Avenue, Building 42, Room 3122, Bethesda, Maryland 20889

[§] Radiation Oncologist, Gibson Cancer Center, 1200 Pine Run Drive, Lumberton, North Carolina 28358

INTRODUCTION

Ionizing radiation damages biological tissues by exciting or ionizing their atoms and molecules. Depending on the radiation dose and the biochemical processes altered, damage may be prompt (expressed minutes to weeks after exposure) or delayed (expressed several months to years later; Figure 9-1).

The exposure dose of gamma or X-rays in air is expressed in roentgens. The dose of any type of radiation absorbed by the tissues was at one time expressed by the rad, which is equivalent to 100 ergs of energy per gram of tissue. The international measure of absorbed dose is the gray, which is equal to 100 rads (conversely, 1 rad equals 1 cGy). Because the biological responses to radiation exposure may vary with the type of radiation, dose equivalents are expressed by the roentgen equivalents mammal (rem), which equal 1 joule per kilogram, or by the sievert, which is an international unit equaling 100 rem. The sievert allows effects from radiations with differing linear energy transfer (LET) values to be compared because 1 Sv of neutron radiation has the same biological effects as 1 Sv of low-LET gamma or X-radiation. Comparisons cannot be made among absorbed-dose measures of different kinds of radiation (for example, 1 Gy of neutron radiation will not have the same effect as 1 Gy of gamma or X-radiation).

Low-level radiation exposure is generally considered to be less than the dose that produces immediate or short-term observable biological effects. In humans, low-LET gamma or X-radiation doses of less than 0.5 Gy do not produce prodromal symptoms or the hematopoietic subsyndrome; however, recent studies suggest that low-level radiation exposure does increase the probability that delayed effects will occur.[1–3] Therefore low-level and delayed radiation effects are frequently discussed together.

There are four types of delayed radiation effects: (1) somatic, (2) genetic, (3) teratogenic, and (4) transgenerational. Irradiation enhances the naturally occurring frequency of the specific effect, and in some cases produces the observable endpoint by a process different than that of a natural process. Certain biological responses have such low thresholds that they are statistically indistinguishable, in many cases, from normal incidence.[3] Even so, current radioprotection guidelines state that all exposures to radiation should be avoided if possible and that exposure should be kept as low as is reasonably achievable.

Background Radiation

Living organisms are continually exposed to ionizing radiation in nature as well as from nuclear weapons testing, occupations, consumer products, and medical procedures. The radiation from all of these sources together is called natural background radiation and is estimated to measure 180 to 200 mrem/person/y. Medical procedures contribute most whole-body background radiation (Figure 9-2).[1,2] In addition, large doses of partial-body radiation may be delivered to the lungs by radon gas (radon-222 and radon-220) produced from the natural decay of radium and thorium.[4] High concentrations of radon gas escape from soil and are released from marble and granite, accumulating in buildings with poor air circulation.[4] Radon exposure is a health concern because its solid daughter products, polonium-214 and polonium-218, decay by alpha particle emission in the human body near the lung tissue and may increase the incidence of lung cancer.[4]

Extraterrestrial radiation includes solar-flare and cosmic radiation. Most cosmic radiation is absorbed by the dense atmosphere before it reaches the earth's surface. A person's exposure to cosmic radiation increases at higher latitudes or altitudes as the atmosphere becomes less dense. For example, a resident of the higher altitude city of Denver receives approximately 100 mrem/y more radiation exposure than does a resident of Washington, DC. A cross-country

Chain of Events

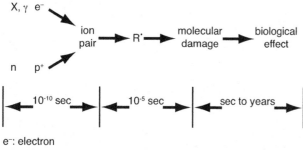

INCIDENT RADIATION

e⁻: electron
n: neutron
p⁺: proton
R˙: free radical

Figure 9-1. Chain of events in radiation exposure. The chain of events involved in radiation exposure is initiated with the exposure. First, an ion pair forms within 10^{-10} seconds. Free radicals are formed after 10^{-5} seconds. Molecular damage occurs within seconds but can take up to years to manifest. Similarly, biological damage occurs within many seconds postradiation but can also take years to manifest.

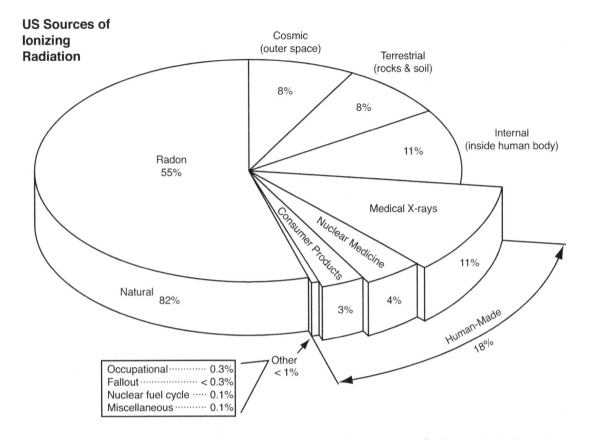

US Sources of Ionizing Radiation

Cosmic (outer space) 8%

Terrestrial (rocks & soil) 8%

Internal (inside human body) 11%

Radon 55%

Medical X-rays 11%

Consumer Products

Nuclear Medicine

Natural 82%

Consumer Products 3%

Nuclear Medicine 4%

Human-Made 18%

Other < 1%

Occupational	0.3%
Fallout	< 0.3%
Nuclear fuel cycle	0.1%
Miscellaneous	0.1%

Figure 9-2. US sources of ionizing radiation. There are many sources of radiation to which an individual may be exposed. The majority of exposure is from natural sources (82%); the remaining exposure is from artificial sources (18%).

airplane flight increases individual exposure by 0.2 mrem/h because the level of cosmic radiation is greater at 36,000 feet than at sea level.[2] As humans venture farther from the protective atmosphere in extremely high-altitude flights, their background occupational exposures to cosmic radiation will increase as well. Spaceflight increases exposure to solar and cosmic radiations; for example, *Apollo* astronauts traveling to the moon received an average of 275 mrem over 19.5 days. Shuttle astronauts receive a similar level of exposure to radiation during spaceflight and may receive a much higher dose during a space walk.[3]

On earth, naturally occurring radioactive elements contribute to background radiation.[1–3] External exposure sources include potassium-40, which may be concentrated in concrete, and radon gas. Internal radiation comes primarily from radioactive isotopes of naturally occurring elements in biological systems, such as potassium-40 and sodium-24. In some areas of Brazil and India, large concentrations of monazite, a mineral containing thorium, are present in the soil or sand. Background radiation exposures there range from 0.008 to 0. 17 Gy/y.[3]

Fallout from nuclear weapons testing peaked in

1964, after 77 atmospheric detonations occurred in 1962. Of the total fallout, 69% was from carbon-14, 4% was from cesium-137, and 3% was from strontium-90. The remaining 24% was from radioactive isotopes of plutonium, rubidium, barium, iodine, iron, manganese, krypton, americium, tritium, and zinc.[4] Carbon-14 will be a long-term contributor to background radiation because it has a half-life of 5,700 years.

Radiation is also emitted from consumer products, such as color television sets (averaging 0.3–1.0 rem/h of use), video screens, smoke detectors (which contain an alpha emitter, usually americium-241), and dinnerware that uses uranium for an orange color.[4–6] Ophthalmic glass, used in prescription lenses, contains trace impurities of thorium-232, and uranium is added to dental porcelain to give dentures a natural fluorescent quality. The latter may result in an alpha radiation dose of 60 rem/y to the gums.

Deterministic Versus Stochastic Events

Radiation effects on the human body are generally divided into two categories: deterministic and stochastic effects. Deterministic effects are those whose

197

severity increases as dose increases. Below a certain level, known as the threshold, the effect is absent. The level of damage particularly depends on the radiation dose received. Deterministic effects depend on the killing of many cells over a relatively short period of time. Examples of this type of damage include organ damage, cataracts, erythema, and infertility.[5–8]

Stochastic effects are independent of absorbed dose and, under certain exposure conditions, the effects may or may not occur. There is no threshold and the probability of having the effects is not proportional to the dose absorbed. Curability of the effect has little to do with the radiation dose received. Stochastic effects modify a limited number of cells following irradiation. Examples of this type of damage include radiation-induced cancer and genetic damage.

Somatic Cells Versus Germ Cells

All cells in the body (except germ cells) are somatic. Germ cells are reproductive cells that pass their genetic material, including mutations, on to the organism's offspring. Somatic cells, on the other hand, do not pass on genetic material.

SOMATIC CELL EFFECTS

Delayed somatic effects of ionizing radiation result from somatic mutations and accumulated damage, and include impaired circulation, necrosis, fibrosis of skin and muscle tissue, loss of hair, loss of taste, impaired bone growth, susceptibility to disease, immunodeficiency, aplastic anemia, cataracts, and increased incidence of cancer. Some organs are more radioresistant than others. Radiation doses exceeding 15 to 50 Gy must be received before damage to the liver or heart is detected.[2] In contrast, other tissues, such as the lens and the sperm, show some detriment from doses as low as 0.15 to 0.30 Gy.[3] Delayed somatic effects of intermediate- or high-level exposures include cataract formation, skin abnormalities, and sterility.

Cataract Formation

The lens tissue of the eye is particularly radiosensitive and radiation exposure can increase its opacity. Radiation cataractogenesis is the most common delayed radiation injury and is thought to result from damage to the anterior equatorial cells of the lens's epithelial tissue.[6,7] These cells normally divide and migrate to the posterior portion of the lens, where they gradually lose their nuclei and become lens fibers.[3] The lens tissue, like that of the testes and the brain, is separated from the rest of the body by a barrier system.[4] As a result, it has no direct blood supply, no macrophages for phagocytosis, and no way to remove accumulated damage. In a study of 446 survivors of the Nagasaki atomic bomb, 45% of the 395 individuals who were 0.1 to 2.0 km from the hypocenter developed cataracts by 1959, whereas only 0.5% (or 2 out of 395) sustained severe visual impairment.[1] Four of the remaining 51 individuals (7.8%) who were 2 to 4 km from the hypocenter developed mild cataract impairment. Even survivors exposed to small doses of radiation were at increased risk for cataract formation. By 1964, the incidence of cataract formation among bomb survivors who received 0.01 to 0.99 Gy of radiation was 1.5% in Hiroshima compared to 1.0% in the control population, and 2.0% in Nagasaki compared to 0.9% in controls.[3] Higher doses tend to increase the degree of opacity and shorten the latency period.[1] Studies have shown that there is a 10% risk of developing a severely imperiling cataract following a single exposure to 2.4 Gy of low-LET radiation, and a 50% risk for a dose of 3.1 Gy. The latency period for cataract formation in humans has been estimated to be 6 months to 35 years; however, fractionation or protracted exposure lowers the incidence and prolongs the latency.[2]

Small radiation doses may increase the lens's opacity, but visually impairing cataract formation results from an accumulation of dead or injured cells and therefore has a threshold. For low-LET radiation, this threshold is 2 Gy, while high-LET neutrons have thresholds of less than 0.2 Gy. The International Commission on Radiological Protection (ICRP) has recommended an occupational exposure limit of 0.15 Sv for the eye.[1,6]

Tissue Fibrosis

Radiation-induced fibrosis (RIF) is one of the most predominant long-term adverse effects of ionizing radiation.[8–14] Typically, fibrotic response occurs due to the progressive onset of extra cellular matrix (ECM) deposition from stromal tissue such as lung, liver, kidney, and intestine.[8] Chronic deposition leads to loss of elasticity and muscular dysfunction or atrophy in extreme cases. The severity of fibrosis depends on radiation dose, quality of radiation, and dose rate.[9,10] Fibrosis may be accompanied by epilation, loss of vascularity, and even necrosis of the tissue.[8] Radiation-induced mutations are also responsible for fibrosis.[11] Cellular response in fibrosis manifestation primarily involves sustained elevation of growth factors or cytokines that trigger a proinflammatory response in fibroblasts, transform epithelial and endothelial cells into ECM-producing myofibroblasts, and infiltrate immune cells into the interstitial spaces.[12] The term "ECM" collectively describes aggregates of fibrous proteins such as fibronectin, collagen, and smooth muscle actin. These aggregates are formed by upregulation of matrix metalloproteinases in myofibroblasts. Severe fibrosis of the lungs can lead to loss of function and, sometimes, mortality.

The mechanism involved in RIF is fairly complicated. Radiation-induced cellular response involves activation of various stress-related signaling pathways, which includes acute responses such as apoptosis, necrosis, and chronic response, such as proinflammatory pathways. Leukocyte infiltration and adhesion into the vessel wall of the irradiated tissue is one of the key factors of progressive inflammatory response. Chronic alteration in signaling pathways can lead to tissue remodeling and fibrosis.[13] One of the key mediators of RIF is transforming growth factor β (TGF-β).[14–17] Early alterations in ECM and TGF-β-gene expression in mouse lungs are indicative of radiation fibrosis.[15] TGF-β signaling involves attachment of peptide to the TGF-I, II, and III receptors. The I and III receptors either homodimerize or heterodimerize and lead to a cascade of events, such as the TGF-β signaling family, S-mothers against decapentaplegic homolog 2 (SMAD2) phosphorylation, nuclear translocation, and transcriptional upregulation of profibrotic proteins.[18] Even though the role of TGF-β in the development of fibrosis is well established, very few studies have attempted to inhibit TGF-β in amelioration of fibrosis. Different strategies developed to reduce fibrosis include systemic administration of superoxide dismutase mimetics, and pentoxyfylline (alone and in combination with alpha tocopherol). Clinical trials have shown beneficial effects of superoxide dismutase in radiation-induced fibrosis.[19–21] Clinical trials using a combination of paclitaxel and arsenic trioxide have somewhat promising results.[21–23] Unfortunately, the US Food and Drug Administration has not yet approved any drug to treat RIF.

Sterility

Males

Germ cells of the human testes are very radiosensitive. Temporary sterility may occur after 1 Gy whole-body or local irradiation, with 50% incidence following exposure to 0.7 Gy. Sperm cells become more resistant as they develop; spermatogonia are more radiosensitive than spermatocytes, which are in turn more radiosensitive than spermatids.[5,24]

Radiogenic aspermia is caused by a maturation depletion process similar to that observed for hematopoietic cells after irradiation. Radiation kills stem cells or delays mitosis so that differentiating cells continue to divide without being replaced. The latency period for aspermia after radiation exposure is approximately 2 months,[1,2] and the time for recovery is several months to years. Chronic and protracted exposures produce greater testicular damage than do acute large exposures. This damage is reflected in the duration of aspermia (approximately 25 wk) and is thought to result from cycling of the radioresistant type-A spermatogonia to the more radiosensitive type-B spermatogonia. A dose of about 0.35 Gy, protracted over 1 to 10 days, produces a 50% incidence of aspermia. At low dose rates, the recovery period depends on the total dose received and can vary significantly. At higher total doses, following the onset of aspermia, it may take up to 3 years for recovery from a 2 to 3 Gy exposure and up to 5 years for 6 Gy exposure.[4]

Females

The ovary is not as sensitive to radiation as are the male testes.[1,2] Temporary sterility may be induced in females by acute radiation doses of 1.5 to 6.4 Gy radiation. Permanent sterility can result from doses of 2 to 10 Gy and depends on the woman's age at the time of irradiation. Older women, particularly those close to menopause, are particularly radiosensitive for sterilization. Permanent sterility may result in 50% of the exposed female population over 40 years of age after 2 Gy of low-LET radiation, compared to an estimated 3.5 Gy for women under 40.[1,6] This is due to the numbers of oocytes present at the time of irradiation. Women have about a half million oocytes at puberty; by menopause, these are almost all depleted through atresia.

Shortly before birth, the oogonia stop multiplying and proceed to prophase I of meiosis. After puberty, meiosis resumes for individual cells by ovulation. Oocytes lose the ability to renew after birth and are unable to replace stem cells that have been damaged or killed by radiation. The oocyte is most radiosensitive as a proliferative stem cell during the fetal stage of gestation, prior to ceasing mitosis and entering meiosis. For fractionated radiation exposure, higher radiation doses of 3.6 to 20.0 Gy are required for sterilization.[1,2]

Radiation Effects on Skin

The acute effects of radiation exposure on skin are well known and result in severe skin burns.[1–6] However, low levels of chronic radiation to skin have been observed as well. Soon after Roentgen's discovery of X-rays, researchers and radiologists became aware of the skin's sensitivity to radiation damage. Eight months after the discovery of X-rays in 1896, a German scientist reported a case of dermatitis and alopecia on the face and back of a 17-year-old male who had been exposed to these rays for 10 to 20 minutes a day for 4 weeks during a scientific investigation.[7] The accompanying erythema, which resembled a burn, was painless; however, chronic radiation dermatitis following repeated exposure is usually extremely painful. Several other anecdotal cases have been noted. In another 1896 case, a man received an hour-long X-ray exposure during an examination for a kidney stone. The patient experienced nausea (a prodromal symptom) 3 hours after irradiation. Following a second exposure lasting 1.5 hours, the patient developed a radiation sequela leading to ulcer formation at the site of exposure, which was not responsive to skin grafting.[7] From 1897 through 1928, additional evidence was collected that demonstrated that low-level radiation exposure caused radiation dermatitis.

Before the introduction of the roentgen in 1928 as a unit to measure exposure dose, the skin erythema dose (SED) was commonly used.[1,2] The SED is the radiation dose required to produce a given degree of erythema and it depends on the quality, energy, and exposure time of the radiation. For X-radiation, the SED is about 8.5 Gy. In 1925, it was proposed that the exposure of radiologists and X-ray machine operators not exceed 1/100th of the SED in a 30-day period.

During a radiation incident, skin may be exposed either by direct blast irradiation or by beta rays from the direct deposition of particulate fallout.[5] The degree of radiation-induced skin damage depends on a number of factors, including the type of radiation, the dose and dose rate, the area of skin irradiated, and skin-quality characteristics, such as texture, age, color, thickness, and location.[5,6] The neck is the most radiosensitive area because its skin is thin and usually not protected by clothing. Additional trauma through burn, abrasion, exposure to ultraviolet light, or extreme temperature variations increase the damage. Environmental factors and inadequate clothing may contribute to hyperthermia, and wool or other coarse fabrics may further abrade the damaged skin. An illness like diabetes or a genetic disease like ataxia telangiectasia may also make the skin more radiosensitive.

In terms of radiation quality, alpha radiation is of little concern for skin damage because the average penetrated dose is usually absorbed by the dead corneocytes of the stratum corneum.[1,6] However, it may present a problem at sites where the skin is thinner and the radiation can penetrate to the basal level. Therefore,

depleted uranium exposure to the skin could not cause significant skin erythema. In contrast, beta particulates in fallout may contain extremely high radiation dose rates (tens of grays per hour). When they land on the skin, their energy may penetrate to the germinal basal cells. This radiation damage (known as a beta burn) was observed in the atomic bomb survivors and the Marshall Islanders who had been exposed to nuclear fallout. The threshold dose of beta radiation for skin damage depends on the average energy of the beta particle, the total absorbed dose, and the dose rate. The average penetrating range of a beta particle is proportional to its energy; thus, higher-energy beta emitters, such as strontium-90 (0.61 MeV average), require lower surface doses to produce wet desquamation than do lower-energy beta particles, such as those from cobalt-60 (0.31 MeV average). Lower-energy beta particles, like sulfur-35 (0.17 MeV energy), are not capable of penetrating to the dermis and cannot induce chronic radiation dermatitis. Most importantly, beta injuries from fallout can be minimized by decontamination and washing.

Five progressive categories of radiation damage are observed in skin: (1) erythema, (2) transepithelial injury (moist desquamation), (3) ulceration, (4) necrosis, and (5) skin cancer.[1–3] Radiation-induced erythema occurs in two stages: (1) mild initial erythema, usually appearing within minutes or hours on the first day after irradiation (occurring earlier with higher doses), and (2) the main erythema, appearing at 2 to 3 weeks and persisting for longer periods. In some cases, a third erythema may occur at 6 weeks. Radiation-induced erythema is a threshold phenomenon. For example, a dose of 6 Gy of low-LET radiation (eg, X-rays) received in less than 1 day, or 10 Gy in 10 days, will induce erythema in 50% of exposed individuals.[3] In contrast, the threshold for neutron radiation is 2 Gy. Because of these variables, and the fact that the threshold dose decreases with an increase in the surface area exposed, erythema is not a good biological dosimeter.

Early erythema arises from the release of mediators and from increased capillary dilation and permeability.[3] Early erythema is equivalent to a first-degree burn or mild sunburn, subsiding within 2 or 3 days. Although indomethacin and other prostaglandin-synthesis inhibitors have been used topically to prevent or reduce erythema caused by sunburn or ultraviolet light, they have not been widely used to treat radiation-induced erythema.

The second onset of erythema is attributed to impaired circulation in the arterioles, producing inflammation and edemas and accompanied by dry desquamation of the epidermal corneocytes. Upper cells are sloughed or abraded off, exposing cells that are not completely keratinized. Cell death and moist desquamation ensue. Both dry and wet desquamation occur about 1 to 4 weeks after irradiation. Regeneration of the stratum corneum requires 2 months to 4 years, and this regenerated tissue will be more sensitive to other skin-damaging agents. The new skin may be thinner than the original, with greater sensitivity to touch and pain. Reduction or loss of the dermal ridges making up the fingerprint has occurred from large or chronic exposures.

Epidermal basal cells are thought to be the targets of early radiation damage.[1-3] Further damage to the surrounding vasculature is an important factor in late radiation injury and necrosis. The blood vessel damage may lead to telangiectasia, and fibrosis and alterations in connective tissue may appear. Hyper- or hypopigmentation may occur after radiation exposure; low doses activate melanocytes and produce hyperpigmentation, and higher doses may result in death of melanocytes and cause hypopigmentation. These biological changes play a role in tissue necrosis and skin cancer development.

CARCINOGENESIS: THE HUMAN DATABASE

Cancer induction is the most important somatic late effect of low-dose radiation exposure. In contrast to other types of late effects, like genetic effects, cancer risk estimates are based on the human experience. There is an association between low-dose radiation exposure and cancer.[1-6] Early reports of this association were anecdotal. Both Marie Curie and her daughter Irene died from leukemia that was thought to have resulted from radiation exposure. One of the earliest reports of radiation-induced cancers occurred in Thomas Edison's laboratory. Edison's assistant died in 1904 from skin cancer contracted while developing a fluorescent light using an X-ray tube.[5] Many early radiologists, researchers, and workers experienced chronic radiodermatitis, increased cancer incidence, and other damage before the dangers of radiation were clarified and protective measures were initiated. Currently, the National Academy of Sciences considers cancer induction to be the most important somatic effect of low-dose ionizing radiation.[1,5]

Cancer development is thought to be a multistep process in which the initial damage leads to a preneoplastic stage, followed by selection and proliferation of the neoplastic cell.[1,2,4] Chromosomal and enzymatic analyses indicate that all of the cancer cells of a tumor and its metastases are derivatives or clones of a single cell. However the multistage theory of cancer development is now believed to involve tumor suppressor genes, oncogenes, and epigenetic effects as well.

Previously the simplistic view of cancer formation involved the three stages in cancer formation: initiation, promotion, and latency (Figure 9-3).[1,2,4] During initiation, fixation of the somatic mutational event occurs, which leads to the development of a neoplasm. Damage can be initiated by various agents, including exposure to radiation or another environmental or chemical carcinogen. During the promotion stage, the preneoplastic cell is stimulated to divide or is given preferential selection. A promoter is an agent that by itself does not cause cancer, but once the initiating carcinogenic event has occurred, it promotes or stimulates the proliferation of the neoplastic cell. Chromosomal and enzymatic analyses indicate that all of the cancer cells of a tumor and its metastases are derivatives or clones of a single cell. During the promotion stage, the preneoplastic cell is stimulated to divide or is given preferential selection.

The mechanism of carcinogenesis is more complicated than a simple initiation-and-promotion model.[1-4] Tissue homeostasis depends on the regulated cell division and self-elimination of each of its constituent members, excluding stem cells. A tumor arises because of uncontrolled cell division and failure for self-elimination. Alterations in genes are responsible for dysregulated growth and self-elimination.

Carcinogenesis appears to be a multistep process with multiple genetic alterations occurring over an extended period of time.[1,2,11] Most genetic alterations that lead to cancer are acquired in the form of somatic mutations (eg, chromosomal translocations, deletions, inversions, amplifications, and point mutations). While the deregulated growth signals by oncogenes are critical to cancer development, other recent findings suggest additional gene alterations. Many cancers seem to possess diminished apoptotic or cell-death programs. The loss of cell cycle control has led to the concept that mutations in protooncogenes and tumor suppressor genes that inhibit apoptosis provide a selective growth advantage to a premalignant cell that allows it to clonally expand. Additionally, mutations in deoxyribonucleic acid (DNA) stability genes increase the rate of acquiring mutations that will result in a malignant tumor. Although tumor cells are considered clonal in origin, most tumors contain heterogeneous populations of cells that differ in their ability to populate the tumor mass or form metastases.

Carcinogenic Process

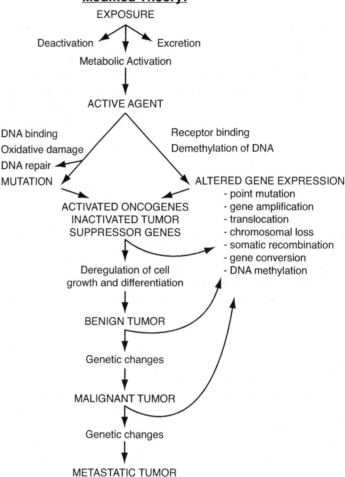

Classic Theory:

Initiation
  (by genotoxic agent)
Promotion
  (by agent that stimulates
  initiated cell to proliferate)
Progression
  (additional genetic damage
  causes malignancy)

Modified Theory:

EXPOSURE

Deactivation   Excretion

Metabolic Activation

ACTIVE AGENT

DNA binding   Receptor binding
Oxidative damage   Demethylation of DNA
DNA repair
MUTATION   ALTERED GENE EXPRESSION
                       - point mutation
                       - gene amplification
ACTIVATED ONCOGENES   - translocation
INACTIVATED TUMOR   - chromosomal loss
SUPPRESSOR GENES   - somatic recombination
                       - gene conversion
                       - DNA methylation
Deregulation of cell
growth and differentiation

BENIGN TUMOR

Genetic changes

MALIGNANT TUMOR

Genetic changes

DNA: deoxyribonucleic acid

METASTATIC TUMOR

Figure 9-3. Carcinogenic process. Carcinogenisis is a multistep process. The classic theory was characterized by initiation, promotion, and progression. In contrast, the modified theory details the involvement of multiple types of molecular DNA (deoxyribonucleic acid) damage (genetic) coupled with alterations in the expression of oncogenes and tumor suppressor genes. Altered gene expression can also occur via an epigenetic process in which the DNA is not damaged.

The Human Database

Information regarding the human experience with radiation-induced cancer comes from four sources (Table 9-1): (1) atomic bomb survivors, (2) medical exposures, (3) occupational exposures, and (4) epidemiological comparisons of geographic areas containing high background radiation.[1–3,5]

The 92,231 survivors of the atomic detonations in Hiroshima and Nagasaki are being monitored by the Radiation Effects Research Foundation for possible radiation-induced health effects.[1,2,5] Of the 37,000 deaths in this population through 2002, 9,110 were attributable to radiogenic and nonradiogenic cancers.[1,2,5]

The foundation is also following 27,000 children of the survivors who were conceived after the detonations to determine if genetic damage induced in their parents and passed on to them resulted in any adverse health effects.[1,2,5] Radiation doses received by a majority of the survivors were initially determined in 1965 and were revised in 1986 after more information on the explosions became available. Revisions in which radiation type (neutrons or gamma radiation) caused the most damage have led to the conclusion that gamma radiation plays a greater role than earlier thought.[5] Therefore, risk estimates for low-LET radiation exposure must be revised, and potential risk estimates may be increased by 50%.

TABLE 9-1

SOURCES OF DATA ON RADIATION EXPOSURE IN HUMANS

Type of Exposure	Population Affected
Atomic bomb	Survivors
	Offspring of survivors
Medical	Treatment of tinea capitis
	X-ray treatment of ankylosing spondylitis
	Prenatal diagnostic X-rays
	X-ray therapy for enlarged thymus gland
	Fluoroscopy treatment for tuberculosis
	Thorotrast treatment
Occupational	Radium dial painters
	Uranium miners and millers
	Nuclear dockyard workers
	Nuclear materials workers
	Participants in nuclear weapons testing
	Construction workers
	Industrial workers
	Reactor personnel
	Civilian aviation personnel
	Astronauts
	Scientific researchers
	Diagnostic and therapeutic radiation personnel

The second group used in human risk estimates is the medically irradiated population for which dosimetry is available: the 14,111 patients in the United Kingdom who received spinal irradiation for treatment of ankylosing spondylitis between 1935 and 1944. Ankylosing spondylitis is a rheumatoid disease primarily affecting the spine and characterized by destruction of the cartilage and ossification of the vertebral joints. An increased incidence of leukemia has been observed in this population. Other medically irradiated groups that are used for risk estimation and who demonstrated increased cancer incidence are children who received head radiation for treatment of tinea capitis and patients who received routine fluoroscopy examinations for postpartum mastitis or during treatment of tuberculosis.

The third category used for determining human risk estimates includes occupational groups who receive very low radiation doses averaging less than 1 rem/y (medical, scientific, and industrial professions). However, depending on the type of radiation, other groups are also sometimes used in determining cancer risk estimates.

The risk of radiation-induced cancer varies considerably with age, with a younger age being associated with increased cancer risk and susceptibility. The exceptions to this are leukemia, which appears to be constant throughout all ages, and respiratory cancers, which increase with age.

Leukemia

Leukemia is one of the most frequently observed radiation-induced cancers.[1-5] It accounts for one sixth of the mortality associated with radiocarcinogenesis, with equal numbers of cancers of the lung, breast, and gastrointestinal tract. Leukemia may be acute or chronic and may take a lymphocytic or myeloid form. With the exception of chronic lymphocytic leukemia, increases in all forms of leukemia have been detected in humans exposed to radiation and in irradiated laboratory animals. More acute than chronic leukemias are induced, although the latencies are roughly equal. Characteristic chromosomal aberrations and alterations in gene expression induced by radiation have been identified in patients with a variety of leukemias.

Leukemia first appeared in the atomic bomb survivors 2 to 3 years after the nuclear detonations and reached a peak incidence 10 to 15 years after irradiation. The average latency period for leukemia is thought to be 2 to 20 years. This estimate is derived from the ankylosing spondylitis patients (6 y) and the atomic bomb survivors (13.7 y). The difference between the two groups may reflect the larger radiation dose (averaging 3.21 Gy) received by the bone marrow of the ankylosing spondylitis patients, compared to an average dose of 0.27 Gy in the atomic bomb survivors.[1,2,5]

Thorotrast exposure has also been linked to leukemia induction. Thorotrast is a contrast medium that contains thorium-22 and decays by alpha particle emission. It was used in diagnostic radiological procedures between 1928 and 1955. An increased incidence of leukemia and liver cancer was observed in patients in whom thorium had concentrated in the liver and bone. The mean radiation dose to the bone marrow from thorotrast ingestion was 3.5 Gy. These data demonstrate that alpha particle exposure, like neutron and gamma radiation exposure, can also induce leukemia.

The incidence of radiation leukemia is influenced by age at the time of exposure. The younger the person at the time of exposure, the shorter the latency and the risk period for developing leukemia. The incidence of leukemia decreases with increasing age at the time of exposure; however, this older individual is at increased risk for a greater period of time. Conversely, as the leukemia risk decreases, the risk of developing a solid tumor increases. There is no apparent difference in the incidences of leukemia in females and males at any age or at any dose.

In terms of military exposure and leukemia risk, over 200,000 US military and civilian personnel have been involved in the testing of nuclear weapons since 1945. This number includes military personnel and civilians who were permitted to view a nuclear detonation from a safe distance, such as those who witnessed testing at the Nevada Test Site and the Pacific Proving Grounds in the Marshall Islands. The average doses received by the participants in those tests were 0.5 rem of gamma radiation and 0.005 rem of neutron radiation. These doses are now considered to be safe; Nuclear Regulatory Commission regulations permit persons in occupations with radiation exposures to receive 3 rem in any calendar quarter, or 5 rem per year. At the request of the Department of Defense, the National Research Council conducted a study of mortality among participants of nuclear weapons tests. The study concluded that "there is no consistent or statistically significant evidence for an increase in leukemia or other malignant disease in nuclear test participants."[5]

Thyroid Cancer

Thyroid cancer is also a concern for low-level exposure and late radiation effects, possibly accounting for 6% to 12% of the mortality attributed to radiation-induced cancers.[1–5] Radiation-induced thyroid cancer is 2.0 to 3.5 times more prevalent in women than in men. This is based on information showing that female atomic bomb survivors sustained thyroid cancer 3.5 times more frequently than male survivors, and as much as 5 times more frequently in one clinical study.[1,2,5] The difference in thyroid tumor inductions in males and females is most likely due to hormonal influences on thyroid function. Variations in thyroid cancer induction also exist for ethnic groups. One study examined thyroid neoplasms in Jewish and gentile women who received radiotherapy (approximately 3.99 Gy) during infancy for enlarged thymus glands.[5] The risk of thyroid cancer in women of Jewish background was four times greater than in gentile women. Both the atom bomb survivor studies and those involving Israelis irradiated for tinea capitis indicate that the incidence of thyroid cancer following radiation is also affected by the age at exposure. The risk is generally greater during the first two decades of life.[5]

Breast Cancer

Breast cancer is the major concern for women exposed to low-level radiation because of its high incidence in the unexposed population.[5] In the United States, one in eleven women will develop breast cancer (the incidence of mortality from breast cancer is almost nonexistent in men). Because of their increased normal incidences of thyroid and breast cancer, women are also at greater risk of developing these cancers as a result of radiation exposure.[1,2,5]

It is important to note that in most cases, radiation exposure increases the incidence of the cancer but does not affect the histology of the tumor nor the prognosis. The risk of breast cancer associated with radiation exposure is age dependent. In female adolescents, breast cancer does not manifest until after puberty. However, studies have shown an increased incidence of breast cancer in atomic bomb survivors who were younger than 10 years old at the time of exposure.[1,2,5] Increases in breast cancer have also been observed in women who received radiotherapy during infancy to treat enlarged thymus glands. The latency period for breast cancer following radiation exposure ranges from 5 to 40 years.[5] Estrogen may promote breast cancer because a woman's age at exposure is associated with increased risk, and because few breast cancers occur before age 30. This is supported by the fact that breast cancer incidence does not increase in men following irradiation. Several investigators have proposed that the actual period in which estrogen is present as a promoter is the important factor in determining cancer incidence and latency. Women irradiated after menopause are less likely to develop radiation-induced breast cancer. A decreased incidence of breast cancer was seen in women who received X-radiotherapy to the ovaries for metropathia hemorrhagica, although the incidence of radiation-induced leukemia did increase, as expected. The radiotherapy induced an artificial menopause, with a corresponding decrease in estrogen production.[1,2]

In terms of dose estimates, the estimated dose of radiation required to double the naturally occurring incidence of breast cancer is 0.8 Gy. Dose fractionation does not appear to reduce the incidence of breast cancer. Damage in breast tissue tends to accumulate rather than to be repaired, so the risk from acute exposure (such as atomic bomb radiation) is the same as the risk from chronic exposure (such as small daily doses from fluoroscopy or treatment for postpartum mastitis).

Other Systemic Cancers

Cancers of the stomach, colon, liver, pancreas, salivary glands, and kidneys are also induced by radiation.[1–3,5] However, these neoplasms are fairly rare. Most radiation-induced solid tumors have a latency of 10 to 30 years and no difference exists in the absolute risks for males and females.

Bone Cancer

The risk of radiation-induced bone, lung, and skin cancers is higher than other systemic cancers.[1,2,5] In the 1920s, workers who hand-painted the fluorescent dials on wristwatches with radium-based paint achieved the necessary fine detail by moistening the tip of the brush into a point with their tongues; in so doing, they ingested small amounts of radium. Because radium is a bone-seeking element with a half-life of 1,600 years, these workers had a higher incidence of bone sarcomas. Increased incidences of breast cancer were also observed.[6]

Lung Cancer

Radiation is one of several carcinogens known to be associated with lung cancer.[1–3,5] Risk estimates have been obtained from atomic bomb survivors, patients with ankylosing spondylitis, and underground miners exposed to uranium and radon.[1,5] In each case an excess was found, even when smoking is considered as a confounder. There is a clear excess of lung cancer in the uranium mine workers of Colorado, the Czech Republic, Sweden, and Newfoundland.[1–3,5] It is difficult to separate the contributory effects of radon, uranium, and smoking in causing the observed lung cancers. There is also some evidence of an excess of lung cancer from domestic radon exposure and it has been estimated that 10% of 150,000 lung cancer deaths are associated with radon exposure.[1,6]

Skin Cancer

Skin cancers are common in those using radiation equipment, although the incidence has decreased due to increased safety standards.[1,5] In general, radiation skin cancers are readily diagnosed and treated at any early stage of development and maintain a high rate of curability.

Dose and Dose-Rate Effectiveness

From the human data that has been collected and evaluated, it seems that high-dose and high-dose-rate radiation exposures are associated with an increased risk of cancer development. The human data from low-dose and low-dose-rate exposures are sparse, and therefore the excess rate is not well defined for humans under these exposure circumstances.

RADIATION EFFECTS IN UTERO

Prenatal exposure to ionizing radiation can interfere with embryonic and fetal development, depending on dose and the gestational age in which exposure occurs.[24] Documented reports show instances of children with severe intellectual disability and microencephaly, as well as other physiological malformations, born to mothers exposed to radiotherapy.[24] Further, experimental data from small mammals are available that indicate that relatively low doses of 0.05 or 0.1 Gy are sufficient to induce sensitivity in the developing embryo. The main factors that determine the outcome of in-utero exposure are the dose, dose rate, and the gestational stage at which exposure occurs.

Developmental Stages

Radiation is highly damaging to rapidly proliferating cells. The biological systems with high cell proliferation rates are extremely radiosensitive. To demarcate the radiation effects at different embryonic/fetal stages, the gestation can be divided into three periods: (1) preimplantation (the period extending from cell fertilization to the time when the embryo attaches to the uterine wall), (2) major organogenesis (the period when the major organs are formed), and (3) fetal stage (from growth of organs to birth).

Preimplantation Stage: In-Vivo Studies

The duration of the preimplantation period is 5 days for mice, 7 days for rats, and 8 days for humans.[25] It is also the stage in which cells are most sensitive to the lethal effects of radiation, resulting in increased prenatal deaths and resorption of the embryo.[26,27] There are no human data (because pregnancy would not have been established at this time), but experimental data in mice, rats, rabbits, and dogs have been collected.[24-32] All animal studies indicate that if the irradiated embryo did not die, it survived without malformation, leading to the "all-or-none" term coined by Russell in 1956 for radiation effects on the conceptus.[1, 26–31] Structural as well as numerical chromosomal aberrations have been implicated in both preimplantation lethality and in subsequent genomic instability. Recent studies on genomic instability in rodents indicate that irradiation at the preimplantation stage resulted in a surprising increase in chromosomal aberrations several cell divisions after the initial exposure.[32] This is of some concern because of reports that genomic instability is inherited by the next generation,[33] which indicates heritable stable mutations.

Organogenesis: In-Vivo Studies

The principal effect of radiation in rodents during this period is the production of congenital abnormalities, growth retardation, and, if the dose is sufficiently high, embryonic or neonatal death. The consequences of exposure depend on the dose, radiation quality, gestational age of the conceptus, oxygen tension, relative biologic effectiveness (RBE), close interactions between cells in the rapidly dividing fetus, and maternal and environmental factors.[34]

Teratogenesis

By far the most common effect of irradiation during organogenesis in rodents is congenital anomalies (Table 9-2). These frequent and highly varied aberrations are intimately related to the developmental stage during exposure, radiation dose and quality, and other compounding factors. Due to the complexities arising from phase-dependent, biological, and other experimental variations, there are discrepancies in the assessment of the lowest or threshold dose at which various malformations have been observed.[35] Neutrons and beta particles are more damaging to the in-utero fetus than low-LET, radiation-like gamma or X-rays.[1,34] Effects of fractionating the radiation dose depend on the critical period. If the critical period has a narrow window, fractionating the dose over that short period of time increases malformations resulting from cell destruction.

The Fetal Stage

The fetal stage extends from the end of major organogenesis until birth (from days 14–20 of gestation in mice and 45–266 in humans). This stage is relatively resistant to radiation lethality and externally detectable malformation at doses below 3 Gy.[32–34] However, anomalies of the central nervous system and sense organs are especially sensitive to the deleterious effects of ionizing radiations. This is accompanied by significant and permanent growth retardation at moderate doses of exposure (~1 Gy). Hematological consequences of fetal irradiation arise from damage to the liver and spleen and manifest as hematological disorders in adults.[35]

Human Studies

Lethality

There are no convincing data in humans regarding lethality of the embryo at the preimplantation period due to the difficulty in determining pregnancy at the initial stages (Table 9-3). However, very few atomic bomb survivors less than 4 weeks of gestational age at the time of the bombing survived, which is an indirect indication of high fetal loss or resorption in the early stages of pregnancies. Higher numbers of stillbirths and neonatal infant deaths were reported for survivors in Nagasaki. Fetal, neonatal, and infant mortality was higher in women who demonstrated radiation sickness and those that were closer to the epicenter of the explosion.[36] Findings following the Chernobyl accident are highly inconsistent; Sweden reported an increase in neonatal mortality, while surrounding Germany, Norway, Finland, and the highly contaminated Kiev region of the former Union of Soviet Socialist Republics showed no changes in perinatal mortality after the accident.[37–40] Studies have focused on stillbirths in 18 European countries and found elevated stillbirths following Chernobyl in the eastern countries of Europe (Poland, Hungary, Sweden, and Greece). In West Germany in May of 1986, mortality among infants within the first 7 days of life was increased, which the authors attributed to Chernobyl fallout in southern Germany.[40,41]

TABLE 9-2

TERATOGENIC EFFECTS OF RADIATION ON RODENTS

Species	Gestational Age (days pc)	Exposure (R)	Effects Observed
Mouse	0.5	5	Increase in resorption
	0.5–1.5	15–20	Exencephaly
	7.5	5	Skeletal malformations
	7.5	5	Decreased litter weight
	8.0	25	Hydrocephalus
	8.5	50	Eye defects
Rat	0.5	5	Growth disturbances
	8.0–9.5	36–40	Ocular and cerebral malformations
	9.0	50	Increase in resorption frequency
	9.0	100	Aortic and urinary malformations
	9.0	50	Brain and spinal malformations
	16–22	10–50	Permanent nerve damage

pc: postconception

TABLE 9–3

TERATOGENIC EFFECTS OF RADIATION ON HUMANS

Effects	Postconception Time (wk)				
	Pre-implantation	Organogenesis	Early Fetal	Mid Fetal	Late Fetal
	1	2–7	8–15	16–25	> 25
Lethality	+++	+	+	——	——
Gross malformation	——	+++	+	+	——
Growth retardation	——	+++	++	+	+
Mental retardation	——	——	+++	+	——
Sterility	——	+	++	+	+
Cataracts	——	+	+	+	+
Other neurology	——	+++	+	+	+
Malignant diseases	——	+	+	+	+

——: no observed effect
 +: demonstrated
++: moderate incidence
+++: high incidence

Growth Retardation

In 1980, the committee for the Biological Effects of Ionizing Radiation compared the average growth pattern over 17 years of 1,613 children exposed in utero at Hiroshima who were closer to the blast center (< 1,500 m) to those who were farther away (> 3,000 m) and thus received lower doses. Children exposed closer to the hypocenter demonstrated significant growth retardation, averaging 2.25 cm shorter, 3 kg lighter, and head diameters 1.1 cm smaller in circumference. Interestingly, the small head circumference did not alter with age, with most children showing no compensatory growth.[42,43]

Teratogenic Effects

Microencephaly and intellectual disability were the main effects observed in the children of the atom bomb survivors. Microencephaly was phase dependent and observed only in those exposed at 0 to 7 and 8 to 15 weeks of gestation, but not among those exposed at 16 weeks or more.[40,41] Studies on children irradiated during medical exposures revealed several kinds of malformations, including eye anomalies, hydrocephaly, ossification of the cranial bones, deformities, alopecia, divergent squint, blindness, and spina bifida (incomplete closure of the spinal column).[38] The gestational age of 8 to 15 weeks is the most sensitive to radiation injury to the central nervous system, followed by the 16- to 25-week period. This is when the highest incidence of intellectual disability was observed in the Hiroshima-Nagasaki cohort, with a threshold of 0.12 to 0.2 Gy.[1,3,5] Studies on cohorts of children exposed in utero to the Chernobyl fallout validates the earlier findings that radiation can impair cognitive ability at doses lower than projected.[40,41] The decline in intelligence quotient could be seen with doses as low as 0.1 Gy at certain sensitive periods. Further, there was increased frequency of a number of congenital malformations, including cleft lip and/or palate ("hare lip"), doubling of the kidneys, polydactyly (extra fingers or toes), anomalies in the development of the nervous and blood systems, amelia (limb reduction defects), anencephaly (defective development of the brain), spina bifida, Down syndrome, abnormal openings in the esophagus and anus, and multiple malformations occurring simultaneously.[40,41]

Cancer Risk and In-Utero Exposure

Data on the effect of postnatal age at irradiation from follow-up studies of the Japanese survivors of the atomic bombings show that relative cancer risks are greatest for younger ages for a number of cancer types, including carcinoma of the colon and stomach.[38,39] Information on cancer risk following in-utero irradiation is available from studies of prenatal diagnostic X-ray exposures, as well as studies of the Japanese survivors. The largest study of the effects of prenatal diagnostic X-irradiation is the Oxford Survey of Childhood Cancers, a national case-control study of childhood cancer mortality carried out in the United Kingdom. Reviewing the available data from the Oxford Survey and other studies, Doll and Wakeford concluded that there is strong evidence that low-dose irradiation of the fetus (about 10 mGy), particularly during the last trimester of pregnancy, causes an increased risk of cancer in childhood (< 15 years of age).[40,41,44–47] However, in 2003, the ICRP drew attention to differences between studies in the relative risks estimated for leukemia and solid cancers and concluded that the data provide an insufficient basis for the specification of risks of in-utero irradiation of individual organs and tissues.[40,47]

GENETIC EFFECTS

A complete discussion of the genetic effects of radiation are beyond the scope of this chapter. However, a summary is provided here as a means to assist the clinician caring for an irradiated individual. Exposure to radiation can cause adverse health effects in descendents as a consequence of mutations in the germ cells of irradiated individuals.[1–5] Hereditary or genetic diseases can result when mutations occurring in the germ cells of irradiated parents are transmitted to progeny. Most cancers occur from mutations in somatic cells.

Although it is a common belief that radiation causes bizarre mutations, radiation exposure does not result in effects that are new or unique but rather it increases the frequency of the same mutations that occur naturally or spontaneously in the general population. Hereditary effects are classified into three categories: (1) Mendelian, (2) chromosomal, or (3) multifactorial (Table 9-4). The frequency of these diseases ranges from 0.15 to 7.1 per million in the general population.

Information of the hereditary effects of radiation comes almost entirely from animal and insect studies. These studies have led to the description of the "doubling dose." The doubling dose is the dose required to double the spontaneous mutation incidence. Based on the mouse studies, the doubling dose in humans is estimated to be 1 Gy. The ICRP has estimated that the hereditary risk of radiation is approximately 0.2% per sievert for the general population, and 0.1% per sievert for occupational exposures based on data derived from rodents and insects.[1,2,5]

Children of the atomic bomb survivors have been studied for a number of adverse health indicators, including congenital defects, gender ratio, physical development, survival, cytogenetic damage, malignant diseases, and oncogenic proteins in blood, as described in the section above. The doubling dose was estimated to be 2 Sv, with a lower limit of 1 Sv.

TABLE 9-4

BASELINE FREQUENCY OF GENETIC DISEASES IN HUMAN POPULATIONS

Disease Class	Frequency (per million)
Mendelian	24,000
Autosomal dominant	15,000
X-linked	1,500
Autosomal recessive	7,500
Chromosomal	4,000
Multifactorial	710,000
Congenital abnormalities	879,200

Data sources: (1) Committee to Assess Health Risks from Exposure to Low Levels of Ionizing Radiation; Board on Radiation Effects Research; Division on Earth and Life Studies; National Research Council of the National Academies. *Health Risks From Exposure to Low Levels of Ionizing Radiation*. Washington, DC: National Academies Press; 2006. (2) Sankaranarayanan K. Ionizing radiation and genetic risks IX. Estimates of the frequencies of mendelian diseases and spontaneous mutation rates in human populations: a 1998 perspective. *Mutat Res.* 1998;411(2):129–178.

TRANSGENERATIONAL EFFECTS

While it is well known that maternal exposure to radiation while pregnant can cause birth defects in children, the effects of paternal exposure prior to conception have only recently been studied. Paternal exposure to radiation has been implicated in the etiology of childhood cancer and seems like a possible factor in the occurrence of clusters of childhood leukemias near some nuclear installations. One interpretation of this phenomenon is that genomic instability has been induced in offspring of irradiated male parents. In a case-control study of leukemia and non-Hodgkin's lymphoma, a higher-than-normal incidence of the diseases occurred in children whose fathers worked at the Sellafield reprocessing plant in West Cumbria,

UK.[44] This study demonstrated that children of men who had been exposed to penetrating ionizing radiation prior to conception were at an increased risk of leukemia, and the authors speculated that cumulative occupational exposure caused a mutation in a father's spermatozoa that could cause the offspring to develop leukemia.[44] A study of children in other health districts of the United Kingdom, whose fathers also worked in the nuclear industry (atomic weapons establishments at Aldermaston and Burghfield, UK), showed a similar elevation in leukemia development.[45,46] However, several retrospective studies were unable to confirm the observations reported in the Gardner study.[47] Taken together, the results of these studies are inconsistent and the cause of the leukemia clusters remains unknown at present. Birth defects and leukemia have not been reported in the offspring of service members exposed to fragments of depleted uranium (an internal emitter used in military munitions).

Several in-vitro studies have demonstrated a mechanism by which radiation induces transmissible genomic instability at the cellular level, expressed in the form of chromosomal aberrations.[48] Using an in-vitro bone marrow assay, the authors observed a high incidence of offspring cells containing chromosomal aberrations after exposure of the parental bone-marrow stem cells to alpha particles from plutonium. Several other studies have demonstrated that chromosomal instability in parental bone-marrow cells can be passed on to offspring cells in the bone marrow.[49,50] Exposure to depleted uranium has also been shown to induce genomic instability in unexposed offspring cells.[51]

Transgenerational mouse studies continue to confirm the hypothesis that paternal radiation exposure can cause genomic instability in unexposed offspring. These studies support the hypothesis that preconceptional parental irradiation of mice can cause transgenerational transmission of factors leading to genomic instability and increased mutations in F1 offspring. Recent studies with depleted uranium using a similar transgenic mouse system have demonstrated that preconceptional, paternal depleted uranium exposure can increase gene mutation frequency in unexposed offspring.[52] The studies with depleted uranium are complicated by the fact that it is not only an alpha-particle emitter but is a toxic heavy metal, so no definite conclusions can be drawn as to whether the offspring effects were due to radiation or chemical toxicity because data support the roles of both radiation and heavy metal effects.

While the epidemiological data are controversial regarding preconceptional paternal radiation effects, numerous studies support both the observation and genomic instability mechanism as being involved in rodent and cellular models. Although the results in animal studies were not obtained at the low-dose level to the male parents (100 mSv) in the epidemiological studies,[44] those data with radiation[53] and depleted uranium[52] suggest that there is evidence for transgenerational transmission of factors leading to genomic instability and increased mutations in F1 offspring. A more definitive answer awaits further studies.

RADIATION-INDUCED IMMUNOSUPPRESSION

Radiation-induced immunosuppression is a critical concern in populations exposed to sublethal to lethal doses of ionizing radiation. Radiation results in a dramatic decrease in peripheral blood cell population, especially granulocytes, lymphocytes, and platelets, due to depletion in hematopoietic stem and progenitor cells.[54,55] However, depletion is often followed by delayed repopulation and recovery as the surviving stem cells reconstitute the hematopoietic system. The delay in repopulation can be correlated to the extent of damage to the stem and progenitor cells, which further depends on the absorbed dose.[56] During this delay, individuals are susceptible to opportunistic infections; thus, accelerated recovery is essential to prevent bone-marrow–related injury and mortality. Radiation-induced stem cell damage was first illustrated in a mouse model by Till and McCulloch; the team demonstrated that bone-marrow stem cells from mice exposed to significant doses of ionizing radiation exhibited lower numbers of stem cell colonies in the spleen and poor capacity to reconstitute the hematopoietic system in recipient animals.[56] Reduction in the reconstitutive capacity of hematopoietic stem cells (HSCs) depended on absorbed dose. Since then, this assay is routinely used to assess stem cell function in animal models and is considered an index of the reconstitutive capacity of HSCs.[57–59]

Bone marrow suppression can be prevented by stimulating hematopoiesis and rapid recovery. In clinical and animal models, such recovery is routinely stimulated by use of various cytokines, cytokine mimetics, and hematopoietic growth factors.[60–64] However, it has become increasingly evident that growth-factor–mediated recovery is not entirely a complete hematopoietic recovery. Radiation-induced damage, such as genotoxic stress, in stem cells is not alleviated by cytokines and growth factors.[65] In contrast, replicative stress is induced upon proliferative stimuli in damaged stem cells that may potentially accumulate genomic instability. Indeed, several studies report higher incidences of malignancies in hematopoietic system in response to ionizing radiation.[66]

Prevalence of long-term immunosuppression is also concerning in patients treated with radio- or chemotherapy years after treatment. It was believed that HSCs have finite capacity to replicate, thus mitotic overload in HSCs potentially leads to accelerated aging and exhaustion of the stem cell pool. However, serial bone-marrow transplant experiments suggest that long-term colony-forming units increased upon serial transplantation in mice, showing practically infinite replicative capacity.[67] Also an increase in telomere length did not increase HSC expansion any further compared to control animals.[68] In some studies involving the effect of oxidative damage in ataxia telangiectasia mutated mice (ATM$^{-/-}$ mice), HSC replicative capacity was inversely correlated to oxidative stress-related DNA damage.[69] Ionizing radiation was also shown to induce expression of senescence markers, such as protein 21 in HSCs in murine models. These studies clearly indicate that preventing DNA damage was the key determining factor in preserving stem cell function.[70,71]

Early onset of leukemogenesis and stem cell aging are major drawbacks of current hematopoietic injury treatments in radiation exposure. More emphasis is required to address the long-term effects of radiation on the hematopoietic system. Current understanding of molecular pathology and more advancement in the regulatory mechanisms of stem cells can help design better drug targets to reduce genomic instability and long-term damage.

REGULATORY GUIDES FOR EXPOSURE

Based on the scientific evidence, the US government (through the National Council on Radiation Protection [NCRP]) has set regulatory guidelines for the occupational exposure of workers and for the general public (Table 9-5). The permissible concentrations for the occupational exposure to radiation workers are 10-fold higher than exposure levels for the general public. It is thought that the presumed detrimental effects on health from exposures at these limits are negligible. Scientific bodies continually reevaluate these risk es-

timates as additional information becomes available on radiation effects in human populations.

The NCRP has defined a dose of 0.01 mSv/y, equivalent to 10 Gy or 1 mrad of low-LET radiation, as the negligible individual risk level.[1,3,5] This implies that almost every dose of radiation carries potential risk; in some cases, the risk is extremely small and difficult to identify. The goal is to keep exposures as low as is reasonably achievable in daily life and in emergency situations.

SUMMARY

The late effects of ionizing radiation can be divided into three major groups: (1) somatic, (2) genetic, and (3) teratogenic. Somatic damage ranges from fibrosis and necrosis of individual organs to cataracts and

cancer (Table 9-6). Most somatic effects require high-threshold doses of radiation; cancer is the main health concern after exposure to low-level radiation. The three most common radiation-induced malignancies

TABLE 9-5

SUMMARY OF RECOMMENDED DOSE LIMITS

Type of Exposure	Dose Limit
Occupational	
Stochastic effects	
Cumulative	10 mSv x age
Annual	50 mSv/y
Deterministic effects (annual dose equivalent limits for tissues and organs)	
Lens of eye	150 mSv/y
Skin, hands, and feet	500 mSv/y
Embryonic/Fetal (effective dose limit after pregnancy declared)	0.5 mSv/mo
Public	
Effective dose limit, continuous or frequent exposure	1 mSv/y
Effective dose limit, infrequent exposure	5 mSv/y
Dose equivalent limits of lens of eye, skin, and extremities	50 mSv/y
Education and Training (annual)	
Effective dose limit	1 mSv/y
Dose equivalent limit for lens of eye	15 mSv/y
Dose equivalent limit for skin and extremities	50 mSv/y
Negligible Individual Dose (annual)	0.01 mSv/y

Data source: National Council on Radiation Protection and Measurements. *Recommendations on Limits for Exposure to Ionizing Radiation.* Bethesda, MD: NCRP; 1993. NCRP Report 116.

are leukemia, breast cancer, and thyroid cancer. The latency periods for the detection of cancer after radiation exposure range from 2 years for leukemia to 30 to 40 years for some solid tumors.

Mathematical models predicting cancer risks based on observations from high radiation exposures imply that 120 to 180 additional cancer deaths will occur for every million individuals receiving 1 cGy of radiation.[1,3,5] This estimate range includes the incidence of all cancers and presumes that no thresholds for induction exist. Some evidence indicates that thresholds for radiation-induced cancer do exist, ranging from 0.01 Gy for breast cancer to 0.2 Gy for leukemia.

Genetic or hereditary effects are the second category of low-level or late effects of radiation. It is estimated that 5 to 65 additional genetic disorders will occur in the next generation for every million individuals receiving 0.01 Gy of gamma or low-LET radiation.[1,3,5] These disorders will be mainly autosomal dominant and gender linked. If each succeeding generation were to receive an additional 0.01 Gy of radiation, equilibrium would be reached in the gene pool, and an average increase of 60 to 1,100 genetic disorders per million individuals would be observed in the population. This would result in a 1.5% increase in the overall incidence of genetic disorders. The normal incidence of genetic disorders in the population is 1 in 10.

The third category of late radiation damage is teratogenic effects. The primary teratogenic somatic effects seen in humans exposed in utero are microencephaly, intellectual disability, and growth retardation. These effects have been observed with an increased incidence in the atomic bomb survivors exposed in utero to doses of less than 0.10 Gy, although a neutron component may have enhanced the radiation effectiveness. In general, thresholds exist for the induction of birth defects by radiation, and effects below 0.10 Gy are negligible. The normal incidence of birth defects is 1 in 10 live births. One concern for low-level exposure to ionizing radiation in utero is the increased incidence of cancer in childhood. An estimated 25 additional cancer deaths are predicted for every million children receiving 1 cGy of radiation in utero.

Preconceptional parental exposures leading to transgenerational effects have recently become a concern. The human data are inconclusive and controversial, so no risk estimates have been established. Further studies in epidemiology and with animal models will provide guidance.

TABLE 9-6

SUMMARY OF DELETERIOUS EFFECTS OF RADIATION*

Endpoint	Risk Estimate
Carcinogenesis (general population; low dose, low dose rate)	5%/Sv
Hereditary effects (general population)	0.2%/Sv
Severe intellectual disability (exposure of embryo/fetus, 8–15 wk)	40%/Sv

*Radiation risk estimates are based upon the human database of radiation-exposed individuals. The relative risk model assumes that radiation increases the spontaneous incidence by a factor. Since the natural cancer incidence increases with age, this model predicts a large number of excess cancers appearing late in life after irradiation. The most recent reassessment of radiation-induced cancer risks by the BEIR V committee was based on a time-related relative risk model. Excess cancer mortality was assumed to depend on dose, age at exposure, time since exposure, and, for some cancers, sex.[1] For example, a 5% risk/Sv means that there is an increased probability of 5 additional cancers per 1,000 individuals exposed per sievert of radiation.
(1) Committee to Assess Health Risks from Exposure to Low Levels of Ionizing Radiation; Board on Radiation Effects Research; Division on Earth and Life Studies; National Research Council of the National Academies. *Health Risks From Exposure to Low Levels of Ionizing Radiation.* Washington, DC: National Academies Press; 1990.

REFERENCES

1. Hall EJ, Giaccia A. *Radiobiology for the Radiologist.* 6th ed. Philadelphia, PA: Lippincott, Williams & Wilkins; 2008.

2. Nias AHW. *An Introduction to Radiobiology.* 2nd ed. New York, NY: Wiley; 1998.

3. Steel GG. *Basic Clinical Radiobiology.* 3rd ed. London, England: Arnold; 2002.

4. Miller AC. *Depleted Uranium: Properties, Uses, and Health Consequences.* Boca Raton, FL: CRC Press/Taylor & Francis; 2007.

5. Buckley PG, Bines WP, Kemball PT, Williams MK. Development of revised Ionizing Radiations Regulations. *J Radiol Prot.* 1997;18(3):115–118.

6. National Council on Radiation Protection and Measurements. *Ionizing Radiation Exposure of the Population of the United States.* Bethesda, MD: NCRP; 2009. NCRP Report 160.

7. Chodick G, Bekiroglu N, Hauptmann M. Risk of cataract after exposure to low doses of ionizing radiation: a 20-year prospective cohort study among US radiologic technologists. *Am J Epidemiol*. 2008;168(6):622–637.

8. O'Sullivan B, Levin W. Late radiation-related fibrosis: pathogenesis, manifestations, and current management. *Semin Radiat Oncol*. 2003;13(3):274–289.

9. Stroian G, Martens C, Souhami L, Collins DL, Seuntjens J. Local correlation between monte-carlo dose and radiation-induced fibrosis in lung cancer patients. *Int J Radiat Oncol Biol Phys*. 2008;70(3):921–930.

10. Evans JC. Time-dose relationship of radiation; fibrosis of lung. *Radiology*. 1960;74:104.

11. Sabatier L, Martin M, Crechet F, Pinton P, Dutrillaux B. Chromosomal anomalies in radiation-induced fibrosis in the pig. *Mutat Res*. 1992;284(2):257–263.

12. Kasai H, Allen JT, Mason RM, Kamimura T, Zhang Z. TGF-beta1 induces human alveolar epithelial to mesenchymal cell transition (EMT). *Respir Res*. 2005;6:56.

13. Rodemann HP, Blaese MA. Responses of normal cells to ionizing radiation. *Semin Radiat Oncol*. 2007;17(2):81–88.

14. Martin M, Lefaix JL, Pinton P, Crechet F, Daburon F. Temporal modulation of TGF-beta 1 and beta-actin gene expression in pig skin and muscular fibrosis after ionizing radiation. *Radiat Res*. 1993;134(1):63–70.

15. Finkelstein JN, Johnston CJ, Baggs R, Rubin P. Early alterations in extracellular matrix and transforming growth factor beta gene expression in mouse lung indicative of late radiation fibrosis. *Int J Radiat Oncol Biol Phys*. 1994;28(3):621–631.

16. Ehrhart EJ, Segarini P, Tsang ML, Carroll AG, Barcellos-Hoff MH. Latent transforming growth factor beta1 activation in situ: quantitative and functional evidence after low-dose g-irradiation. *FASEB J*. 1997;11(12):991–1002.

17. Burger A, Löffler H, Bamberg M, Rodemann HP. Molecular and cellular basis of radiation fibrosis. *Int J Radiat Biol*. 1998;73(4):401–408.

18. Martin M, Lefaix J, Delanian S. TGF-beta1 and radiation fibrosis: a master switch and a specific therapeutic target? *Int J Radiat Oncol Biol Phys*. 2000;47(2):277–290.

19. Machtay M, Scherpereel A, Santiago J, et al. Systemic polyethylene glycol-modified (PEGylated) superoxide dismutase and catalase mixture attenuates radiation pulmonary fibrosis in the C57/bl6 mouse. *Radiother Oncol*. 2006;81(2):196–205.

20. Delanian S, Baillet F, Huart J, Lefaix JL, Maulard C, Housset M. Successful treatment of radiation-induced fibrosis using liposomal Cu/Zn superoxide dismutase: clinical trial. *Radiother Oncol*. 1994;32(1):12–20.

21. Delanian S, Lefaix JL. Current management for late normal tissue injury: radiation-induced fibrosis and necrosis. *Semin Radiat Oncol*. 2007;17(2):99–107.

22. Delanian S, Porcher R, Rudant J, Lefaix JL. Kinetics of response to long-term treatment combining pentoxifylline and tocopherol in patients with superficial radiation-induced fibrosis. *J Clin Oncol*. 2005;23(34):8570–8579.

23. Delanian S, Porcher R, Balla-Mekias S, Lefaix JL. Randomized, placebo-controlled trial of combined pentoxifylline and tocopherol for regression of superficial radiation-induced fibrosis. *J Clin Oncol*. 2003;21(13):2545–2550.

24. Rugh R. The impact of ionizing radiations on the embryo and fetus. *Am J Roentgenol Radium Ther Nucl Med*. 1963;89:182–190.

25. Streffer C, Molls M. Cultures of preimplantation mouse embryos: a model for radiological studies. *Adv Radiat Biology*. 1987;13:169–213.

26. Russell LB, Russell WL. The effect of radiation on the preimplantation stages of the mouse embryo. *Anat Rec*. 1950;108:521.

27. Russell LB. X-ray-induced developmental abnormalities in the mouse and their use in the analysis of embryological patterns. II. Abnormalities of the vertebral column and thorax. *J Exp Zool*. 1956;131:329–395.

28. Streffer C, Shore R, Konermann G. Biological effects after prenatal irradiation (embryo and fetus). A report of the International Commission on Radiological Protection. *Ann ICRP*. 2003;33:5–206.

29. Friedberg W, Hanneman GD, Faulkner DN, Darden EB Jr, Deal RB Jr. Prenatal survival of mice irradiated with fission neutrons or 300kVp x-rays during the pronuclear-zygote stage: survival curves, effect of dose fractionation. *Int J Radiat Biol Relat Stud Phys Chem Med*. 1973;24:549–560.

30. Michel C, Blattmann H, Cordt-Riehle I, Fritz-Niggli H. Low-dose effects of X-rays and negative pions on the pronuclear zygote stage of mouse embryos. *Radiat Environ Biophys*. 1979;16:299–302.

31. Pampfer S, Streffer C. Prenatal death and malformations after irradiation of mouse zygotes with neutrons or x-rays. *Teratology*. 1988;37:599–607.

32. Pampfer S, Streffer C. Increased chromosome aberration levels in cells from mouse fetuses after zygote X-irradiation. *Int J Radiat Biol*. 1989;55:85–92.

33. Pils S, Müller WU, Streffer C. Lethal and teratogenic effects in two successive generations of the HLG mouse strain after radiation exposure of zygotes—association with genomic instability? *Mutat Res*. 1999;429:85–92.

34. United Nations Scientific Committee on the Effects of Atomic Radiation. *Sources and Effects of Ionizing Radiation: UNSCEAR 2000 Report to the General Assembly, With Scientific Annexes*. Vol II. New York, NY: United Nations; 2000.

35. Uma Devi P, Satyamitra M. Protection against prenatal irradiation-induced genomic instability and its consequences in adult mice by Ocimum flavonoids, orientin and vicenin. *Int J Radiat Biol*. 2004;80:653–662.

36. Yamazaki JN, Wright SW, Wright PM. Outcome of pregnancy in women exposed to the atomic bomb in Nagasaki. *AMA Am J Dis Child*. 1954;87:448–463.

37. Little J. The Chernobyl accident, congenital anomalies and other reproductive outcomes. *Pediatr Perinat Epidemiol*. 1993;7:121–151.

38. Grosche B, Irl C, Schoetzau A, van Santen E. Perinatal mortality in Bavaria, Germany, after the Chernobyl reactor accident. *Radiat Environ Biophys*. 1997;36:129–136.

39. Miller RW, Mulvihill JJ. Small head size after atomic irradiation. *Teratology*. 1976;14:355–357.

40. Doll R, Wakeford R. Risk of childhood cancer from fetal irradiation. *Br J Radiol*. 1997;70:130–139.

41. Goldstein L, Murphy DP. Etiology of ill-health in children born after postconceptional maternal irradiation. *Am J Roentgenol*. 1990;22:322–331.

42. Committee to Assess Health Risks from Exposure to Low Levels of Ionizing Radiation; Board on Radiation Effects Research; Division on Earth and Life Studies; National Research Council of the National Academies. *Health Risks From Exposure to Low Levels of Ionizing Radiation*. Washington, DC: National Academies Press; 1990.

43. Schull WJ. Late radiation responses in man: current evaluation from results from Hiroshima and Nagasaki. *Adv Space Res*. 1983;3(8):231–239.

44. Gardner MJ, Snee MP, Hall AJ, Powell CA, Downes S, Terrell JD. Results of case-control study of leukaemia and lymphoma among young people near Sellafield nuclear plant in West Cumbria. *BMJ*. 1990;300:423–429.

45. Roman E, Beral V, Carpenter L, et al. Childhood leukaemia in the West Berkshire and Basingstoke and North Hampshire District Health Authorities in relation to nuclear establishments in the vicinity. *Br Med J (Clin Res Ed)*. 1987;294:597–602.

46. Roman E, Watson A, Beral V. Case-control study of leukaemia and non-Hodgkin's lymphoma among children aged 0-4 years living in West Berkshire and North Hampshire health districts. *BMJ*. 1993;306:615–621.

47. Doll R, Evans HJ, Darby SC. Paternal exposure not to blame. *Nature*. 1994;367:678–680.

48. Kadhim MA, Macdonald DA, Goodhead DT, Lorimore SA, Marsden SJ, Wright EJ. Transmission of chromosomal instability after plutonium alpha-particle irradiation. *Nature*. 1992;355:738–740.

49. Sabatier L, Dutrillaux B, Martin MB. Chromosomal instability. *Nature*. 1992;357:548.

50. Holmberg K, Meijer AE, Auer G, Lambert B. Delayed chromosomal instability in human T-lymphocyte clones exposed to ionizing radiation. *Int J Radiat Biol*. 1995;68:245–255.

51. Miller AC, Brooks K, Stewart M, et al. Genomic instability in human osteoblast cells after exposure to depleted uranium: delayed lethality and micronuclei formation. *J Environ Radioact*. 2003;64(2–3):247–259.

52. Miller AC, Stewart M, Rivas R. Preconceptional paternal exposure to depleted uranium: transmission of genetic damage to offspring. *Health Phys*. 2010;99(3):371–379.

53. Luke GA, Riches AC, Bryant PE. Genomic instability in haematopoietic cells of F1 generation mice of irradiated male parents. *Mutagenesis*. 1997;12:147–152.

54. Kumar KS, Ghosh SP, Hauer-Jensen M. Gamma-tocotrienol: potential as a countermeasure against radiological threat. In: Watson RR, Preesy VR, eds. *Tocotrienols: Vitamin E Beyond Tocopherols*. Boca Raton, FL: CRC Press; 2008: Chap 7.

55. Drouet M, Mourcin F, Grenier N, et al. The effects of ionizing radiation on stem cells and hematopoietic progenitors: the place of apoptosis and the therapeutic potential of anti-apoptosis treatments [in French]. *Can J Physiol Pharmacol*. 2002;80(7):700–709.

56. McCulloch EA, Till JE. Regulatory mechanisms acting on hemopoietic stem cells. Some clinical implications. *Am J Pathol*. 1971;65(3):601–619.

57. Down JD, Boudewijn A, van Os R, Thames HD, Ploemacher RE. Variations in radiation sensitivity and repair among different hematopoietic stem cell subsets following fractionated irradiation. *Blood*. 1995;86(1):122–127.

58. Botnick LE, Hannon EC, Vigneulle R, Hellman S. Differential effects of cytotoxic agents on hematopoietic progenitors. *Cancer Res*. 1981;41(6):2338–2342.

59. Milenkovic P, Ivanovic Z, Stosic-Grujicic S. The in vivo effect of recombinant human interleukin-1 receptor antagonist on spleen colony forming cells after radiation induced myelosuppression. *Eur Cytokine Netw*. 1995;6(3):177–180.

60. Andrews RG, Knitter GH, Bartelmez SH, et al. Recombinant human stem cell factor, a c-kit ligand, stimulates hematopoiesis in primates. *Blood*. 1991;78(8):1975–1980.

61. Talmadge JE, Tribble H, Pennington R, et al. Protective, restorative, and therapeutic properties of recombinant colony-stimulating factors. *Blood*. 1989;73(8):2093–2103.

62. Blumenthal RD, Sharkey RM, Quinn LM, Goldenberg DM. Use of hematopoietic growth factors to control myelosuppression caused by radioimmunotherapy. *Cancer Res*. 1990;50(3 Suppl):1003s–1007s.

63. Talmadge JE, Herberman RB. The preclinical screening laboratory: evaluation of immunomodulatory and therapeutic properties of biological response modifiers. *Cancer Treat Rep*. 1986;70(1):171–182.

64. Yamamoto N, Sekine I, Nakagawa K, et al. A pharmacokinetic and dose escalation study of pegfilgrastim (KRN125) in lung cancer patients with chemotherapy-induced neutropenia. *Jpn J Clin Oncol*. 2009;39(7):425–430.

65. Ziegler BL, Sandor PS, Plappert U, et al. Short-term effects of early-acting and multilineage hematopoietic growth factors on the repair and proliferation of irradiated pure cord blood (CB) CD34+ hematopoietic progenitor cells. *Int J Radiat Oncol Biol Phys*. 1998;40(5):1193–1203.

66. Hempelmann LH. Epidemiological studies of leukemia in persons exposed to ionizing radiation. *Cancer Res*. 1960;20:18–27.

67. Iscove NN, Nawa K. Hematopoietic stem cells expand during serial transplantation in vivo without apparent exhaustion. *Curr Biol*. 1997;7(10):805–808.

68. Allsopp RC, Morin GB, Horner JW, DePinho R, Harley CB, Weissman IL. Effect of TERT over-expression on the long-term transplantation capacity of hematopoietic stem cells. *Nat Med*. 2003;9(4):369–371.

69. Ito K, Hirao A, Arai F, et al. Regulation of oxidative stress by ATM is required for self-renewal of haematopoietic stem cells. *Nature*. 2004;431(7011):997–1002.

70. Wang Y, Schulte BA, Zhou D. Hematopoietic stem cell senescence and long-term bone marrow injury. *Cell Cycle*. 2006;5(1):35–38.

71. Wang Y, Schulte BA, LaRue AC, Ogawa M, Zhou D. Total body irradiation selectively induces murine hematopoietic stem cell senescence. *Blood*. 2006;107(1):358–366.

Chapter 10

RADIOLOGICAL CONSIDERATIONS IN MEDICAL OPERATIONS

JOHN P. MADRID, MS*

*Captain, United States Army; Health Physicist, Military Medical Operations, Armed Forces Radiobiology Research Institute, 8901 Wisconsin Avenue, Building 42, Bethesda, Maryland 20889

INTRODUCTION

From the time that the first nuclear weapon was used against Japan during World War II to the end of the Cold War during the early 1990s, the use of nuclear weapons in strategic nuclear war with rival nations was the primary radiological concern facing the US military. US defense strategies involved planning for the possibility that military installations and large elements of troops in theater would be targeted during large-scale nuclear attacks involving the launch of multiple nuclear weapons.

It would be naive to completely disregard the threat of strategic nuclear war; however, following the conclusion of the Cold War and after more recent incidents, such as the Oklahoma City bombing (1995) and the attacks on the World Trade Center and Pentagon (2001), the focus on the use of radiological and nuclear weapons has shifted toward the threat of use by terrorist organizations. This has greatly changed the way our society must plan to respond to radiological and nuclear attacks. Radiological and nuclear terrorism is more likely to occur on US soil, as opposed to being directed toward troops in theater. Attacking civilians to produce fear and panic is one of the primary goals of terrorist organizations, and both radiological and nuclear weapons could be used to accomplish this goal. A single, well-planned attack involving a dirty bomb could potentially result in hundreds of trauma casualties, as well as psychological casualties, contaminated victims, and concerned citizens numbering in the thousands. An even more ominous possibility, the detonation of an improvised nuclear device in a major city could result in numbers of casualties orders of magnitude greater than those expected to be caused by a dirty bomb.

Managing the consequences of such an incident would require the rapid coordination of extensive personnel, engineering, transportation, communications, and medical support, among other resources. No organization in the world is able to mobilize such capabilities as quickly and in such quantity as the US military. Because of the possibility that radiological or nuclear weapons could be used against the United States or its allies, our military forces, including medical support, must be prepared to provide assistance to both combatant commanders and civilian authorities if such an incident should occur.

Military medical resources will be involved, either directly or indirectly, with several important aspects of the response to a large-scale radiological or nuclear incident. These could include the search for and extraction of casualties; site survey and determination of hazard zones; decontamination of casualties; triage and treatment of casualties suffering from blast, burn, and radiation injuries; and evacuation of casualties to higher levels of care. Medical personnel will need to understand the radiological hazards associated with these activities so they can minimize the danger to victims and to themselves.

RADIATION FUNDAMENTALS

Radiation and its properties are concepts of which few truly have a thorough understanding. Radiation is not tangible; it makes no characteristic sound or smell, and radioactive materials have no distinct taste. Unlike the popular misconception, radioactive materials generally do not glow, except when produced by a handful of materials under certain conditions. Some high-level radioactive sources will give off heat, but the presence or absence of heat neither confirms nor rules out the possibility of radiation being present. Because we are not able to sense radiation, it can be a difficult concept to comprehend. This can lead to fear, which is often unwarranted. Hollywood and the media have capitalized on our fears of radiation by exaggerating the effects radiation produces, further distorting the general public's understanding of it. Without a doubt, high doses of radiation can cause serious health effects and death, but by taking the appropriate precautions to protect ourselves, we can minimize the risk presented by radiation hazards. Understanding the basic physical properties and biological effects of radiation will help people develop a respect for radiation while demystifying unfounded misconceptions.

Radiation is the emission of energy in the form of waves or particles. Radiation that is emitted as a wave (or ray) is called electromagnetic radiation. Examples of electromagnetic radiation include (in order of increasing energy) radio waves, microwaves, infrared light, visible light, ultraviolet light, X-rays, and gamma rays. Physically, all types of electromagnetic energy are composed of the same thing—photons—but vary in frequency, wavelength, and energy, giving the different types their characteristic physical properties. Radiation that is emitted in particulate form typically occurs as alpha particles, beta particles, or neutrons. There are other, less common types of particulate radiation, but they are not relevant to the topic of this chapter.

All types of radiation fall into one of two categories: ionizing and nonionizing, depending on how much energy the radiation has. Ionizing radiation includes only radiation that is energetic enough that a single particle or wave is able to break the bonds of a molecule or strip a bound electron from an atom or molecule. It is of particular interest because it can damage molecules in cells, such as DNA (deoxyribonucleic acid), resulting in damage or death to those cells. The focus of this chapter is on medical operations in which there is a hazard caused by ionizing radiation. In this chapter, the term "radiation" pertains exclusively to ionizing radiation. X-rays and gamma rays are the only two types of electromagnetic energy that are considered ionizing radiation. Each of the types of particulate radiation previously mentioned is considered ionizing radiation.

Types of Radiation

X-rays. X-rays are electromagnetic radiation emitted when energy is transferred to an electron of the orbitals surrounding the nucleus of an atom, or when charged particles in motion are decelerated. When energy is transferred to a bound electron of an atom, the electron can temporarily achieve a higher bound energy state. Eventually it will lose the excess energy to go back to its original, more stable energy state by emitting a photon, which will often be in the X-ray frequency range. If a moving charged particle, such as an electron, hits a surface, it will interact with the other electrons and nuclei of the atoms in the material, causing the particle to slow down and lose energy. Some of the energy it loses will be emitted in the form of photons and, in some cases, photons generated by this method will also be in the X-ray frequency range. X-rays can travel many meters through air and require dense materials, such as lead or concrete, to provide adequate shielding. They are often machine generated by equipment such as medical imaging devices and industrial radiography devices.

Gamma Rays. When certain types of nuclei are in an unstable energy state, they will eventually achieve a more stable energy state by emitting excess energy in the form of a photon, known as a gamma ray. This is sometimes accompanied by the emission of particulate radiation as well. Like X-rays, gamma rays can travel many meters through air and require dense materials for shielding. They are produced by many types of radioactive materials and are also produced during the detonation of a nuclear weapon.

Alpha Particles. A type of particulate radiation emitted from the nucleus of an atom that consists of two protons and two neutrons bound together is known as an alpha particle. The two protons result in a net charge of + 2 for alpha particles. Because of this net charge, alpha particles interact strongly with the

electrons and nuclei of other atoms as they are passing through a material. They do not penetrate very deeply because of this strong interaction, traveling a distance of only a couple centimeters through air, and being completely shielded by material as thin as a sheet of paper. They do not pose a significant health threat when outside the body, since the alpha particles will be absorbed in the body's outer layer of dead skin cells; however, alpha particles can do substantial damage when inside the body, where there is no protective layer of skin cells. Nuclear fuel used in reactors and nuclear weapons contains alpha-emitting sources, as do some materials that could be used in radiological dispersal devices.

Beta Particles. Another type of particulate radiation emitted from the nucleus of an atom is known as a beta particle. These are either an electron (beta –) or a positron (beta +). A positron is physically identical to an electron, but has a charge of + 1 instead of – 1. Like alpha particles, the net charge on beta particles causes them to interact strongly with surrounding electrons and nuclei as they pass through a material. Therefore, they do not require dense material for shielding. Glass or plastic several millimeters thick is typically adequate for shielding beta radiation. These particles can travel distances on the order of several meters through air and they can penetrate several millimeters deep through the skin, so beta-emitting materials in direct contact with the skin can result in a skin burn (known as a beta burn) if there is enough of the material on the skin for a long enough period of time. Because clothing provides a protective barrier to beta particles, only exposed skin is vulnerable. The fission process that occurs in nuclear reactors and during a nuclear detonation creates beta-emitting radioactive materials, which are a component of nuclear fallout. Radiological dispersal devices and radiological exposure devices are also likely to involve beta emitters.

Neutrons. Neutrons are uncharged particles that are primarily produced during the fission process that occurs in nuclear reactors and during a nuclear detonation, although there are a few types of radionuclides that emit neutrons by undergoing spontaneous fission. Since they have no net charge, neutrons can travel many meters through air and require dense material for shielding. Neutron exposure presents a risk only after the initial pulse of radiation during a nuclear detonation, or in situations in which humans could be exposed to neutron flux during criticality incidents (eg, responding to a damaged nuclear reactor core). However, neutrons can cause nonradioactive materials to become radioactive. This phenomenon, known as induced radiation activation, occurs when the nuclei of nonradioactive material absorb some of the neutrons, thereby becoming unstable and resulting in the production of beta- and gamma-emitting radioactive materials.

Radiation Terms and Units

Radiation can be generated by machines, as is the case with linear accelerators, most diagnostic medical X-ray equipment, and some industrial radiography devices. The radiation generated by these machines, though ionizing, is generally produced by electromechanical means, not by radioactivity. The term "radioactivity" is reserved exclusively for materials that have atoms whose nuclei spontaneously emit radiation.

Atoms that are radioactive are called radionuclides. Both radioactive and nonradioactive atoms having a specific number of protons and a specific number of neutrons are indicated by specifying the chemical species, X, along with the mass number, A, and are written as ^AX or $X - A$, where X is determined by the number of protons in the nucleus and A is equal to the sum of the protons and neutrons in the nucleus. For example, if there are 27 protons in the nucleus, the chemical species is cobalt (Co). If each nucleus also has 33 neutrons, the mass number (A) is $27 + 33 = 60$. This particular atom, cobalt-60, is radioactive and is represented by the symbol ^{60}Co or Co-60.

Atoms of the same chemical species (ie, having the same number of protons) can have differing numbers of neutrons. These atoms are called isotopes. For example, the isotopes of cobalt include Co-56, Co-57, Co-58, Co-59, and Co-60. All cobalt atoms have the same number of protons (27) in the nuclei of their atoms; however, these isotopes each have a different number of neutrons. The number of neutrons affects the stability of a particular isotope. Isotopes that are radioactive are called radioisotopes. The term "radioisotope" is often used synonymously with the term "radionuclide."

The rate at which a radioactive source emits radiation is known as activity. Activity is measured in units of bequerels (Bq) or curies (Ci), where 1 Ci equals 37 billion Bq. One bequerel is equivalent to one emission of radiation per second (Table 10-1).

As the nuclei of a radioactive material emit radiation, the material becomes less radioactive over time. This process is called radioactive decay. Radioactive decay can be expressed in terms of the physical half-life of the material. The physical half-life is the amount of time after an initial measurement of activity that it

TABLE 10-1

RADIATION UNITS AND CONVERSIONS

Physical Property	Description	Traditional Unit	SI Unit	Conversion
Activity	Amount of radiation emitted per unit of time for a given amount and type of radioactive material	Ci	Bq	1 Ci = 37,000,000,000 Bq
Exposure	Amount of ionization produced by X-rays or gamma rays in a given volume of air at a given time	R	C/kg	1 R = 0.000258 C/kg of air
Absorbed dose	Amount of radiation energy absorbed per unit of mass of material	rad	Gy	1 rad = 0.01 Gy
Dose equivalent	Absorbed dose multiplied by a weighting factor taking into account the biological effects caused by the particular type of radiation involved	rem	Sv	1 rem = 0.01 Sv

Bq: becquerel
C: coulombs
Ci: curie
Gy: gray
R: roentgen
rad: radiation absorbed dose
rem: roentgen equivalent in mammal
SI: international system of units
Sv: sievert

takes for a radioactive source to decay to half of the activity that was measured initially. After two half-lives have elapsed, a source will have decayed to one fourth the initial activity. After three half-lives, it will have decayed to one eighth, and so on. Each type of radioisotope has its own characteristic physical half-life, and half-lives can vary from fractions of a second to billions of years, depending on the type of radioisotope.

The activity of a source, *A(t)*, at a specific time after an initial measurement of activity is given by the following relationship:

$$A(t) \approx A(0) \cdot e^{-0.693 \cdot t / T_{P\frac{1}{2}}}$$

In this equation, *A(0)* is the activity that was initially measured, *t* is the amount of time that has elapsed since the activity was initially measured, and $T_{P\frac{1}{2}}$ is the physical half-life of the isotope. This equation can be used to determine how long it will take for a known source to decay to a safe level.

As radioactive materials decay, they do not vanish; they are converted into some other type of atom. The resulting atom is called a daughter product or a decay product. In some cases, the daughter product will be stable; in other cases, the daughter product will be radioactive. If it is radioactive, it will subsequently decay to form its own daughter products. This process can involve many subsequent generations of daughter products, resulting in a decay chain until a stable daughter product is produced, or it could involve just a single generation, depending on the original radionuclide.

When in the presence of radioactive materials, the magnitude of the hazard depends on more than just the type of radionuclide and its activity. The health threat depends on the amount of radiation to which one is exposed. Radiation exposure is a measure of the amount of ionization produced by the radiation in a given volume of air. The unit of measure of exposure is called the roentgen (R), and is equivalent to 0.000258 coulombs per kilogram of air. Some types of radiation detection equipment measure the exposure rate (exposure per unit time) present at a given location and time. Direct measurements of exposure are valid for only X-ray and gamma radiation, but not particulate forms of radiation (see Table 10-1).

A quantity that is more directly related to the magnitude of the health threat presented by radiation is the absorbed dose. The absorbed dose is a measure of the radiation energy absorbed by a material per unit mass of the material (see Table 10-1). It applies to all types of radiation and materials. The unit of absorbed dose is the gray (Gy) or the rad, where 100 rad equals 1 Gy. In the context of medical operations following a

TABLE 10-2

RADIATION QUALITY FACTORS

Type of Radiation	Quality Factor
X-rays, gamma rays, beta particles	1
Alpha particles	20
Neutrons of unknown energy	10

Data source: US Army Center for Health Promotion and Preventive Medicine. *The Medical CBRN Battlebook*. Aberdeen Proving Ground, MD: USACHPPM; 2008. USACHPPM Technical Guide 244.

radiological or nuclear incident, a measurement of 1 R of exposure can be assumed to be equal to 0.01 Gy (1 rad) of absorbed dose when measuring X-ray or gamma radiation.

Not all types of radiation are equally damaging to the cells of the body. Because of their physical properties, alpha particles and neutrons transfer much more energy than beta particles, X-rays, or gamma rays. Therefore, alpha particles and neutrons have the potential to do more damage to the cells with which they interact. A quantity known as the dose equivalent takes into account both the amount of radiation to which one is exposed and the relative amount of damage to the body associated with the type of radiation causing the exposure (see Table 10-1). The dose equivalent, *H*, is calculated using the following equation:

$$H = Q \cdot D$$

In this equation, *Q* is a weighting factor (quality factor) corresponding to the type of radiation, and *D* is the absorbed dose. When calculated using *D* in rads, the units of *H* are roentgen equivalents mammal (rem); when calculated using *D* in grays, the units of *H* are sieverts (Sv; 100 rem = 1 Sv). Note that for X-ray, gamma, and beta radiation, *Q* equals 1 (Table 10-2), so there is a one-to-one relationship between the value of the dose equivalent and the value of the absorbed dose for these types of radiation. However, this is not the case for types of radiation that have a *Q* value that is not equal to 1 (see Table 10-2).

Radiation Protection

Whenever there exists the possibility of exposure to radiation, the amount of exposure should be kept as low as reasonably achievable (ALARA). In radiation safety, this concept is known as the principle of ALARA. In other words, people should not subject themselves or others to any more exposure to radiation than is absolutely necessary to accomplish the task resulting in the exposure. During a radiological or nuclear incident, many of the victims will be exposed to radiation, and exposure to workers during the response effort will be unavoidable. However, there are some basic tenets of radiation safety that, if followed, will minimize the doses of radiation received by both the victims and the response personnel. These tenets include time, distance, shielding, and contamination control.

Time. Absorbed dose is a cumulative quantity that increases with the amount of time for which one is exposed. The less time a person spends in a radioactively contaminated environment or near other sources of radiation, the lower the dose received.

Distance. The amount of radiation to which one is being exposed decreases as the distance from the source of radiation increases. For point sources (sources with dimensions that are small compared to the distance between the source and the location at which the dose rate is to be determined), the dose rate and the distance are related by the following relationship, known as the inverse square law:

$$D_1' X_1^2 = D_2' X_2^2$$

In this equation, X_1 and X_2 represent two separate distances from a point radiation source, and D_1' and D_2' represent the corresponding absorbed dose rates at X_1 and X_2, respectively. This relationship is not a valid approximation for sources that are not point-like, but for non-point-like sources, the dose rate will still decrease as the distance from the source increases. By maximizing the distance from radiation sources, radiation dose rate can be minimized.

Shielding. As radiation passes through a material, it becomes attenuated in intensity as the particles or waves of radiation interact with the electrons and nuclei of the material. Various materials can be used as shielding to reduce the amount of radiation exposure. Shielding materials should be selected based on the type of radiation. Dense materials, such lead, concrete, or the ground, will shield radiation more effectively than less dense materials, and hydrogenous materials, like water, are effective at shielding neutrons. Additionally, the amount of shielding provided by a given material increases with the thickness of the material.

Contamination Control. Radiological and nuclear incidents are likely to result in the spread of radioactive materials. Radioactive material located in an area in which its presence is not intended is known as contamination, and it can occur in the environment or on equipment, buildings, and vehicles, and both outside and inside the human body. It is important to clarify the difference between contamination and exposure. Exposure occurs when a person or object is in the field of radiation being emitted by a source. Radiation exposure can damage the cells of the body; however, it does not result in the person or object that was exposed becoming radioactive (except in the case of a large dose of neutrons). Therefore, exposure to radiation does not cause a person or object to become a radiological hazard, and the exposed person or object is not necessarily contaminated. A person or object can be considered contaminated only if it has radioactive materials on or inside of it; thus, the contaminated person or object receives a certain amount of exposure from the contamination. Additionally, the contamination could cause exposure to anything else that is in the vicinity, and it could lead to cross-contamination (contaminating something that was not previously contaminated). Therefore, people and objects that become contaminated must be decontaminated to prevent unnecessary exposures and further spread of contamination.

Human contamination will occur in one of two types: external or internal. External contamination is defined as contamination located outside the body, either on the skin, clothing, or hair. Removing external radiological contamination is relatively straightforward. Removing clothing will eliminate most of the external contamination. Rinsing with warm water and soap will typically remove the rest. Warm water is preferred over cold because cold water can cause pores to constrict, trapping radioactive materials in the skin.[1] Similarly, warm water is preferred over hot because hot water can cause pores to expand, allowing contamination to be absorbed into the skin more readily.[1] Washing with water and shampoo will remove contamination in the hair, but conditioner should be avoided.[2] If contamination is still present in the hair, hair can be clipped, but in most cases this will not be necessary.

It should be noted that field decontamination methods, such as the M291 Individual Skin Decon Kit and the M295 Individual Equipment Decon Kit issued to service members, are intended to neutralize contamination from chemical agents, not radiological agents. They will be ineffective against radiological contamination. Radioactivity is a property of the nuclei of the atoms and cannot be neutralized. Using these chemical decontamination kits and similar methods in which a substance is rubbed over exposed body parts and equipment to neutralize chemical agents will only result in further spreading radiological contamination. Radiological contamination must be physically removed from the body and from equipment.

Internal contamination is defined as contamination

located within the body. Humans can become internally contaminated through several routes of exposure, including inhalation, ingestion, injection, absorption of soluble radionuclides through the skin or wounds, and radioactive fragments becoming embedded in the body following an explosion involving radioactive materials. Methods of removing internal contamination from the body vary depending on the type of radioactive material involved and the route of exposure.

Radioactive fragments that are embedded in the body can have high levels of activity, resulting in a significant, potentially life-threatening dose to both the victim and others who are near the victim.[1] While this scenario would be relatively rare, if it is determined that a patient has been contaminated with highly radioactive fragments, the fragments must be immediately removed and placed in a secure location away from others so as not to present a hazard.

For soluble radionuclides that have been absorbed into the skin, normal external decontamination procedures might not fully remove the contamination. Applying sweat-inducing materials to the contaminated portions of the body or having the contaminated individual perform light exercise can reduce the amount of contamination remaining in the skin by causing it to be sweated out.

Radioactive materials inhaled, ingested, or injected into the body, and soluble radioactive materials that get into the bloodstream via absorption through the skin or wounds will either be distributed uniformly throughout the body or will accumulate in one or more target organs, depending on the chemical configuration of the radionuclide. For example, strontium is chemically analogous to calcium, so it deposits primarily in the bones, whereas cesium is chemically analogous to sodium and potassium, which are found in the components of all cells; therefore, cesium becomes distributed throughout the body. Radionuclides deposited in the body will be excreted over time at a rate related to the biological half-life of the radioactive material. The biological half-life is similar to the physical half-life in that it is equal to the amount of time it takes for half of an initial amount of a substance to be excreted from the body. The amount of activity of a radionuclide incorporated into the body decreases over time as a function of both the physical half-life and the biological half-life of the radionuclide. The effective half-life is defined as:

$$T_{Eff \frac{1}{2}} = (T_{P \frac{1}{2}} \bullet T_{B \frac{1}{2}}) / (T_{P \frac{1}{2}} + T_{B \frac{1}{2}})$$

In this equation, $T_{P1/2}$ is the physical half-life and $T_{B \frac{1}{2}}$ is the biological half-life. The amount of activity of a radionuclide in the body will decrease according to the effective half-life. The activity in the body, $A_i(t)$, at a given time, t, after the initial uptake can be calculate from the equation:

$$A_i(t) \approx A_i(0) \bullet e^{-0.693 \bullet t / T_{Eff \frac{1}{2}}}$$

Here, $A_i(0)$ is the initial amount of the radionuclide incorporated into the body.

In the event of internal contamination, there are treatments that can be administered to patients to increase the rate of excretion or to minimize the uptake in target organs (for example, chelating agents, such as diethylenetriamine pentaacetic acid [DTPA; used for plutonium]; ion exchange resins, such as ferric hexacyanoferrate (II) [Prussian blue; used for cesium and thallium]; and blocking agents, such as potassium iodide [KI; used to prevent uptake of radioactive isotopes of iodine]).

RADIOLOGICAL AND NUCLEAR SCENARIOS

This chapter focuses on medical operations following a large-scale radiological or nuclear incident resulting in many injuries or contamination to the population. There are several generic scenarios by which this could occur, and these scenarios are briefly discussed to distinguish the types and magnitude of casualties expected to result from each scenario, as well as identifying other factors that will affect medical operations during each type of scenario.

Radiological Exposure Device

The radiological exposure device (RED) is the simplest method of using radioactive material to cause injury and panic. An RED is a high-level radioactive source hidden so as to cause exposure to those who are in its vicinity. The sources used for these devices will most likely be gamma emitters, since gamma rays can travel a great distance and can penetrate through material concealing the RED, whereas alpha and beta particles do not have as great a range and would most likely be shielded by materials used for concealment. REDs can cause acute radiation syndrome (ARS) if the activity of the source is high enough and if nearby individuals are exposed for long enough. REDs will not result in contaminated casualties, since there would be no radioactive material on the victims. If an RED were concealed under a chair or desk in an office, it would likely affect only a handful of individuals who work in the vicinity of the location where it was hidden.

However, if an RED were hidden on a bus or passenger train, it could potentially result in many more casualties, and the casualties would not come from an isolated location. Radiation exposure due to an RED would likely be initially overlooked unless the presence of the RED was already known. This is because prodromal symptoms of ARS are similar to many other illnesses, and the lack of contamination on victims means that radiation detection equipment would not provide any indication of their potential exposure. Once news of an RED hits the media, a large number of concerned individuals, many of whom will not have received any exposure at all, will seek medical screening for health effects caused by radiation exposure.

Radiological Dispersal Device

A radiological dispersal device (RDD) is any type of device that is used to spread radioactive contamination. The most likely method of developing an RDD is to combine radioactive materials with a conventional explosive and then detonate it, thereby spreading radioactive contamination. This type of RDD is also called a dirty bomb. The magnitude of the explosion produced by a dirty bomb would not be any greater than if it were caused by the explosives alone. Adding radioactive materials does not increase explosive power, but the radioactive material will introduce additional factors that will affect the response effort. The number and types of physical injuries associated with a dirty bomb attack would be about the same as those for a conventional bomb and, in addition, both victims and responders would be potentially vulnerable to inhaling airborne radioactive materials. There is also the possibility of radioactive fragments being embedded in victims who were near the explosion. Contamination on the ground and on the skin and clothes of victims will not likely present an immediate health hazard because spreading the contamination over a large area will reduce the concentration to relatively low levels; however, contaminated individuals will still require decontamination even for low levels of contamination.

Another type of RDD scenario is the dispersal of airborne radioactive materials via crop duster or other methods by which aerosolized particulates are introduced into the atmosphere. This method could affect a very large area—possibly many square miles. As is the case with dirty bombs, spreading the radioactive material over a large area would most likely reduce the concentration of the contamination enough so that it is not an immediate external hazard, but would still require decontamination and would present an inhalation hazard to anyone in the affected area.

These two examples are not the only possible methods by which an RDD can be employed, but they are two of the most commonly suggested designs and they illustrate the radiological concerns associated with an RDD attack. In addition to the spread of radiological contamination and the potential for the contamination to become an internal hazard, it is also important to point out that for every person who becomes contaminated after an RDD attack, there will likely be many more people who were not contaminated who will seek monitoring for contamination and screening for health effects. This is the factor that makes RDDs desirable as a weapon of terror, since the use of radioactive materials can produce widespread panic and result in a surge that rapidly overwhelms medical and other resources.

Nuclear Reactor Incident

One of the most infamous radiation accidents in history was the reactor accident at Chernobyl in Ukraine in April 1986. An experimental test at one of the Chernobyl reactors caused steam in the reactor core to build up. The increase in steam pressure caused the core to burst and produced a fire that burned for several days, releasing large amounts of radioactive material into the atmosphere in the plume of smoke. More recently, in March 2011 an earthquake and subsequent tsunami caused severe damage to the reactor containment and spent fuel storage tanks at the Fukushima Daiichi nuclear power plant in Japan, resulting in an extensive release of radioactive material into the environment. These two incidents demonstrate how wide-ranging the effects of a major reactor accident can be. The population within a 20-km radius surrounding the Fukushima plant had to be evacuated, and a 30-km evacuation radius was implemented around the Chernobyl plant; that area is still uninhabited today. It has also been speculated that nuclear reactors might be targeted by terrorists, either by crashing aircraft into a reactor or spent fuel storage area, or by using explosives to attack a reactor and spent fuel storage from inside the walls. There are design precautions and security measures in place to deter attacks such as those described; however, consideration should still be given to the consequences of such an incident when planning for radiological response.

Unspent reactor fuel, which consists primarily of isotopes of uranium (U) or plutonium (Pu), is a relatively minor external hazard and is nonexplosive. Nuclear detonation can be achieved only through the use of a nuclear weapon. Rather, nuclear fuel is used in a reactor to generate heat during a process called fission, in which U-235 nuclei or Pu-239 nuclei split into two or more smaller nuclei, called fission products. A large amount of energy is released during fission, including the emission of gamma rays and neutrons. Additionally, the resulting fission products consist of a composite of numerous isotopes, many of which are highly radioactive beta and gamma emitters. For this reason, spent nuclear fuel (fuel that has undergone fission) can present a serious radiological hazard.

After an attack on a reactor or spent fuel storage area, there would likely be trauma and burn injuries from the attack, and workers and responders could receive high doses of radiation resulting in ARS if the reactor core or spent fuel storage is compromised. If a reactor incident results in a fire or an explosion, radioactive fission products and unspent fuel could be released into the atmosphere, affecting the local population. The radioactive contamination released into the atmosphere is known as fallout, and it is both an external hazard, which can cause large whole-body doses and beta burns, and an internal hazard if inhaled or ingested. The affected population will have to be advised to shelter in place or evacuate, depending on which course of action will result in a lower radiation dose, and decontamination of humans, equipment, and the environment will be necessary. Contamination can have long-term effects by accumulating in crops intended for consumption by humans and animals. After the Chernobyl incident, there was an extremely high additional incidence of thyroid cancer in children who drank milk from cows who had ingested crops that had an uptake from the fallout. Radioactive isotopes of iodine are one of the fission products found in abundance in fallout, so the affected population and responders may be advised to take potassium iodine tablets early on to block accumulation of radioactive iodine in the thyroid.

Nuclear Weapon Incident Without Nuclear Detonation

If a nuclear weapon becomes damaged, either due to an accident or as a result of malicious activity, it can cause injuries and contamination even if a nuclear detonation does not occur. A nuclear detonation is produced by first detonating conventional explosives to compress highly enriched nuclear material in the weapon, but damage to the weapon can cause these conventional explosives to detonate without initiating the nuclear detonation. The resulting explosion would spread contamination consisting of highly enriched uranium or plutonium and possibly tritium. The consequences of such an incident would be very similar to those produced by a dirty bomb attack, resulting in the spread of radioactive material and injuries primarily caused by the blast. There could also be significant chemical hazards associated with this type of incident.

The radioactive materials used in nuclear weapons are not an immediate external hazard, but they can present an internal hazard. The primary route of exposure would most likely be inhalation of particles suspended in the air following an explosion. Some Department of Defense (DoD) publications discuss specific guidelines for responding to an incident involving a damaged nuclear weapon.[3]

Nuclear Detonation

An attack involving detonation of a nuclear weapon would be far more devastating than any of the other scenarios previously described. Nuclear weapons could be used by either an enemy nation or in an attack in which a terrorist organization obtains a nuclear weapon or acquires the materials and technology to construct their own weapon, known as an improvised nuclear device.

The magnitude of a nuclear detonation is measured in terms of how many tons of trinitrotoluene (TNT) it would take to produce an equivalent explosion. For example, a nuclear weapon that produces a 10-kt nuclear yield would have an explosive power equivalent to that produced by 10,000 tons of TNT. A detonation caused by terrorists would most likely produce a yield of approximately 10 kt or less; however, an attack using a military nuclear weapon could result in yields on the order of megatons (millions of tons of TNT).[4]

When a nuclear weapon detonates, it produces a powerful blast wave followed by forceful winds. The blast wave and winds will drag people across the ground or throw them into objects, resulting in contusions, abrasions, and puncture injuries. Other objects can be thrown through the air, causing projectile injuries. Injuries caused by broken glass are expected to be very common. Additionally, structures will collapse under the pressure from the blast, crushing those in buildings or trapping them inside, resulting in injuries similar to those caused by an earthquake (for more information on blast injuries, see Chapter 3, Triage and Treatment of Radiation and Combined-Injury Mass Casualties).

A rapidly expanding fireball will be produced at the center of the detonation. The fireball radius will not travel nearly as far out as the blast wave, but virtually any object within the fireball will be incinerated. In addition to the fireball, there will be a thermal pulse consisting of intense ultraviolet, visible, and infrared energy that radiates outward and will produce effects even farther out than the blast. The thermal pulse will result in flash burns to humans directly exposed to it, and it can start fires in buildings, resulting in secondary flame burns to humans. The intense flash of visible light can cause retinal burns and temporary flash blindness, which can indirectly cause injuries such as car crashes (for more information on thermal injury, including flash and flame burns, see Chapter 3, Triage and Treatment of Radiation and Combined-Injury Mass Casualties).

Neutrons and gamma rays will be emitted from a nuclear detonation, traveling out farther than the fireball, but not as far as the thermal pulse. Humans directly exposed to the initial flux of gamma rays and neutrons could receive doses of radiation high enough to cause ARS. For ground bursts or very low altitude air bursts, the area in the immediate vicinity of the detonation can become radioactive as a result of beta-gamma–emitting activation products produced by the neutron flux. This region can pose a significant hazard to response personnel who enter the highly radioactive area in search of casualties.

Additionally, there will be a large quantity of dust and debris that is pulled up into the air in the low-pressure region produced following a ground burst or low altitude air burst. This plume of dust and debris will also include fission products generated during the detonation, activation products created by the release of neutrons, and weapons-grade uranium or plutonium that was not consumed during the detonation. The plume can disperse highly radioactive fallout over tens or even hundreds of square miles, and the affected population will need to be advised to shelter or evacuate. Exposure to the fallout can cause whole-body gamma doses resulting in ARS, and direct contact with the skin can cause beta burns. Fallout is also an internal hazard if inhaled or ingested. Response to fallout produced from a nuclear detonation would be similar to the response to fallout from a nuclear reactor incident.

The energy released during a nuclear detonation will cause atoms and molecules in the atmosphere to become ionized. This separation of charges will result in a powerful, short-lived, electric field known as an electromagnetic pulse (EMP). The EMP will not produce direct physiological effects in humans; however, it can induce a voltage spike in long power lines, which can overload electronic devices that are connected to the power grid. This can result in malfunction or inoperability of communication devices, water distribution that operates off electric pumps, electronic medical equipment, and other systems that involve electronics. The EMP could even damage some electronic devices that are not connected directly to the power grid, such as the control modules of vehicles. It can have effects ranging out several miles from a ground burst. For a high-altitude (100–200 miles) burst, it is estimated that there could be effects hundreds of miles away. Emergency planners and medical officers should have contingency plans in place to take into account the effects of EMP.

OPERATIONS

Radiation Detection Equipment

Because our senses are not able to measure the magnitude of radiation or even detect its presence, we must rely on various types of detection equipment to provide this information. Different types of radiation detection equipment will be needed, depending on the application for which it is required. For example, survey meters—including ion chambers, Geiger-Müller counters, proportional counters, and scintillation counters—are used to measure the levels of radiation present at a given location and time. These instruments will typically measure radiation in terms of exposure rate (ie, roentgens per hour), or count rate (ie, counts per minute). Ion chambers are usually the best instruments to use when measuring levels of radiation for the purpose of setting up radiation control boundaries. A Geiger-Müller counter with a pancake-style probe is usually preferred for detecting beta-gamma contamination on people or equipment. For contamination caused by alpha emitters, scintillation counters designed specifically for detecting alpha particles are preferred.[5]

Dosimeters are worn to measure the amount of radiation to which one has been exposed over a given time period when working around sources of radiation. Electronic personal dosimeters (EPDs) are ideal for emergency responders going into areas where high levels of radiation could be found, since EPDs provide a direct measurement of either the exposure rate or the absorbed dose (sometimes both), and most EPDs have alarms that can be set to go off when specified dose levels or exposure rates are exceeded. Pocket ion-chamber dosimeters will also provide a direct measurement of the absorbed dose; however, they do not measure exposure rate and most do not have alarms that can be set.

A thermoluminescent dosimeter (TLD) is a type of passive dosimeter often used to measure occupational exposure to low levels of radiation. It does not provide a direct measurement of dose or exposure rate. After the wear period, a TLD must be processed with specialized equipment to determine the accumulated radiation dose. After the TLD is processed, the data can be used to provide a record of the wearer's exposure history. If the availability of dosimeters is limited during a radiological or nuclear emergency, priority for dosimetry should go to those who are likely to be exposed to the highest levels of radiation. When distributing dosimeters, EPDs are preferred if real-time data is required, followed by pocket ion-chamber dosimeters, followed by TLDs. If radiation dose rates are relatively low, or if a high level of confidence in the accuracy of data is needed for regulatory purposes, TLDs are the industry standard.

A spectrometer is a type of device that can be used to identify the particular type of radioisotope involved. Radioactive materials emit radiation at characteristic discrete energy levels, depending on which radioisotope is producing it. A type of spectrometer known as a multichannel analyzer measures the energy of radiation emitted and compares the measured energy to a database of energies from known radioisotopes to determine the most likely radioisotope involved. In addition to identifying unknown sources of radiation, many multichannel analyzers work in combination with instruments that measure exposure rates or dose rates.

For any radiological or nuclear incident in which there is an inhalation hazard, it will be necessary to determine the extent of airborne radioactive material. Air sampling equipment designed to measure the quantity of radioactive material present in the air will have to be used to obtain this data. Once this data has been collected, it should be used to make corrections to computer-simulated dispersal models.

Radiation Dose Limits to Workers

Federal regulations specify the doses of radiation allowed to both the general public and radiation workers in the United States (Table 10-3). For members of the general public, defined as those who have not willingly accepted a risk of exposure to radiation as a consequence of their occupations and are not under medical surveillance for radiation exposure, the radiation dose limit is 0.1 cSv (0.1 rem) annually.[6] For adult radiation workers, defined as those over 18 years of age who have willingly accepted a risk of exposure to radiation as a consequence of their occupations and are under medical surveillance for radiation exposure, the annual whole-body dose limit is 5 cSv (5 rem).[6] For radiation workers who are minors, the annual limit is 0.5 cSv (0.5 rem), and declared pregnant radiation workers are limited to a dose of 0.5 cSv (0.5 rem) over the duration of the declared pregnancy.[6]

Following a radiological or nuclear incident, first responders will likely have to go into areas that are contaminated with radioactive material to search for and stabilize casualties, medical personnel will receive casualties who are radiologically contaminated, and cleanup crews will have to go into the contaminated region during the recovery phase to clear debris and remove contamination. It will not be possible for these workers to perform their duties without incurring exposure to radiation, and it is recognized that during response to a large-scale radiation emergency, the dose limits to the general public and the occupational dose limits might be too restrictive. Therefore, various agencies have developed recommendations for dose limits applicable to emergency situations (see Table 10-3).

In situations in which the dose limits to the general public and occupational dose limits are not practical, the US Environmental Protection Agency recommends limiting responder dose to 10 cSv (10 rem) if incurring such a dose is necessary to protect critical facilities that are essential to the welfare of the community (eg, power generation stations, water treatment plants, hospitals).[6] For lifesaving operations, the Environmental Protection Agency suggests a dose limit of 25 cSv (25 rem), with higher doses permitted on a voluntary basis.[4,6]

The EPA also recommends that if responders are subjected to these higher doses, they should be informed beforehand of the risk. For doses less than approximately 100 cSv (100 rem), the primary risk is an increased chance of getting cancer. However, exposure to radiation causes a much smaller increase in cancer risk than many people realize; especially when compared to baseline cancer rates, which are comparatively very high.[7]

The threshold dose necessary to cause ARS is around 100 cSv (100 rem). The National Council on Radiation Protection and Measurements suggests a factor of safety of 2 to avoid exceeding this threshold, recommending a dose of 50 cSv (50 rem) as the turnback dose limit for responders.[2]

If a high level of risk is acceptable during critical missions or if an extremely high level of risk is acceptable during priority missions, the DoD's recommended operational exposure guidance (OEG) to commanders is to limit forces to 75 cGy (75 rad). If an extremely high level of risk is acceptable during critical missions, 125 cGy (125 rad) is the recommended OEG. Commanders must remember to take into account a unit's previous exposure when determining the appropriate OEG for a particular mission.[8]

It is important to note that the emergency dose limits to responders suggested by the various agencies are only recommendations and are not intended to limit the authority of the commander. It is the commander's responsibility to define dose limits for responders

TABLE 10-3

REGULATORY DOSE LIMITS AND RECOMMENDATIONS FOR EMERGENCY DOSE LIMITS

Population or Body Region	Dose Limit
General public	0.100 cSv (0.100 rem) total effective dose equivalent per calendar year
Adult occupational radiation workers	5 cSv (5 rem) total effective dose equivalent per calendar year
Lens of eye	15 cSv (15 rem) effective dose equivalent per calendar year
Individual organ	50 cSv (50 rem) deep dose equivalent plus committed dose equivalent per calendar year
Skin or extremity	50 cSv (50 rem) shallow dose equivalent per calendar year
Declared pregnant worker	0.5 cSv (0.5 rem) for duration of pregnancy, not to exceed 0.05 cSv (0.05 rem) per month
Occupational exposure to minors	0.5 cSv (0.5 rem) total effective dose equivalent per year
EPA recommendation for saving valuable property in emergencies	10 cSv (10 rem)
EPA recommendation for lifesaving in emergencies	25 cSv (25 rem), higher doses on voluntary basis after being informed of risk
NCRP recommendation for turn-back decision during emergencies	50 cSv (50 rem)
OEG to military commanders when high risk is acceptable for critical missions or when extremely high risk is acceptable for priority missions	75 cGy (75 rad)
OEG to military commanders when extremely high risk is acceptable during critical missions	125 cGy (125 rad)

EPA: Environmental Protection Agency
NCRP: National Council on Radiation Protection and Measurements
OEG: operational exposure guidance
Data sources: (1) US Army Center for Health Promotion and Preventive Medicine. *The Medical CBRN Battlebook.* Aberdeen Proving Ground, MD: USA CHPPM; 2008. USACHPPM Technical Guide 244. (2) National Council on Radiation Protection and Measurements. *Key Elements of Preparing Emergency Responders for Nuclear and Radiological Terrorism.* Bethesda, MD: NCRP; 2005. NCRP Commentary 19. (3) US Homeland Security Council Interagency Policy Coordination Subcommittee. *Planning Guidance for Response to a Nuclear Detonation.* Washington, DC: DHS; 2009. (4) US Department of the Army, US Department of the Navy, US Department of the Air Force, US Coast Guard, US Marine Corps. *Operations in Chemical, Biological, Radiological, and Nuclear (CBRN) Environments.* Washington, DC: DA, DN, DAF, USCG, USMC; 2008. Joint Publication 3-11.

under his or her command, and that decision must be based on the risk associated with exposure versus the benefit gained from carrying out the tasks that result in the exposure. The commander should follow the principle of ALARA in defining dose limit goals, setting the limits at the lowest level practical for a given mission.

If at all possible, worker doses should be recorded. This is best accomplished by providing each worker with a physical dosimeter, such as an EPD, a pocket dosimeter, or a TLD. If dosimetry is not available, health physics personnel can assist in determining a reasonable dose estimate. Consideration should be made to avoid assigning pregnant workers to tasks that will result in radiation exposure.[1]

Surveying Patients for Contamination

Both injured and noninjured individuals involved in a nuclear or radiological incident could have external contamination on their clothing or bodies. To determine if and where contamination is located on a person, a contamination survey should be performed. Ideally, a detector with a pancake-design Geiger-Müller probe will be the best type to use for detecting localized contamination from beta-gamma–emitting isotopes. For contamination by alpha emitters, a probe designed specifically for detecting alpha radiation should be used.

The calibration date of the detector should be verified before performing the contamination survey. The calibration date will most likely be indicated on the side of the instrument. Typically, detectors must be calibrated at least every 2 years.[5] A detector that is not due for calibration is preferred; however, during emergencies, instruments that are not calibrated may have to be used, since an out-of-calibration detector is better than having no detector at all. After verifying the calibration date, the battery check function should be inspected to ensure that there is sufficient battery life (not all detectors will have a battery check function). Spare batteries should be readily available. If a check source is available, the instrument should be turned on and the probe brought near the check source to verify that the instrument is working properly. Next, background levels of radiation should be measured and recorded. Background levels must be measured in an area that is known to be free of sources of radiation.

When surveying someone for contamination, it is important to hold the probe very close to the surface being surveyed so it will be able to detect low levels of contamination. For beta-gamma contamination, the probe window should be held approximately 1 inch from the surface,[9,10] whereas for alpha contamination, it may have to be held even closer. Care should be taken not to touch the probe to the contaminated surface, since this could result in the transfer of contamination to the probe that would cause false-positive readings and could be difficult to remove. If the contamination is known to contain beta-gamma emitters, a protective cover, such as a thin plastic bag or rubber glove, can be placed over the probe.[5] The probe will still detect the contamination and if the protective bag or glove becomes contaminated, it can be easily removed and replaced. This technique will not work for detecting alpha emitters because a protective cover will prevent the instrument from detecting alpha particles. The rate of travel at which the probe is used to survey a surface must not be too rapid to avoid missing small, localized areas of contamination. Typically, the probe should travel at a rate of about 1 to 2 inches per second.[9,10]

If able, an individual being surveyed should stand with arms out and feet slightly wider than shoulder width (Figure 10-1). The probe should be scanned over all surfaces on the anterior of the person's body, beginning with the top of the person's head and continuing

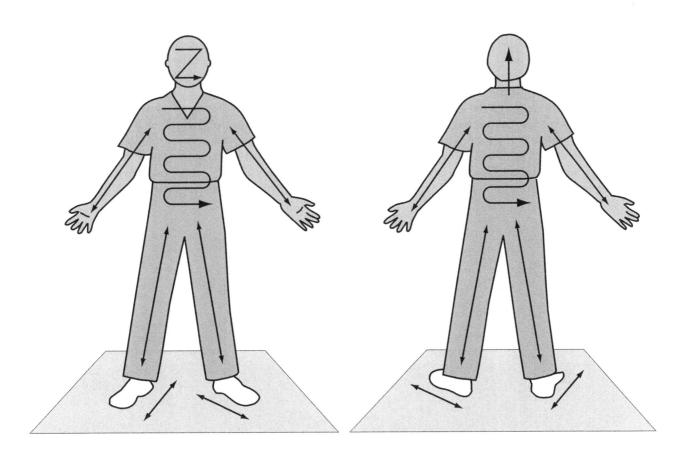

Figure 10-1. Path of detector travel during ambulatory patient contamination survey.
Reproduced with permission from: Radiation Emergency Assistance Center/Training Site, Oak Ridge, TN.

to the face, neck, and shoulders; front of the arms, palms of the hands, and fingertips; armpits; chest; abdomen; sides; crotch; front, inside, and outside of the legs; and finishing with the top of the feet. Then the individual should be asked to turn around and the probe should be scanned over all posterior surfaces of the body, again beginning with the top of the head and ending at the feet. Lastly, the bottom of the individual's shoes should be checked for contamination. Variations in this procedure can be implemented for nonambulatory patients.

It can take a long time to survey a person's entire body by this method. Therefore, in situations in which the number of individuals requiring contamination surveys is so great that the time required to survey all of them by this method will have an adverse impact on other operational aspects of the mission, a more expedient contamination survey can be implemented.[5] The expedient method consists of surveying the person's face, shoulders, hands, and bottom of the shoes, since these are the areas that are most likely to be contaminated if there is contamination present. If other parts of the body are contaminated, the levels of contamination will most likely be very low, and when clothing is removed, the contamination will likely be removed along with it.

Search and Rescue

It is highly probable that emergency response personnel will have to go into the affected area to perform search and rescue operations after a large-scale radiological or nuclear incident. Reaching victims quickly will be important, since many may have life-threatening injuries and could be trapped in locations with dangerously high radiation levels. However, re-sponders must use caution to ensure that they do not rush into high-level radiation areas indiscriminately and become casualties themselves.

Following a release of radioactive material, response units should immediately begin coordinating with agencies that have computer-modeling capabilities to obtain models of the affected area. There are software programs that can provide overlays of estimates for blast, thermal, initial radiation, and fallout distribution, as well as casualty estimates for these effects based on the type and magnitude of the incident. The models generated can be used to get a preliminary estimate of radiation levels and the most probable locations of victims who will require extraction. Some local response agencies can produce these models, and National Guard Weapons of Mass Destruction Civil Support Teams have modeling capability for domestic incidents. The US Department of Homeland Security's Interagency Modeling and Atmospheric Advisory Center is responsible for modeling large-scale domestic incidents for the federal government,[4] and the DoD's Defense Threat Reduction Agency has advanced modeling capability for both foreign and domestic incidents.

Computer models should be used only as an initial estimate and must not be assumed to represent real conditions with complete accuracy. As soon as possible, field data must be obtained using radiation detection equipment to accurately plot the levels of radiation. The National Council on Radiation Protection and Measurements recommends identifying two radiation control perimeters that define an inner extreme caution zone and an outer low radiation zone (Figure 10-2). The inner perimeter corresponds to an exposure rate of 10 R/h (approximately 0.1 Gy/h), and operations within this perimeter should be limited to

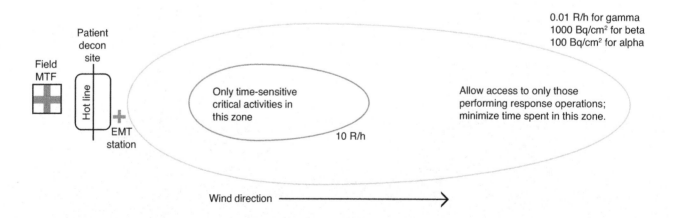

Figure 10-2. Recommended radiation control zones. Figure not drawn to scale.

only time-sensitive critical activities, such as lifesaving.[2] The outer perimeter corresponds to an exposure rate of 0.01 R/h (approximately 0.0001 Gy/h), or 1,000 Bq/cm^2 for beta-gamma contamination, or 100 Bq/cm^2 for alpha contamination, whichever is farther out. Access to the area within this perimeter should be limited to those performing response operations.[2] Depending on the size of the area effected, the radiation control perimeters might be too large to completely surround with markers, such as warning tape or flags; in which case, the perimeters might need to be defined using landmarks such as roads and terrain features. If the affected area is large enough, additional intermediate radiation control perimeters can be implemented, if warranted. The markers defining these zones must be clearly communicated to all response personnel, including those who will remain outside these zones.

Personnel performing search and rescue operations in a radiologically contaminated environment must use personal protective equipment (PPE; Table 10-4). Standard firefighting gear (bunker gear), including self-contained breathing apparatus (SCBA), helmet, and thermally insulated coat, pants, boots, and gloves will provide adequate protection for responders entering the controlled zones.[2,11] If radioactive materials are the only hazard present, the level of PPE can be downgraded to an anticontamination suit, protective boots and gloves, and either a nonpowered, full-face, air-purifying respirator, or, preferably, a powered air-purifying respirator. A powered air-purifying respirator is preferred because many powered models do not require fit testing. Combination high-efficiency particulate air (HEPA) or P-100 filters and organic vapor/acid gas cartridges should be used with these respirators.[11] Either type of air-purifying respirator will be equally as effective as SCBA, since the inhalation hazard presented by the radioactive materials will be almost entirely in the form of airborne particulates, which are readily filtered out by air-purifying respirators. Additionally, the wear time for SCBA is limited by the amount of air contained in the tank, whereas air-purifying respirators do not have this limitation.

TABLE 10-4

RECOMMENDED PERSONAL PROTECTIVE EQUIPMENT FOR VARIOUS OPERATIONAL FUNCTIONS

Type of Operation	Recommended Protective Equipment
Responders entering radiation control zones when fires are present	Dosimetry (EPDs preferred) and standard firefighting gear: SCBA, helmet, thermally insulated coat, pants, boots, and gloves
Responders entering radiation control zones when radioactive materials are the only hazard	Dosimetry (EPDs preferred) and level C HAZMAT gear: anticontamination suit, protective boots and gloves, powered air-purifying respirator (preferred) or full-face, nonpowered air-purifying respirator, combination HEPA or P-100 filter and organic/acid gas cartridges
Crew members transporting contaminated patients in vehicles	
Medical and decontamination personnel on the contaminated side of the patient decontamination hot line	
Workers on the clean side of the patient decontamination hot line	Dosimetry and standard hospital infection control precautions: disposable gowns, hospital gloves, shoe covers, hair covers, and N95 respirators (preferred) or surgical masks
Workers at field MTFs	
Hospital workers	

EPD: electronic personal dosimeter
HAZMAT: hazardous material
HEPA: high-efficiency particulate air
MTF: medical treatment facility
SCBA: self-contained breathing apparatus
Data sources: (1) National Council on Radiation Protection and Measurements. *Key Elements of Preparing Emergency Responders for Nuclear and Radiological Terrorism*. Bethesda, MD: NCRP; 2005. NCRP Commentary 19. (2) Centers for Disease Control and Prevention; Smith JM, Spano MA. *Interim Guidelines for Hospital Response to Mass Casualties from a Radiological Incident*. Atlanta, GA: CDC; 2003. (3) US Army Center for Health Promotion and Preventive Medicine. *Personal Protective Equipment Guide for Military Medical Treatment Facility Personnel Handling Casualties from Weapons of Mass Destruction and Terrorism Events*. Aberdeen Proving Ground, MD: USACHPPM; 2003. USACHPPM Technical Guide 275. (4) Occupational Safety and Health Administration. *OSHA Best Practices for Hospital-Based First Receivers of Victims from Mass Casualty Incidents Involving the Release of Hazardous Substances*. Washington, DC: OSHA; 2005. (5) Departments of the Army, Navy, and Air Force. *NATO Handbook on the Medical Aspects of NBC Defensive Operations*. Washington, DC: DA, DN, DAF; 1996. AMed P-6(B), FM 8-9, NAVMED P-5059, AFJMAN 44-151.

However, SCBA must be used when entering areas with some types of chemical hazards, fires, confined spaces, unknown hazards, or in any situation in which the environment could be depleted of oxygen.

Anticontamination suits and respirators will minimize external and internal contamination to the wearer, but they do not shield the wearer from exposure to gamma or neutron radiation. Responders going into the radiation control zones should wear dosimeters to monitor the amount of radiation to which they have been exposed. Ideally, EPDs are the dosimeters of choice because they provide a real-time measure of the radiation exposure rate and the accumulated radiation dose. The dose alarm and the exposure rate alarm should be set based upon the dose limits defined by the incident commander. For responders entering areas that could have very high dose rates, the National Council on Radiation Protection and Measurements recommends setting the EPDs to alarm at a dose of 0.50 Gy (50 rad), and an exposure rate of 10 R/h (approximately 0.10 Gy/h).[2] If EPDs are not available, the next best choice is a pocket dosimeter, which will still provide an immediate measure of accumulated radiation dose (although it will not measure exposure rate and most do not have alarms that can be set). If neither EPDs nor pocket dosimeters are available, TLDs can be used. Ideally, each responder should have a dosimeter, and the dose to that responder should be recorded and included in the individual's medical history. If there are not enough dosimeters for each responder, one dosimeter can be given to each team of workers and the dose measured by the dosimeter can be assigned to every team member.

As responders exit the outer radiation control perimeter, they should be surveyed for contamination and, if necessary, decontaminated. A separate decontamination site exclusively for responders coming out of the radiation control zones can be set up to expedite the process. Responders can usually decontaminate themselves by carefully doffing protective clothing, making sure not to contaminate previously uncontaminated parts of their clothes and bodies. Any remaining contamination can usually be removed by brushing it off or by spot decontamination with tape or soap and water. Equipment being brought out of the radiation control zones should also be surveyed and decontaminated, if necessary.

Radiologically contaminated injured casualties should be evacuated by ambulance or other vehicle. If casualties have serious injuries, transportation to higher levels of care always takes priority over contamination control. The amount of contamination on a casualty being transported will not be an immediate hazard to either the casualty or to others in the vehicle, whereas the injuries the victim has sustained could very well be immediately life threatening. The only way to confirm whether a casualty is radiologically contaminated is to use detection equipment. If contamination is confirmed or suspected, the casualty should be lightly dusted off and, if necessary, he or she should be wrapped in a sheet or blanket before being loaded into the vehicle for transport.[11,12] This will minimize the amount of contamination transferred from the victim to the vehicle. It is recommended that workers who are in the vehicle with the contaminated casualty wear protective outer garments, gloves, boots, and either nonpowered, full-face, air-purifying respirators, or, preferably, powered air-purifying respirators (see Table 10-4). After contaminated casualties are transported, the vehicle can be decontaminated by vacuuming it, scrubbing surfaces with soap and water, and collecting the runoff. When the level of contamination is equal to or less than two times background levels, the vehicle can be considered free of contamination.

Nuclear Weapon Damage Zones

A system for estimating the most likely location of casualties with severe but survivable injuries has been developed for use in the event of a nuclear detonation (see also Chapter 3, Triage and Treatment of Radiation and Combined-Injury Mass Casualties). Three zones are defined based on the extent of physical damage to the infrastructure (Figure 10-3).[4] The innermost zone, known as the "no-go" or severe damage zone, is the region surrounding the hypocenter of the detonation. It will be characterized by buildings that are completely destroyed. Radiation levels will be very high in this zone, possibly preventing responder access. The number of casualties with survivable injuries in this zone will be minimal.

Surrounding the no-go zone is the moderate damage zone. This zone will be characterized by substantial building damage and rubble, fires, overturned vehicles, and downed utility poles. There will be many casualties with serious injuries in this zone, but many of the injuries will be survivable with prompt medical attention. Lifesaving efforts should focus on this zone.

Surrounding the moderate damage zone will be the light damage zone. This zone will be characterized by damage consisting mostly of broken windows and light damage to buildings. Most injuries sustained in this zone will be relatively minor and can be treated by self-care or outpatient care.

It must be noted that these three zones do not provide a reliable measure of the levels of radiation present and are independent of the radiation control

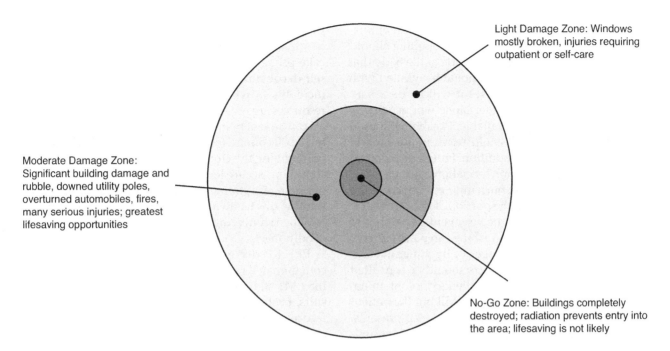

Light Damage Zone: Windows mostly broken, injuries requiring outpatient or self-care

Moderate Damage Zone: Significant building damage and rubble, downed utility poles, overturned automobiles, fires, many serious injuries; greatest lifesaving opportunities

No-Go Zone: Buildings completely destroyed; radiation prevents entry into the area; lifesaving is not likely

Figure 10-3. Nuclear weapon damage zones.

zones described earlier. These zones are used only to get an estimate of the location where there will be the greatest number of casualties with serious but survivable injuries. One must also take into account the area affected by fallout and the threat the fallout presents to response operations, as well as the impact that radiation exposure from fallout will have on the survivability of injuries.

Patient Decontamination Site

To receive potentially contaminated casualties, patient decontamination sites should be positioned upwind from the site of the incident at a point near the outer radiation control perimeter (see Figure 10-2).[5] Immediately downwind of the patient decontamination station there should be an emergency medical technician (EMT) station where patients first arrive to receive initial triage and basic lifesaving first aid while waiting to go through decontamination (see Figure 10-2). During initial triage, those who are in the greatest need of medical care should receive priority for decontamination. If the patient's condition is such that taking time for surveying and decontamination prior to providing urgent care will result in regression to a more severe medical state, decontamination should be bypassed and the patient should be transferred directly to the medical treatment facility (MTF). Much of the contamination originally on the patient will have shaken off or have been brushed off by this time, and

the patient might have already received initial mass decontamination by first responders. Therefore, the amount of contamination left on the patient upon arrival at the MTF will not present an immediate hazard to either the patient or medical personnel. The radiological contamination on the patient can eventually present a hazard if one is exposed to it for a long enough period of time, but the more immediate concern will be the patient's physical injuries. Treatment of life-threatening injuries always takes priority over radiological decontamination.

Patients who are stable enough to go through decontamination before going to the MTF should proceed from the EMT station to the patient decontamination site. There, a contamination control line (hot line) should be designated and clearly marked, with the contaminated side being established downwind and the clean side upwind. While on the contaminated side, the patient should first be surveyed for contamination. Prior to decontamination, nasal swabs should be taken from each nostril of all patients suspected of being internally contaminated as a result of inhalation. When using a Geiger-Müller pancake probe, count rates of 100,000 counts/min around the head, face, and shoulders are a strong indicator of possible internal contamination.[5]

If localized contamination is found during the survey, spot decontamination can be performed by removing clothing that is contaminated and either using adhesive tape to remove contamination or washing affected areas of the skin. If the contamination is over the person's entire body, clothing should be completely removed and the parts of the body that were not covered by clothing should be washed with soap and water. In some cases it will be necessary to wash the entire body. Water alone will usually be adequate if soap is not available. Scrubbing should not be too vigorous or it could result in abrasion of the skin, allowing for an additional route of exposure for internal contamination. Special precautions must be taken for patients with burn injuries. No scrubbing should be performed on the portion of the skin that is burned, and rinsing must be very gentle so as not to remove the burned tissue. Washing can place patients with extensive burns in danger of hypothermia and hypotension, so medical officers should be consulted before decontaminating these patients.[1] Decontamination should not be performed if it will put the patient at greater risk than the contamination itself presents. The contamination will remain in burned skin because there is no circulation and most of it will eventually slough off with the burn eschar.[1,7]

Contaminated clothing should be collected and brought to a secure location away from the decontamination site. If possible, personal items belonging to the patient should be decontaminated, placed in a plastic bag, and kept with the patient. After decontamination, the patient should be surveyed again to ensure that contamination has been reduced to acceptable levels. As a rule of thumb, count rates of two times background or less are desired.[1] Under some circumstances, levels up to 10 times background can be considered acceptable if achieving lower levels of contamination is not practical. After repeated washing, if the count rates do not drop, external decontamination should cease and internal contamination should be suspected. Once external decontamination is complete, the patient should be transferred across the hot line and should proceed to the MTF. Information suggesting possible internal contamination should be recorded, and this data, along with any nasal swabs that were collected, should be kept with the patient as he or she is transferred to the MTF.

During a radiological mass casualty situation, the patient decontamination site can quickly become overwhelmed by casualties with varying degrees of injuries and levels of contamination. Those who are externally contaminated but are uninjured and are not suspected of having internal contamination should be directed to an alternate decontamination site dedicated exclusively to the external decontamination of people who do not need medical care.[5] The alternate decontamination site should be at a location where radiation levels are near background, and it should also be upwind

from the incident site. If contamination on a patient is less than 1,000 counts/min on a Geiger-Müller pancake probe, the patient can be given instructions on self-decontamination and sent home.[5] For large-scale incidents in which decontamination personnel and resources are severely limited, contaminated individuals can be sent home to self-decontaminate at levels up to 10,000 counts/min.[5] Self-decontamination consists of removing the clothing and placing it in a bag to be stored in a secure location, such as the furthest corner of a garage, a storage shed, or in an isolated portion of the house as far away from the inhabitants as possible, and then showering with soap and shampoo (without conditioner).

PPE for decontamination team members on the contaminated side of the hot line, including workers at the EMT station, should consist of anticontamination suits, protective boots and gloves, and either a full-face air purifying respirator or, preferably, a powered air-purifying respirator with a minimum protection factor of 1,000.[11,13] Combination P-100 or HEPA filters and organic vapor/acid gas cartridges should be used with these respirators (see Table 10-4).[11] Workers on the contaminated side should be surveyed and decontaminated as necessary before crossing over to the clean side. Workers can usually decontaminate themselves by carefully doffing their protective clothing on the contaminated side, making sure not to contaminate themselves further. Contaminated clothing and equipment should remain on the contaminated side of the hot line until it has been decontaminated. For workers on the clean side of the hot line, standard precautions, including the use of disposable gowns, hospital gloves, hair covers, and shoe covers, are adequate (see Table 10-4).[11] If available, respiratory protection, such as N95 respirators, should be used on the clean side. If N95 respirators are not available, surgical masks will typically provide adequate protection.[10] Dosimeters should be used by workers on both the contaminated side and clean side; however, if the supply of dosimeters is limited, priority should go to those on the contaminated side.

It is important to ensure that there are enough workers to receive nonambulatory patients on both the clean and contaminated sides of the hot line. Additionally, patient decontamination can be very tiring and the protective clothing can be hot. During prolonged operations, it will be necessary to implement rotating work–rest cycles for decontamination personnel.

Modesty can be a concern among those who require decontamination, so patients who are able to decontaminate themselves unassisted should be allowed to do so. Written instructions can be provided to guide them through decontamination procedures and, if necessary, a decontamination team member of the same sex can observe to ensure thoroughness of decontamination.

Logistical coordination will need to take place in advance to ensure that an adequate number of towels and gowns are available for those who are decontaminated. Additionally, operations might have to be carried out in cold weather or in the evening, so blankets, heating, and lighting might be necessary as well.

When setting up the decontamination site, consideration should be made as to how to contain contaminated runoff from decontamination operations, and reasonable efforts should be made to collect the runoff, if feasible. However, collecting contaminated water should not detract from resources needed for emergency lifesaving operations. While protecting the environment is an important consideration, lifesaving operations take priority. Personnel and other resources will be severely limited and time will be precious during a large-scale radiological or nuclear incident. Therefore, resources should first be used for emergency operations that support lifesaving and protecting critical facilities essential to the welfare of the community. As the situation stabilizes and resources become more readily available, additional resources can be shifted toward environmental protection.[2,10,13]

Field Medical Treatment Facility

After a large-scale radiological or nuclear incident, many nearby hospitals could be destroyed or in the dangerous fallout plume, or if the incident occurs away from a city, there might not be any preexisting hospitals in the vicinity. In any of these cases, it might be necessary to establish an MTF near the incident site. If a field MTF is to be established, it should be located about 30 to 50 meters upwind of the patient decontamination site (see Figure 10-2).[13] In addition to injured patients who have been decontaminated, the field MTF must be prepared to receive contaminated casualties who have bypassed the decontamination site upon direction of the EMT station triage officer. Although the level of contamination on casualties who bypass decontamination will not present an immediate hazard, protective measures should still be implemented to minimize cross-contamination and keep exposure levels as low as reasonably achievable. Separate entrances to the MTF can be designated for contaminated and noncontaminated patients and, if feasible, contaminated patients should be treated in a separate section from uncontaminated patients. Traffic flow through the MTF should be directed such that contaminated patients do not pass through uncontaminated areas and uncontaminated patients do not pass through contaminated areas.[14] If possible, contaminated equipment should be segregated from uncontaminated equipment.

Standard precautions used on the clean side of the patient decontamination hot line also constitute adequate PPE for workers in the field MTF (see Table 10-4).[2,11] Individual dosimeters should be worn if they are available. Workers should be surveyed for contamination before going from contaminated sections of the MTF to clean sections. Maintaining good hygiene and changing out protective clothing when going from contaminated sections to clean sections of the MTF will minimize the spread of contamination. Contaminated protective clothing should be collected and kept in containers clearly marked as containing radioactive waste. When containers become full, they should be transferred to a designated radioactive waste storage area that is in a secure location away from people.

Radiological contamination on a patient will not present an immediate threat to either the patient or medical staff, so decontamination procedures should not impede injury treatment. Patients should be surveyed for contamination and decontaminated if necessary; however, this can likely be carried out at the same time that the patient is being treated without interfering with treatment procedures. Removing the patients' clothing will eliminate most of the contamination. Sponges and moist wipes can be used to remove remaining contamination on the skin, and contaminated wounds should be gently irrigated. After decontamination, the patient should be surveyed again to ensure contamination levels have been reduced to appropriate levels. Levels two times background are usually considered acceptable.[1] Contaminated wipes, sponges, clothing, and other wastes should be collected, marked as radioactive, and brought to the radioactive waste storage area. A reasonable effort should be made to collect liquids that contain contamination.

Although it is unlikely for radioactive fragments to become embedded in a victim's body, it is a possibility. Fragments could be highly radioactive and could result in dangerously high doses to both the patient and medical staff;[1] they should be removed immediately, placed in a container that will provide shielding, marked as radioactive, and brought to the radioactive waste storage area. Workers should maximize their distance and minimize the amount of time they spend near these fragments.

Nasal swabs collected at the decontamination site or at the field MTF should be tested at the MTF using the appropriate type of detector (beta-gamma or alpha) to determine the possible presence of internal contamination due to inhalation. The time after exposure that the nasal swabs were collected should be recorded and the nasal swabs should be saved and eventually processed by a laboratory that has the analytical capabilities to obtain a more quantitative measure of internal contamination. When using a Geiger-Müller pancake probe, count rates of 100,000 counts/min around the head, face, and shoulders prior to decontamination are also an indicator of possible internal contamination.[5] For cesium-137, a radioisotope likely to be used in RDDs and a fission product generated during nuclear reactions, an exposure rate of 0.1 mR/h measured at the surface of the victim's chest after decontamination indicates probable internal contamination from inhalation.[5] If possible, bioassays, such as urine and fecal samples, can be collected at the field MTF and sent to an appropriate laboratory to determine if the patient is internally contaminated. The presence of both external and internal contamination should be documented in the patient's records. Treatments for internal contamination should be administered at the field MTF, if available. If bioassay capabilities or treatments for internal contamination are not available at the field MTF, these steps might have to be performed at a higher level of care.

Higher Level Medical Treatment Facilities

Many casualties will report to nearby hospitals on their own, while others will be transferred to hospitals by medical evacuation following large-scale radiological or nuclear incidents. Often those who self-refer to hospitals will have minor injuries or no injuries at all, but will be concerned about exposure to radiation.[10] Hospitals can become quickly overwhelmed by the surge of people seeking medical care. As soon as hospitals receive word of a radiological or nuclear emergency, they should activate their emergency management plans and begin preparing for mass casualties. Mutual aid agreements with other hospitals will most likely need to be invoked to compensate for the excess patient load. Specific entrances should be designated for hospital staff and for patients arriving from the incident site in order to control patient flow into the building. All other entrances should be locked down.[10]

Many people will go directly to hospitals without having received mass decontamination by first responders or technical decontamination at the field decontamination site. The hospital decontamination team should be activated immediately and positioned at the entrance designated to receive patients. Operation of the hospital decontamination site should be similar to the operation of the field decontamination site, with

patient flow first being directed to an EMT station on the contaminated side of the hot line for triage and basic lifesaving first aid. Additional security measures might have to be implemented to control the flow of patient traffic. To accommodate the massive surge of patients, an alternate decontamination and assessment facility might need to be established for those who do not have serious injuries.[14,15] Those who are uninjured or have minor injuries should be directed by the EMT station to the alternate decontamination and assessment facility. The location and staffing of potential alternate facilities should be coordinated in advance during the emergency-planning phase.

If patients' injuries are severe, they may be directed by the EMT station triage officer to bypass decontamination and go directly to the emergency department. Lifesaving treatment always takes priority over radiological decontamination. Patient decontamination procedures should be similar to those used at the field decontamination site. Protective equipment for workers on both the clean and contaminated sides of the hot line should also be generally the same as those used by workers on the clean and contaminated sides of field decontamination sites, respectively (see Table 10-4).[11]

Hospital worker PPE should generally be the same as that used at field MTFs (see Table 10-4),[2,11,13] as should contamination control procedures. Additionally, the floor over which contaminated patients will be traveling can be covered with paper or plastic sheeting.[1] If contaminated patients must pass through uncontaminated areas of the hospital, they should be wrapped in a sheet to minimize the spread of contamination.[1,12] Equipment that is not in use should be removed or covered to reduce the likelihood that it will need to be decontaminated later.[12]

Nuclear medicine, radiology, and radiation therapy clinics might have specialized equipment that can be used to detect both internal and external contamination. This equipment might include whole-body counters, gamma cameras, and survey meters. Hospital workers specializing in medical physics, radiation safety, nuclear medicine, and radiation oncology can offer advice relating to the management of external and internal contamination and treatment of radiation injuries.

Several specialized government organizations, including the Armed Forces Radiobiology Research Institute's Medical Radiobiology Advisory Team, the US Army's Radiological Advisory Medical Team, and the Department of Energy's Radiation Emergency Assistance Center/Training Site can be contacted to provide expertise related to medical effects of radiation and medical management of radiation casualties.

SUMMARY

The radiological and nuclear threat poses several potential scenarios in which medical personnel might find themselves caring for victims who have been exposed to high levels of radiation or who have been contaminated with radioactive material. These patients may also have conventional trauma and burn injuries. In caring for these victims, workers must ensure that they minimize the spread of contamination and do not expose themselves to any more radiation than is necessary.

Specialized radiation detection equipment will be needed to identify the presence or absence of radiation and determine the magnitude of the radiological hazard. Selecting the appropriate detection equipment will depend on the application for which it is to be used. Some types of detection equipment are designed to measure the amount of radiation present at a given location, some measure the amount of radiation to which one was exposed over a given time period, some are used to identify the type of radioisotope producing the radiation, and some are used to measure the amount of radioactive material in the air.

Regulatory radiation dose limits should not be exceeded by workers if possible. However, under emergency conditions, commanders are authorized to set higher dose limits for workers if regulatory dose limits must be exceeded to save lives and protect critical facilities that are essential to the welfare of the community. Various agencies have their own recommendations for emergency radiation dose limits, but it is ultimately the incident commander's responsibility to determine acceptable dose limits for workers.

Responders might have to go into potentially contaminated areas with high levels of radiation to perform search and rescue missions. To protect these responders, radiation control zones should be identified around the incident site and PPE should be implemented. Standard firefighting gear will protect search and rescue workers from most hazards, and dosimetry should be issued to each responder.[2,11] If radiation is the only hazard, the primary concerns to workers will be minimizing contamination and preventing inhalation of radioactive materials. In this case, dosimetry, air-purifying respirators, anticontamination suits, and protective gloves and boots will be adequate.[11]

Victims will need to be surveyed for contamination; those who are contaminated will require decontamination. Therefore, a patient decontamination site must be established, along with an EMT station for patient triage and lifesaving first aid prior to decontamination. Dosimetry and PPE for workers on the contaminated side of the hot line should be the same as that for search and rescue workers operating in an area where radiation is the only hazard.[11,13] PPE equivalent to standard hospital infection control precautions, along with dosimetry, will be adequate for workers on the clean side.[11] Radiological decontamination is usually accomplished by removing contaminated clothing and performing spot decontamination using tape or soap and water or, for more extensive contamination, completely showering with soap and water. Contamination levels are usually considered acceptable if they are equal to or less than two times background levels.[1] If patients have serious life-threatening injuries, they should bypass decontamination and be transferred directly to an MTF. Major trauma and burn injuries will be more of a threat to the patient's life than radiological contamination, and the patient can usually be decontaminated while receiving medical attention.

In some cases, a field MTF will need to be established; in other cases, patients will be transferred directly to nearby hospitals. In either case, contaminated patients who have been directed to bypass decontamination because of the severity of their injuries will not present a significant hazard to workers. However, contaminated patients will still require decontamination at some point, and methods of controlling the spread of contamination should still be implemented as long as they do not interfere with medical care. This can include designating separate treatment areas for clean patients and contaminated patients, covering floors with paper or plastic sheets, and controlling the flow of traffic to avoid cross-contamination. Patients can be decontaminated during treatment by removing clothing and using sponges or moist wipes to clean affected areas. PPE, such as that used for standard infection control precautions, is sufficient, and dosimetry should be used if available.[2,11]

High levels of radiation can present a hazard to both victims and response workers, and even low levels of radiological contamination will require time and resource-intensive contamination control efforts. These factors can have a negative impact on medical operations if preparations are not made. However, by understanding radiation and ensuring readiness to handle these issues, we can still function safely and effectively following a radiological or nuclear incident.

REFERENCES

1. National Council on Radiation Protection and Measurements. *Management of Terrorist Events Involving Radioactive Material*. Bethesda, MD: NCRP; 2001. NCRP Report 138.

2. National Council on Radiation Protection and Measurements. *Key Elements of Preparing Emergency Responders for Nuclear and Radiological Terrorism*. Bethesda, MD: NCRP; 2005. NCRP Commentary 19.

3. US Department of Defense. *Nuclear Weapon Accident Response Procedures*. Washington, DC: DoD; 2005. DoD 3150.08-M.

4. US Homeland Security Council Interagency Policy Coordination Subcommittee. *Planning Guidance for Response to a Nuclear Detonation*. Washington, DC: DHS; 2009.

5. Conference of Radiation Control Program Directors, Inc. *Handbook for Responding to a Radiological Dispersal Device. First Responder's Guide–The First 12 Hours*. Frankfort, KY: CRCPD, Inc; 2006.

6. US Army Center for Health Promotion and Preventive Medicine. *The Medical CBRN Battlebook*. Aberdeen Proving Ground, MD: USACHPPM; 2008. USACHPPM Technical Guide 244.

7. Armed Forces Radiobiology Research Institute; Goans RE. *Medical Management of Radiological Casualties*. Ft Lauderdale, FL: Quick Series Publishing; 2009.

8. US Department of the Army, US Department of the Navy, US Department of the Air Force, US Coast Guard, US Marine Corps. *Operations in Chemical, Biological, Radiological, and Nuclear (CBRN) Environments*. Washington, DC: DA, DN, DAF, USCG, USMC; 2008. Joint Publication 3-11.

9. US Army Center for Health Promotion and Preventive Medicine. *Basic Radiological Dose Estimation–A Field Guide*. Aberdeen Proving Ground, MD: USACHPPM; 2001. USACHPPM Technical Guide 236A.

10. Centers for Disease Control and Prevention; Smith JM, Spano MA. *Interim Guidelines for Hospital Response to Mass Casualties from a Radiological Incident*. Atlanta, GA: CDC; 2003.

11. US Army Center for Health Promotion and Preventive Medicine. *Personal Protective Equipment Guide for Military Medical Treatment Facility Personnel Handling Casualties from Weapons of Mass Destruction and Terrorism Events*. Aberdeen Proving Ground, MD: USACHPPM; 2003. USACHPPM Technical Guide 275.

12. International Atomic Energy Agency. *Manual for First Responders to a Radiological Emergency*. Vienna, Austria: International Atomic Energy Agency; 2006.

13. Occupational Safety and Health Administration. *OSHA Best Practices for Hospital-Based First Receivers of Victims from Mass Casualty Incidents Involving the Release of Hazardous Substances*. Washington, DC: OSHA; 2005.

14. Departments of the Army, Navy, and Air Force. *NATO Handbook on the Medical Aspects of NBC Defensive Operations*. Washington, DC: DA, DN, DAF; 1996. AMed P-6(B), FM 8-9, NAVMED P-5059, AFJMAN 44-151.

15. International Commission on Radiological Protection. *Annals of the ICRP. Protecting People Against Radiation Exposure in the Event of a Radiological Attack*. New York, NY: Elsevier; 2005. ICRP Publication 96.

Chapter 11

PERSPECTIVES IN RADIOLOGICAL AND NUCLEAR COUNTERMEASURES

K. SREE KUMAR, PhD[*]; JULIANN G. KIANG, PhD[†]; MARK H. WHITNALL, PhD[‡]; AND MARTIN HAUER-JENSEN, MD, PhD, FACS[§]

[*]Senior Research Scientist, Radiation Countermeasures Program, Scientific Research Department, Armed Forces Radiobiology Research Institute, Uniformed Services University of the Health Sciences, 8901 Wisconsin Avenue, Bethesda, Maryland 20889

[†]Program Advisor, Combined Injury Program, Scientific Research Department, Armed Forces Radiobiology Research Institute, Professor of Radiation Biology and Medicine, Uniformed Services University of the Health Sciences, 8901 Wisconsin Avenue, Bethesda, Maryland 20889

[‡]Program Advisor, Radiation Countermeasures Program, Scientific Research Department, Armed Forces Radiobiology Research Institute, Uniformed Services University of the Health Sciences, 8901 Wisconsin Avenue, Bethesda, Maryland 20889

[§]Professor of Pharmaceutical Sciences, Surgery, and Pathology; Associate Dean for Research, College of Pharmacy; Director, Division of Radiation Health, University of Arkansas for Medical Sciences, 4301 West Markham, Slot 522-10, Little Rock, Arkansas 72205

INTRODUCTION

Medical Management of Radiation Events

Threat from a nuclear event can occur due to a radiologic (dispersal or use of radioactive material) or nuclear (improvised nuclear device) exposure. A comprehensive response plan to meet such events can be found on the Web site http://www.remm.nlm.gov, and was summarized by Coleman et al.[1] The components of this response plan consist of underpinnings from basic radiation biology, tailored medical responses, delivery of medical countermeasures for postevent mitigation and treatment, referral to expert centers for acute treatment, and long-term follow-up. The emphasis of this plan is emergency management of a nuclear event.

Protection of First Responders

Radiation countermeasures have been classified as radioprotectants (administered before radiation exposure), mitigators (given during or shortly after exposure, before overt symptoms appear), and treatments (given after overt symptoms appear).[2] One important application of radiation countermeasures is to protect first responders deployed in a radiation exposure field for rescue and other military operations. This is an urgent need for the military and for US Department of Homeland Security scenarios involving nuclear terrorist threats. Radiation exposure can result in short-term lethality and long-term consequences, like cancer and pulmonary fibrosis. Currently, there are no countermeasures against these threats that can be used in humans, which is a serious capability shortfall. This is a critical issue for commanders in planning and executing military operations. Developing radiation countermeasures for use prior to exposure has been identified as one of the highest priority areas for research.[3] Postirradiation treatment is also an important aspect of radiation countermeasure development, but that is beyond the scope of this chapter and is discussed elsewhere in this volume.

Historically, studies on radiation countermeasures began in 1949, testing the radioprotective efficacy of cysteine in mice.[4] Since that time, many diverse compounds have been shown to have protective characteristics (Table 11-1). More recently, several medical protocols have been proposed,[5] but a safe and effective radiation countermeasure is not available for acute radiation syndrome (ARS). The one approved radiation countermeasure (to be given in a clinic setting before therapeutic irradiation), amifostine (see Radiation Countermeasures, Aminothiols and Other Thiol Derivatives, below), causes several toxic manifestations[6] that could impair task performance, which is critical for military and first-responder operations. Radiation countermeasure development has focused on protecting against acute, high-dose radiation injury and protecting the normal tissues of cancer patients who are undergoing radiotherapy. Additional areas that need to be studied involve protecting against low-dose and chronic radiation exposure scenarios, such as in potential terrorist events using nuclear devices ("dirty bombs" or improvised nuclear devices) and during extra-vehicular activity associated with space missions, including proposed manned flights to Mars by the National Aeronautics and Space Administration.

With new advances in immunology, biochemistry, radiobiology, and pharmacology, the development of a safe and effective radiation countermeasure may be at hand. Over the longer term, newer concepts and techniques in molecular biology may provide exciting approaches for developing specific and effective means to prevent, mitigate, or treat radiation injury. The primary objective of prophylactic studies is to develop an agent or combination of agents that will substantially increase survival and enhance the postincidence effectiveness of first-responder military personnel on a nuclear battlefield. These treatments must be easily self-administered shortly before or after radiation exposure to reduce early molecular, cellular, and tissue damage. This chapter briefly reviews the relevant radiobiological concepts, presents strategies and mechanisms, and discusses some of the more promising agents being investigated.[7]

RADIATION INJURY

To understand the various strategies being used to prevent, mitigate, and treat ionizing radiation injury, it is first necessary to define ionizing radiation and to consider the events that occur in the development of ARS (also see Chapter 2, Acute Radiation Syndrome in Humans).

Ionizing Radiation

Ionizing radiation can be defined as any type of electromagnetic radiation (such as gamma or X-rays) or particulate radiation (such as neutrons or alpha particles) that has sufficient energy to ionize atoms or mol-

TABLE 11-1

SELECTED RADIATION COUNTERMEASURE AGENTS

Compounds	Protective Efficacy (scale of 1–4, 4 being the best)	Probable Mechanism of Action
Aminothiols		Free-radical scavenging, hydrogen donation
Cysteine[1]	2	
WR-2721[2–4]	4	
N-acetylcysteine[5]	3	
Diethyl dithiocarbamate[5]	2	
Immunomodulators		Hematopoietic system regeneration
Glucan[6,7]	3	
Trehalose dimycolate[8]	3	
Endotoxin[9]	3	
5-AED[*10,11]	3	
Cytokines		Hematopoietic system regeneration
Interleukin 1[12]	3	
Tumor necrosis factor[12]	2	
Antioxidants/Nutraceuticals		Free-radical scavenging
Vitamin E[13,14]	3	
Vitamin A (β-carotene)[15]	2	
Superoxide dismutase[16,17]	3	
Selenium[18,19]	2	
γ-tocotrienol[20–22]	4	
Eicisanoids		Uncertain
DiPGE$_2$[23]	3	
Iloprost, Misoprostol[24]	3	
Unknown/Proprietary		
BIO-300[*†]	2	
Ex-RAD[*‡25]	2	Antiapoptotic
CBLB502[*§26]	3	TLR agonist
17-DMAG (geldanamycin derivative)[27]	2	Antiapoptotic

*Approved by US Food and Drug Administration as investigational new drug
†BIO-300 is manufactured by Humanetics Corporation (Eden Prairie, MN).
‡Ex-RAD is manufactured by Onconova Therapeutics, Inc (Newtown, PA).
§CBLB502 is manufactured by Cleveland BioLabs, Inc (Buffalo, NY).
5-AED: androst-5-ene-3beta,17beta-diol (5-androstenediol)
DiPGE$_2$: 16,16-dimethyl prostaglandin E$_2$
17-DMAG: 17-(dimethylaminoethylamino)-17-demethoxygeldanamycin
TLR: toll-like receptor
Data sources: (1) Patt HM, Tyree E, Straube RL, Smith DE. Cysteine protection against X-irradiation. *Science* 1949;110:213–214. (2) Yuhas JM. Biological factors affecting the radioprotective efficiency of S-2-(3-aminopropylamino)ethylphosphorothioic acid (WR-2721): LD$_{50(30)}$ doses. *Radiat Res.* 1970;44:621–628. (3) Glover DJ, Glick JH, Weiler C, Hurowitz S, Kligerman M. WR-2721 protects against the hematologic toxicity of cyclophosphamide: a controlled phase II trial. J *Clin Oncol.* 1986;4:584–588. (4) Weiss JF, Kumar KS, Walden TL, Neta R, Landauer MR, Clark EP. Advances in radioprotection through the use of combined agent regimens. *Int J Radiat Biol.* 1990;57:709–722. (5) Landauer MR, Davis HD, Dominitz JA, Weiss JF. Comparative behavioral toxicity of four sulfhydryl radioprotective compounds in mice: WR-2721, cysteamine, diethyldithiocarbamate, and N-acetylcysteine. *Pharmacol Ther.* 1988;39:97–100. (6) Patchen ML, Brook I, Elliott TB, Jackson WE. Adverse effects of pefloxacin in irradiated C3H/HeN mice: correction with glucan therapy. *Antimicrob Agents Chemother.* 1993;37:1882–1889. (7) Patchen ML, MacVittie TJ, Weiss JF. Combined modality radioprotection: the use of glucan and selenium with WR-2721. *Int J Radiat Oncol Biol Phys.* 1990;18:1069–1075. (8) Madonna GS, Ledney GD, Elliott TB, et al. Trehalose dimycolate enhances resistance to infection in

(*Table 11-1* **continues**)

Table 11-1 **continued**

neutropenic animals. *Infect Immun.* 1989;57:2495–2501. (9) Ainsworth EJ. From endotoxins to newer immunomodulators: survival-promoting effects of microbial polysaccharide complexes in irradiated animals. *Pharmacol Ther.* 1988;39:223–241. (10) Whitnall MH, Villa V, Seed TM, et al. Molecular specificity of 5-androstenediol as a systemic radioprotectant in mice. *Immunopharmacol Immunotoxicol.* 2005;27:15–32. (11) Whitnall MH, Wilhelmsen CL, McKinney L, Miner V, Seed TM, Jackson WE III. Radioprotective efficacy and acute toxicity of 5-androstenediol after subcutaneous or oral administration in mice. *Immunopharmacol Immunotoxicol.* 2002;24:595–626. (12) Neta R. Role of cytokines in radioprotection. *Pharmacol Ther.* 1988;39:261–266. (13) Srinivasan V, Jacobs AJ, Simpson SA, Weiss JF. Radioprotection by vitamin E: effects on hepatic enzymes, delayed type hypersensitivity, and postirradiation survival of mice. In: Prasad KN, ed. *Modulation and Mediation of Cancer by Vitamins.* Basel, Switzerland: Karger; 1983: 119–131. (14) Kumar KS, Srinivasan V, Toles R, Jobe L, Seed TM. Nutritional approaches to radioprotection: vitamin E. *Mil Med.* 2002;167:57–59. (15) Seifter E, Rettura G, Padawar J, Stratford F, Weinzweig J, Demetriou AA, Levenson SM. Morbidity and mortality reduction by supplemental vitamin A or beta-carotene in CBA mice given total-body-radiation. *J Natl Cancer Inst.* 1984;73:1167–1177. (16) Petkau A. Radiation protection by superoxide dismutase. *Photochem Photobiol.* 1978;28:765–774. (17) Srinivasan V, Doctrow S, Singh VK, Whitnall MH. Evaluation of EUK-189, a synthetic superoxide dismutase/catalase mimetic as a radiation countermeasure. *Immunopharmacol Immunotoxicol.* 2008;30:271–290. (18) Davis TA, Clarke TK, Mog SR, Landauer MR. Subcutaneous administration of genistein prior to lethal irradiation supports multilineage, hematopoietic progenitor cell recovery and survival. *Int J Radiat Biol.* 2007;83:141–151. (19) Patchen ML, MacVittie TJ, Weiss JF. Combined modality radioprotection: the use of glucan and selenium with WR-2721. *Int J Radiat Oncol Biol Phys.* 1990;18:1069–1075. (20) Kumar KS, Ghosh SP, Hauer-Jensen M. Gamma-tocotrienol: potential as a countermeasure against radiological threat. In: Watson RR, Preedy VR, eds. *Tocotrienols: Vitamin E Beyond Tocopherols.* Boca Raton, FL: CRC Press; 2009: 379–398. (21) Ghosh SP, Kulkarni S, Hieber K, et al. Gamma-tocotrienol, a tocol antioxidant as a potent radioprotector. *Int J Radiat Biol.* 2009;85:598–606. (22) Berbée M, Fu Q, Boerma M, Wang J, Kumar KS, Hauer-Jensen M. Gamma-tocotrienol ameliorates intestinal radiation injury and reduces vascular oxidative stress after total-body irradiation by an HMG-CoA reductase-dependent mechanism. *Radiat Res.* 2009;171:596–605. (23) Walden TL Jr, Patchen M, Snyder SL. 16,16-Dimethyl prostaglandin E₂ increases survival in mice following irradiation. *Radiat Res.* 1987;109:440–448. (24) Kumar KS, Srinivasan V, Palazzolo D, Kendrick JM, Clark EP. Synergistic protection of irradiated mice by a combination of iloprost and misoprostol. *Adv Exp Med Biol.* 1997;400B: 831–839. (25) Ghosh SP, Perkins MW, Hieber K, et al. Radiation protection by a new chemical entity, Ex-Rad: efficacy and mechanisms. *Radiat Res.* 2009;171:173–179. (26) Burdelya LG, Krivokrysenko VI, Tallant TC, et al. An agonist of toll-like receptor 5 has radioprotective activity in mouse and primate models. *Science.* 2008;320:226–30. (27) Fukumoto R, Kiang JG. Geldanamycin analog 17-DMAG limits apoptosis in human peripheral blood cells by inhibition of p53 activation and its interaction with heat shock protein 90 kDa after ionizing radiation. *Radiat Res.* 176:333-345, 2011.

ecules; that is, to eject electrons from their outer orbits.

In considering the effects of radiation on biological systems, it is important to distinguish the different types of ionizing radiation according to their linear energy transfer (LET). This term describes the amount of energy deposited by a particular type of radiation per unit of path length. Low-LET radiation (gamma and X-rays) is sparsely ionizing because it causes few ionizations per micron of path length, whereas high-LET radiation (neutrons and alpha particles) is densely ionizing because it produces many ionizations per micron of path length. Generally, high-LET radiation produces more biological damage than low-LET radiation.[7,8]

Biological Damage

Death from radiation injury is the result of a sequence of events that occurs over a period of less than a billionth of a second to several weeks (Figure 11-1).[9,10] The first step in this sequence is the transfer of radiation energy from the photon or particle to atoms and molecules in its path through a process of direct (eg, alpha or beta particles) or indirect (eg, X-rays, gamma rays, or neutrons) ionization. This results in the ejection of a particle (such as an electron) that causes the first discrete lesion in the sequence: direct or indirect damage to macromolecules that are critical for biological function. Direct and indirect ioniza-

tion are separate from, and occur prior to, direct or indirect damage to macromolecules (see below). If a critical biological molecule is in the radiation path, it can become chemically altered by direct interaction by radiation energy (direct damage). If that molecule is not in the radiation path, it can still become chemically altered indirectly via reactions with free radicals, reactive oxygen species, and reactive nitrogen species produced primarily from the radiolysis of water, and by interactions of free radicals.[9] Although the importance of membrane damage is still being evaluated, damage to deoxyribonucleic acid (DNA) and proteins are important factors in cell death, with DNA strand breaks commonly thought to be the primary lesions.[9,10]

Reactive oxygen species are important in the overall scheme of radiation injury because their lifetime in solution is sufficiently long to allow them to diffuse and extend the damage beyond the primary path of radiation. In this way, the effects of ionizing radiation within the cell are greatly amplified. Most radiation injury from low-LET radiation is the result of indirect damage, while that from high-LET radiation is from direct damage.[11] The net effect of direct and indirect damage is the disruption of molecular structure and function, leading to dysfunctional cells and organ systems and resulting in altered cell division, cell death, depletion of stem-cell pools, and, if the radiation dose is high enough, death of the organism.

Types of Radiation Injury

ARS (sometimes called acute radiation *sickness*) develops after exposure of the whole body or a major part of the body to ionizing radiation with doses in excess of 1 to 2 Gy. A useful concept for understanding ARS is the 50% lethal dose, or LD_{50}. This is the radiation dose that will lead to death of 50% of uniformly exposed individuals, assuming no medical intervention.[12] In reality, the lethal dose is influenced by a number of confounding factors, such as the type of radiation, uniformity of radiation exposure, dose rate, penetration, combined injury with biological or chemical damage, and health status of the exposed individual. Supportive therapy exerts a substantial influence on survival after radiation exposure. Hence, the LD_{50} in humans is about 3.5 to 4.0 Gy when no or only minimal supportive care is provided. On the other hand, with the use of standard supportive therapy, the LD_{50} is estimated to be in the 6 to 7 Gy range.[12,13] With optimal pretreatment, availability of an appropriate bone marrow match, and successful bone marrow transplantation, doses in the 9 to 14 Gy range may be survivable.[14] Partial shielding of the active bone marrow, such as occurs when the exposure is nonuniform, also exerts a major effect on survival. For example, shielding of just 10% of the active bone marrow will lead to close to 100% survival after a total-body dose that is otherwise at the LD_{50}.

Several systems have been proposed to classify ARS according to severity and prognosis based on the radiation dose received. For example, the Radiation Injury Severity Classification was proposed by an international group in 2008.[15] Another system, published by the International Atomic Energy Agency, classified ARS in five categories: (1) mild (1–2 Gy), (2) moderate (2–4 Gy), (3) severe (4–6 Gy), (4) very severe (6–8 Gy), and (5) lethal (more than 8 Gy).[16] It should be noted, however, that exposed individuals may survive doses up to 12 Gy for 6 to 12 months with optimal supportive therapy.

Clinically, ARS after exposure to whole-body irradiation generally progresses through four phases. The prodromal period is characterized by nausea, vomiting, and, at higher radiation doses, diarrhea. A latency period of variable duration comes next. The third phase of radiation illness includes various manifestations, depending on the radiation dose received. Last is the period of recovery or demise.

ARS affects, at increasing doses, the hematopoietic, gastrointestinal, cardiovascular, and central nervous systems (CNS). It is common practice to divide ARS into subsyndromes depending on the organ systems that are predominantly responsible for the symptoms.

Hematopoietic Subsyndrome

The bone marrow is the most important organ of the hematopoietic system, but several other organs, such as the thymus, lymph nodes, and spleen, contribute to maintaining homeostasis of the immune responses. The hematopoietic system contains pluripotent and multipotent stem cells that give rise to lineage-committed progenitor cells and subsequently to mature

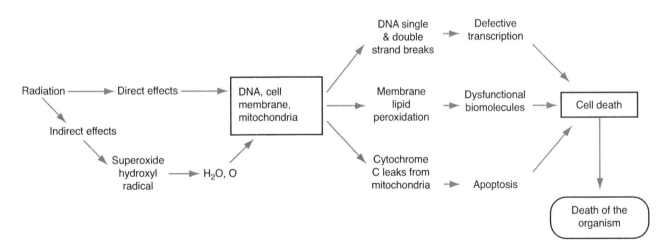

Figure 11-1. Direct and indirect radiation effects on key biological molecules leading to cell and organism death.
DNA: deoxyribonucleic acid
H_2O: water
O: oxygen

peripheral blood cells. The hematopoietic stem cell is central to maintaining hematopoiesis and in recovery after exposure to ionizing radiation. While previously considered a single "target cell," it has now become increasingly recognized that, rather than viewing hematopoietic stem cells in isolation, they should be considered in context with their microenvironment. Hence, the stem cell niche consists of multiple cell types, tissue matrix, and paracrine factors, as well as metabolic products that play essential roles in the ultimate regulation of stem-cell survival, proliferation, and differentiation.[17,18] The entire hematopoietic and immune systems can be regenerated from hematopoietic stem cells. While the majority of hematopoietic stem cells are located in the bone marrow, a few also circulate in the body. The exact role of these circulating stem cells and the extent to which they home to specific locations is still unclear.

All cells of the immune system originate from bone-marrow–derived hematopoietic stem cells. It is customary to classify the immune system into primary, secondary, and tertiary organs. The thymus is the production site of naive T cells that subsequently migrate to the secondary lymphoid organs, such as lymph nodes, spleen, and Peyer's patches in the intestine. Once activated, lymphocytes can enter tertiary, nonlymphoid sites, such as the skin and intestinal mucosa, and contribute to infection clearing. The immune system of the intestine is the largest in the body, containing 50% to 80% of all the body's immunoglobulin-producing cells and 40% of its T cells.

Because of the rapidly proliferating hematopoietic progenitor cell compartment in the bone marrow, the hematopoietic system is extraordinarily radiosensitive. Radiation doses as low as 0.5 to 1 Gy elicit clear changes, and significant hematopoietic and immune system dysfunction occur after radiation doses in excess of 2 Gy. Clinically, hematopoietic injury is characterized by decreased numbers of white cells, red cells, and platelets in the peripheral circulation.

The temporal development of hematopoietic radiation injury is well known.[19] As a general rule, lymphocytes are depleted within hours of radiation exposure, granulocytes and platelets over days, and erythrocytes over weeks. Small lymphocytes, although they do not divide, are extremely radiosensitive and are known to undergo apoptosis (acute cell death, described later in this chapter) after exposure to radiation doses as low as 0.2 to 0.3 Gy. In fact, how fast and low the lymphocyte count drops after radiation has been proposed as a way to predict the level of exposure.[19] Granulocytes and platelets also have rather short life spans; thus granulocytopenia and thrombocytopenia develop early after radiation exposure.

Death from infectious and bleeding complications generally occurs after acute radiation exposure (because of granulocytopenia and thrombocytopenia) within 14 to 28 days after irradiation. Successful treatment depends almost entirely on the ability to enhance the recovery of the hematopoietic stem and progenitor cells within a reasonable period of time. Immune system dysfunction is another important part of the hematopoietic subsyndrome. Naive T cells may take up to a year to regenerate, which puts the patient at increased risk for infections.

Gastrointestinal Subsyndrome

The epithelial lining of the intestine covers an area roughly 200 times that of the surface of the skin and is the most rapidly renewing cell system in the body. Epithelial cells proliferate in the crypts, migrate along the villi, and eventually get shed into the intestinal lumen. The cell cycle time in the human intestine is approximately 30 hours.[20] Therefore, radiation injury to the intestine becomes clinically manifest within days of exposure. In unirradiated humans, intestinal villus cells are replaced by proliferating progenitor crypt cells, which originate from the bottom of the villi. But on radiation exposure, villus cells are no longer replaced by crypts, since crypt cells undergo clonogenic (mitotic) death or apoptosis. The relative importance of clonogenic death versus apoptosis of intestinal crypt cells in the context of the gastrointestinal subsyndrome is unclear. It appears that, while the propensity of the intestinal microvascular endothelium to undergo apoptosis affects the intestinal radiation response,[21] apoptosis of intestinal crypt cells does not play a major role.[22]

The gastrointestinal tract plays a prominent role in the response to total-body irradiation in several ways. First, it is responsible for the prodromal symptoms (nausea, vomiting, and diarrhea) seen even after very low (1 Gy) radiation doses. These symptoms present within minutes to hours of radiation exposure, before structural injury occurs. The time to onset, severity, and duration of the prodromal symptoms are considered a reasonably reliable indication of the radiation dose received. However, because of a high false-positive rate, prodromal symptoms as predictors of radiation dose should be used with caution.[23] Second, the classical gastrointestinal subsyndrome, as described by Quastler, develops in humans after exposure to radiation doses in excess of 6 Gy.[24] It is associated with extensive destruction of the mucosa and characterized by severe diarrhea with pronounced loss of fluids and electrolytes, leading to dehydration and electrolyte imbalance. Treatment with electrolytes and fluids may postpone death, but there are few specific therapeutic options available and survival is extremely unlikely with full-fledged gastrointestinal radiation subsyndrome. Death occurs 3 to 14 days after exposure, usually before day 10, and mostly around day 5 to 7. Although bacteremia does occur in the classical gastrointestinal subsyndrome, it is infrequent and antibiotics do not generally reduce lethality. Third, and perhaps most importantly, gastrointestinal injury plays a prominent role in the response to radiation doses in the hematopoietic dose range (2–6 Gy in humans). Radiation doses in this range do not result in development of full-fledged gastrointestinal subsyndrome. However, breakdown of the mucosal barrier converts the intestine into a large proinflammatory organ that releases cytokines and other inflammatory mediators into the circulation. Moreover, translocation of bacteria from the bowel lumen to the systemic circulation and remote organs occurs, and sepsis from enteric microorganisms (usually Enterobacteriaceae) is an important cause of death after exposure to radiation in this dose range.

Neurovascular Subsyndrome

The mature CNS consists of neurons, glial cells, astrocytes (oligodendrocytes), and blood vessels. Mature neurons are postmitotic (ie, specialized cells that are unable to divide). In contrast, most glial cells retain their capacity to divide under specific circumstances, albeit with slow turnover rates.[25] Microglia, so named because they were once classified as glial cells, develop from monocytes and have phagocytic properties similar to macrophages elsewhere.

Despite the fact that neurons and neuroglial cells are resistant to irradiation in terms of cell death, and that the neurovascular syndrome develops only after very high radiation doses, it is interesting to note that changes in neurological function occur after very low radiation doses. For example, electroencephalographic abnormalities are detectable after doses as low as 0.01 Gy.[26] True neurovascular subsyndrome occurs after exposure to more than 50 Gy, with an expected survival time of generally less than 48 hours. The symptoms of acute CNS injury include disorientation, apathy, and ataxia. Seizures, triggered by minimal external stimuli, are also common. Death results from meningomyeloencephalitis and acute vascular leakiness, resulting in increased fluid accumulation and pressure on critical structures. Cerebral and brainstem edema, caused by fluid leakage, may also result in increased pressure

on critical structures, in turn affecting essential physiological functions, such as blood-pressure regulation, respiration, and temperature regulation. Therapy-resistant cardiovascular shock ("radiogenic shock") sometimes develops in individuals exposed to doses in this range. The mechanism underlying the inability to maintain blood pressure under these circumstances appears to involve a combination of factors, such as massive fluid extravasation, endothelial apoptosis and disruption of tight junctions between endothelial cells, autonomic nervous system dysfunction with loss of blood-pressure control, vasodilatation because of histamine release and other vasoactive mediators by mast cells, and other factors.[27]

The exact pathogenesis of the neurovascular subsyndrome remains unclear, and the issue of whether the target is vascular, parenchymal, or a combination is still unresolved. The prevailing notion at this time is that endothelial cell apoptosis, rather than oligodendrocyte apoptosis, is the primary event responsible for the acute disruption of the blood-brain barrier after irradiation, while oligodendrocyte apoptosis occurs as a secondary consequence.

Radiation-Induced Multiple Organ Dysfunction Syndrome

To convey principles of radiation toxicity in a particular organ effectively, it is useful to consider the radiation response of that organ separately. Moreover, after exposure to total-body irradiation, depending on the radiation dose received, symptoms that can be ascribed to specific organ systems predominate, hence the terms hematopoietic, gastrointestinal, and neurovascular subsyndromes. However, it is important to recognize that reference to the individual subsyndromes of ARS simply indicates that toxicity in those organ systems predominate clinically, but that the pathophysiological manifestations depend heavily on interactions among multiple cell types and organ systems in the body.

In other words, to develop a proper understanding of acute radiation toxicities in response to total-body irradiation, it is imperative that this reductionistic view be supplemented with pertinent principles based on systems biology. The importance of these interacting factors has led to the concept of radiation-induced multiple organ dysfunction syndrome.[28] Hence, total-body irradiation affects all tissues and organ systems in the body, and there are critical interactions among many of these tissues and organ systems. For example, although intestinal irradiation is necessary and sufficient to produce what is commonly referred to as the gastrointestinal subsyndrome (in fact, surgical removal of the exposed bowel prevents the syndrome from occurring),[29] it is firmly established that lethality from bowel toxicity is heavily influenced by radiation injury to other organ systems, such as the hematopoietic system.[30] Conversely, it is also well known that intestinal injury, even after radiation doses in the hematopoietic dose range, influences lethality from hematopoietic and immune system failure.

PROTECTION, MITIGATION, AND TREATMENT

Characteristics of a Radiation Countermeasure

An ideal radiation countermeasure must have several characteristics that are necessary for its applicability to first responders. It must

- be stable at ambient temperature,
- be easily administered either as an intramuscular injection or orally,
- be free from toxic side effects that will compromise behavior and performance, and
- be free from abuse potential, and
- lack toxicity on repeat administration.

In addition to these characteristics, it is necessary to consider any countermeasure's therapeutic index. The therapeutic index, as used here, refers to the ratio between the toxic LD_{50} and the protective drug dose used to produce a specific dose reduction factor (DRF). It would also be advantageous to include information on acute side effects produced by potential agents at protective doses.

Several strategies have been developed to obtain a radiation countermeasure with these desirable characteristics to reduce radiation injury and mortality. These strategies are based on the mechanisms of pharmacological agents to protect against indirect damage, repair damage once it occurs, or stimulate the regeneration of depleted cell populations (Figure 11-2).

Spanning these strategies are new genetic approaches that are just beginning to be used in the development of advanced pharmacological agents. Combinations of agents that exploit the operative mechanisms in at least two of these strategies may substantially improve drug effectiveness. Barring the conventional physical approaches of time, distance, and shielding, almost nothing can be done pharmacologically to protect against the initial transfer of radiation energy to either water or critical biological molecules. The transfer occurs too rapidly (within 10^{-14} seconds after irradiation) and is a purely physical process.[9]

The failure of radioprotective agents to protect against direct damage to critical molecules indicates an inherent upper limit to the degree of protection that can be achieved pharmacologically. Because injury from high-LET radiation is due primarily to direct damage, and because the relative yields of radiolytic products of water and reactive oxygen species decreases with increasing LET, protection against high-LET radiation injury with free-radical scavengers will be less effective.[7]

The earliest point at which a protective effect from pharmacological agents can be detected is around 10^{-12} seconds after irradiation.[10] At that time, pharmacological agents can begin to prevent chemical damage by directly scavenging the free radicals produced by radiolysis of water or by interaction among themselves.[9] The next level of protection can occur by repairing the chemical damage produced in critical biological molecules and also by reacting with the chemical intermediates that indirectly damage these molecules.

Mechanisms

The damage induced by the products of radiation and water interactions can be reduced either by inhibiting the formation of these reactive radical intermediates or by eliminating them from the cellular environment. This can be accomplished using agents that induce hypoxia or scavenge toxic products.

Hypoxia

The formation of reactive oxygen species can be inhibited by the induction of hypoxia. The extent of radiation damage in a tissue is directly related to the degree of oxygenation of that tissue; agents capable of reducing oxygenation will mitigate the injury.[7,31] Many of these chemical agents are known to induce transient systemic or localized hypoxia.[7,8] Systemic hypoxia can be achieved in several ways: through induction of hemodynamic cardiovascular alterations, interference with hemoglobin function, increased tissue oxygen use, and depressed respiratory-center function. At the cellular and molecular levels, localized hypoxia can be achieved by agents that take part in the chemical and biochemical reactions that use oxygen.

Induction of hypoxia is a widespread protective mechanism that accounts, at least in part, for the protective action of many different chemicals, drugs, and physiological mediators. In spite of that, the usefulness

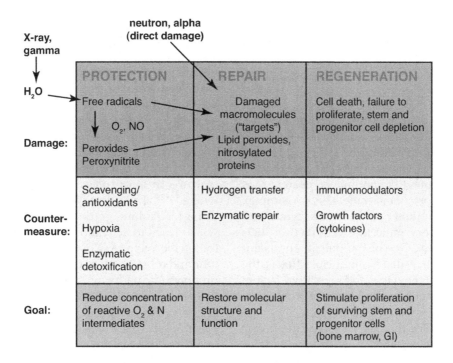

Figure 11-2. Three major possible mechanisms of radiation countermeasures. **Protection**: Preventing damage by scavenging free radicals (eg, H·, OH·, O₂·) or reducing formation of reactive oxygen or nitrogen intermediates such as hydrogen peroxide and peroxynitrite. Representative agents: aminothiol compounds (eg, amifostine) and antioxidants (such as γ-tocotrienol). **Repair**: Repairing molecular damage caused by free radicals. Representative agents: aminothiols. **Regeneration**: Stimulating function or proliferation of stem cells and progenitor cells in organs that rely on stem-cell proliferation for normal functioning, especially the hemopoietic system. Representative compounds: immunomodulators and cytokines. Cytokines are generally given after radiation; immunomodulators before. Steroid immunomodulator 5-androstenediol and antioxidant γ-tocotrienol stimulate cytokine expression and enhance survival after radiation.
GI: gastrointestinal
N: nitrogen
NO: nitric oxide
O₂: oxygen

of this mechanism must be considered with caution because of the potential effects of hypoxia on normal physiological function. This caution may apply more to agents that induce a systemic hypoxic state than to those that create localized hypoxia.

Scavenging

Free-radical scavenging and enzymatic detoxification refer to the ability of chemicals and endogenous enzymes to remove products of water radiolysis and highly reactive oxygen species before they can damage molecules of biological importance.[32,33] In essence, these are competitive reactions between protective agents and biological molecules. In aqueous solutions, protective agents and enzymes react with free radicals and oxygen species to form relatively stable, nontoxic end products, thereby reducing the concentration of

these reactive species and sparing the biological target. Many protectants are very efficient scavengers of water-derived free radicals.

Chemical Repair by Hydrogen Transfer

Radiation damage to a critical biological molecule results in the transformation of that molecule into an organic free radical. In this form, the molecule can then react with oxygen or other free radicals and become permanently chemically altered. However, if a suitable hydrogen donor is in the vicinity of the damaged molecule, it can compensate for the damage by donating or transferring a hydrogen atom.[7,33] Hydrogen atom transfer can be thought of as an instant repair process in which the original molecular structure is restored before the damaged critical molecule becomes permanently altered by further chemical reaction. Many of the agents that function as free-radical scavengers, particularly sulfhydryl agents, can also donate a hydrogen atom (eg, the aminothiols).[7]

Genetic Repair

Similar chemical alterations may also be induced by natural biological processes and disease states that generate free radicals. In the case of DNA, mammalian cells have evolved an elaborate and remarkably efficient system of enzymes that continually repair lesions in that critically important molecule. This is a complex system involving a number of different enzymes and a variety of regulatory molecules that control their synthesis and activity. One of the potentially useful features of this system is that it is inducible; that is, the synthesis of the repair enzymes and regulatory factors is activated when the need arises. Strains of prokaryotic organisms exist that are capable of surviving very high doses of radiation. One that has received attention is *Deinococcus radiodurans*, which is an extremely radio-resistant strain of bacteria.[34] Although a study of these relatively simple prokaryotic systems may provide some insight into the genetic mechanisms involved in radiation sensitivity, relatively little progress has been made to unravel the radioprotective mechanisms in these bacteria to exploit for radiation countermeasure drug development.

Antiapoptotic Mechanisms

Much of the tissue injury occurring after exposure to ionizing radiation is due to apoptosis, either of mature cells (eg, lymphocytes), or progenitor cells necessary for tissue replenishment.[35–37] The two classes of progenitors that have received the most attention in countermeasure development are those in bone marrow responsible for regenerating blood cells and platelets and those in gastrointestinal crypts responsible for regenerating the gastrointestinal mucosa.[38,39] Since much radiation-induced apoptosis takes place in the hours after exposure, it has been recommended that delivery of antiapoptotic countermeasures should take place as early as possible.[40–43]

Radiation-induced apoptosis is caused by signaling pathways in the cell triggered by damage to macromolecules, or sensors that respond to radiation-induced free radicals. These signaling pathways comprise networks of interacting molecules that can alter the balance between repair and survival on one hand and programmed cell death on the other. The goal of antiapoptotic strategies is to activate or inhibit signaling molecules in such a way as to alter this balance in favor of survival.[44] In some cases, blocking apoptosis

could make populations of cells more vulnerable to specific challenges. For example, inhibition of apoptosis with pifithrin improved survival in mice exposed to radiation doses that cause hematopoietic syndrome. However, in animals exposed to higher radiation doses, deletion of protein 53 (p53) was associated with increased mitotic catastrophe in the gastrointestinal mucosa and decreases in survival compared to vehicle-injected irradiated mice.[45]

Radiation-induced signal transduction pathways leading to apoptosis have been reviewed elsewhere.[44,46,47] The primary event is usually considered to be DNA damage detected by sensing proteins, which leads to activation of the ataxia telangiectasia mutated protein (ATM), which triggers both proapoptotic and prosurvival pathways. A central signal in the proapoptotic pathway is p53, which activates protein 21 (p21), cell cycle arrest, and eventual DNA repair and survival or apoptosis. Protein-53–independent proapoptotic pathways are also activated by irradiation,[48] and these pathways lead to effector caspases. In addition, ATM activates nuclear factor κ-light-chain-enhancer of activated B (NFκB) cells, a prosurvival factor. NFκB induces or activates a number of target genes that promote resistance to ionizing radiation, including cytokines; human epidermal growth factor receptor 2 (HER-2); manganese superoxide dismutase (MnSOD); cyclins; 14-3-3 proteins; growth arrest- and DNA-damage–inducible, alpha gene (GADD45β); human inhibitor of apoptosis protein-1 (HIAP-1); Ku (a protein involved in nonhomologous end joining of DNA); B-cell lymphoma 2 (Bcl-2); B-cell lymphoma-extra large (Bcl-XL); X-linked inhibitor of apoptosis protein (XIAP); and caspase 8 and fas-associated protein with death domain-like apoptosis regulator (c-FLIP).[49] Many of the radiation countermeasures under development inhibit p53 and/or activate NFκB. For example, growth factors and cytokines activate NFκB and inhibit apoptosis, and are themselves induced by NFκB.[50] Countermeasures that activate toll-like receptors also inhibit apoptosis via induction of NFκB.[51] Ex-RAD (Onconova Therapeutics, Inc, Newtown, PA) down regulates proapoptosis proteins such as p53 and its downstream regulators p21, Bcl-2–associated X protein (BAX), c-Abl, and protein 73.[52] Glycogen synthase kinase (GSK) 3 promotes cell death caused by the mitochondrial intrinsic apoptotic pathway, and GSK inhibitors have been proposed as radiation countermeasures.[53] Octadecenyl thiophosphate (OTP), a mimic of the proapoptotic signal lysophosphatidic acid (LPA), has also been shown to protect against radiation injury.[54] Another lipid pathway considered a possible target for mitigating radiation-induced apoptosis is the acid sphingomyelinase (ASMase)/ceramide pathway.[22]

Less is known about radiation-induced pathways triggered by events other than DNA damage. Reactive oxygen species and reactive nitrogen species inhibit protein tyrosine phosphatase, which can result in increased activation of signaling molecules, including receptors that promote activation of mitogen-activated protein kinase (MAPK) and phosphatidylinositol 3-kinases (P13K) pathways.[55,56] Some have proposed that oxidized proteins constitute a more important factor than DNA damage in radiation injury.[57] Recently, there has been interest in the possible role of oxidized proteins in the endoplasmic reticulum (ER), inducing autophagy or apoptosis in irradiated cells (ER stress, or unfolded protein response).[47,58] Unfolded proteins in the ER are detected by the sensors protein kinase RNA-like endoplasmic reticulum kinase (PERK), inositol-requiring 1 (IRE1), and activating transcription factor 6 (ATF6). These sensors in turn can activate downstream proapoptotic signals, such as controlled amino acid therapy/enhancer binding protein homologous protein (CHOP), c-Jun N-terminal kinases (JNK), and Bcl-2 proteins. Unfolded protein response can also lead to autophagy via these sensors. Activation of the PI3K/Akt/mammalian target of rapamycin (mTOR) pathway can promote survival via effects on autophagy and apoptosis.[47,59] There are indications of a balance between these two modes of cell death such that inhibition of apoptosis may lead to autophagy and vice versa.[47] Whether these signaling pathways and their effects on apoptosis and autophagy will have any influence on the long-term consequences of radiation is not clearly known. Importantly, blocking apoptosis can actually lead to an increase in radiosensitivity related to a concomitant promotion of autophagy.[60] An understanding of these relationships will be essential to developing radiation countermeasures based on inhibition of apoptosis or autophagy.

Regeneration After Radiation Injury

The aim of this strategy is to increase survival by stimulating the function and regeneration of stem and progenitor cell populations that have decreased in number due to radiation injury. Conceptually, this strategy can be applied to any organ system (such as the hematopoietic and gastrointestinal systems) that relies on stem-cell proliferation to provide mature differentiated cells for proper functioning. Only regeneration of the hematopoietic system is discussed here. Regeneration is a feasible strategy for mitigating radiation injury at doses below the threshold dose that would result in 100% death of hematopoietic stem cells. Exactly which cell type becomes stimulated depends on the type of agent involved. Nonspecific immuno-

modulators are exogenous agents that can bind to and stimulate a variety of different cell types. These agents are thought to induce the stimulated cells to release a variety of peptides (cytokines) that act specifically on immunopoietic and hematopoietic progenitor and stem cells to stimulate their growth and differentiation into mature, functional cells.[61]

Figure 11-3 examines hematopoietic progenitor cell survival as measured by the number of colony-forming units (CFUs) found in the spleens (endogenous CFU [e-CFU]/spleen) of irradiated mice. Some of the mice were treated with the regenerating agent glucan. In the radiation-control animals that were not given glucan, the number of e-CFU/spleen decreased with increasing radiation dose. Similarly, the effectiveness of glucan in increasing the survival of these cells also decreased with increasing radiation dose. This indicates that the effectiveness of these agents depends on the number of surviving progenitor cells. Above the threshold radiation dose that results in 100% progenitor-cell death (greater than 8.5 Gy in Figure 11-3), regeneration becomes ineffective.

Partial-Body Irradiation and Regeneration

The contribution of these protective measures was evident in the Chernobyl accident victims, in whom bone-marrow grafts apparently failed. These failures were due, at least in part, to host-versus-graft reactions

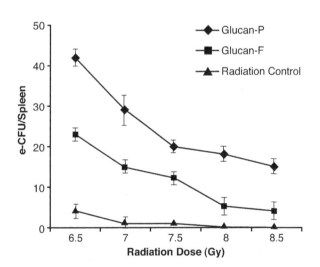

Figure 11-3. Hematopoietic progenitor cell survival as a function of radiation dose treated or not treated with glucan, a radiation countermeasure agent that promotes progenitor cell regeneration in irradiated mice. Glucan efficacy decreases as increased numbers of progenitor cells are killed by higher doses of radiation.

e-CFU: endogenous colony-forming unit

TABLE 11-2

SUPPORTIVE THERAPY IN SURVIVAL OF IRRADIATED PRIMATES*

	No Supportive Therapy	Antibiotics, Fluids, Platelets	Allogeneic Bone Marrow Transplant[†]	Partial Shielding[‡]
Total primates	4	4	5	4
Survivors	0	0	5	4
Mean survival (days)	12.5	16.3	> 30	> 30

*Irradiated with a dose of 8 Gy
[†]Also given antibiotics, fluids, and platelets
[‡]Less than 1% surviving stem cells
Data source: Giambarresi L. Prospects for radioprotection. In: Walker RI, Cerveny TJ, eds. *Medical Consequences of Nuclear Warfare*. In: Zajtchuk R, Jenkins DP, Bellamy RF, Ingram VM, eds. *Textbook of Military Medicine*. Washington, DC: Department of the Army, Office of The Surgeon General, Borden Institute; 1989. Chap 11: 245–273.

initiated by surviving stem cells, even in patients who were exposed to doses of radiation much greater than that expected to completely deplete stem cells.

The effectiveness of minimal local shielding in protecting even small numbers of stem cells is demonstrated in experiments done with monkeys (Table 11-2).[62] Supportive therapy (fluid, platelets, and antibiotics) significantly increased the dose of radiation expected to cause death to 50% of an exposed population within

30 days ($LD_{50/30}$) of irradiated animals. In monkeys exposed to a lethal dose (8 Gy) of whole-body cobalt-60 radiation, supportive therapy extended survival for a few days but had no effect on 30-day survival rates because the radiation dose completely depleted the stem-cell population. However, when the tibias of these animals were shielded so that less than 1% of their bone-marrow stem cells survived, regeneration occurred and many of the animals survived.

RADIATION COUNTERMEASURES

Single Agents

Some of the agents currently under various stages of research as candidates for protection are given in Table 11-1.

Aminothiols and Other Thiol Derivatives

Aminothiols make up the vast majority of agents that have been developed and tested in laboratory models for their ability to increase survival after irradiation.[63] These compounds are chemical analogues of cysteine, the sulfur-containing amino acid. Like cysteine, they have a sulfhydryl group separated by two or three carbon atoms from a strongly basic nitrogen group. As a group, the aminothiols are very effective protectants and they must be present in the system during irradiation. Optimal protection in laboratory animals is generally obtained by intraperitoneal injection 15 to 30 minutes before irradiation. The aminothiols function primarily through free-radical scavenging[9] and hydrogen-transfer mechanisms.[64,65] Hypoxia induction may also play a part in their functioning.[8,64]

One of the most significant events in the development of radioprotective agents was the synthesis of

an aminothiol derivative in 1969 known as amifostine (previously known as WR-2721).[66] This drug was developed through a program sponsored by the Walter Reed Army Institute of Research and is the most thoroughly studied of over 4,000 compounds developed and tested to date. Amifostine has reportedly shown a high degree of protection, with a radiation dose factor of 2.7 when given to mice intraperitoneally 30 minutes before exposure to gamma radiation.[67,68] This is the highest DRF against mouse lethality at 30 days reliably reported for a single injection of a conventional radioprotectant.

In addition to providing radioprotection, amifostine significantly reduces the toxicity of the tumor chemotherapeutic agents cyclophosphamide and cisplatin,[69,70] apparently without altering their chemotherapeutic effectiveness. There are also reports indicating that amifostine preferentially protects normal tissues but not solid tumors against radiation.[68] For these reasons, amifostine is used under clinical supervision as an adjunct to tumor radiation and chemotherapy.

Amifostine remains unavailable as a field-useable radioprotective agent because it induces nausea, vomiting, and hypotension.[71,72] Although no cumulative or irreversible toxicity has been observed in humans or experimental animals receiving this drug (even at relatively high doses), the animals did show significant performance degradation after its parenteral administration.[73,74] Another problem that must be overcome is the drug's poor oral bioavailability, due primarily to first-pass metabolism by the intestinal mucosa during absorption.[75] In addition, the drug is hydrolyzed in the acidic environment of the stomach, a factor that is aggravated by its ability to slow gastric emptying.[76] Because amifostine is a hypocalcemic agent, another clinical side effect of this drug is inhibition of parathyroid hormone secretion.[6] Due to these limitations, amifostine is not a drug of choice for radioprotection of first responders or astronauts in whom performance decrement is not acceptable. Although a DRF of about 1.2 has been obtained with amifostine administered intraperitoneally to mice at a dose that produced no observable side effects or performance degradation,[74] an equivalent dose in large animals and humans had unacceptable side effects.

Several other radioprotective derivatives of amifostine were developed through the Army's program. WR-3689 and WR-151327 were the most effective among these thioates (WR-2721 is considered the gold standard for radiation protection studies in mice). However, none of them was free from toxicities. Some studies indicate the efficacy of WR compounds against high-LET radiation, such as neutrons, either by radiation alone[77,78] or when combined with infection.[79] Other thiol compounds that have shown radioprotective effect include mercaptopropionyl glycine (MPG) and N-acetyl cysteine. Effective doses of these drugs for significant protection were close to the maximum tolerated dose.[80] Some of the thiols, such as aminoethyl thiouronium bromide (AET), are protective against high-LET radiation.

Nutraceuticals, Antioxidants, and Endogenous Antioxidant Systems

Certain naturally occurring compounds function as antioxidants, such as vitamins and minerals, enzymes, and enzyme mimetics. These are part of a natural biochemical defense system that has evolved to protect cells against free radicals and reactive oxygen species arising from normal metabolic processes. This defense can be divided into two components: (1) compounds of low molecular weight that scavenge free radicals, and (2) enzymes that detoxify reactive oxygen species.[81]

The low-molecular–weight compounds that function as free-radical scavengers in this defense system include vitamins A and E, which are lipophilic, and ascorbic acid (vitamin C), which is hydrophilic. The enzymatic arm of this system includes superoxide dis-

mutase, which catalyzes the conversion of superoxide anions to hydrogen peroxide and molecular oxygen. The hydrogen peroxide produced by this reaction is removed from the system by two other enzymes: catalase and glutathione peroxidase. Selenium contributes to this scheme in that it is a cofactor for glutathione peroxidase.

Vitamin E has been shown to increase survival after irradiation when mice were fed a diet supplemented with three times the normal daily mouse requirement of vitamin E (dl-alpha-tocopherol) for 1 week before an 8.5 Gy dose of cobalt-60 gamma radiation and for 30 days after exposure. This regimen provided a survival protection of 90% and resulted in a decrease in radiation-induced, delayed-type hypersensitivity.[82] A single subcutaneous injection of vitamin E provided greater protection than administration in the diet.[83] Topical treatment of exteriorized intestine or oral treatment of rats with vitamin E increased the survival of intestinal crypts.[84] Both vitamin E and ascorbic acid reduced radiation-induced micronucleus formation and chromosomal aberrations in mice; vitamin E was more efficacious than ascorbic acid.[85]

Tocotrienols are superior to α-tocopherol in their radioprotective efficacy, perhaps because they are better antioxidants than α-tocopherol. Another effective option is γ-tocotrienol, a radioprotectant with a DRF of 1.3 that protects mice from hematopoietic failure, gastrointestinal injury, and lethality (Figure 11-4).[86–88] Unpublished results indicate that δ-tocotrienol is almost as effective as γ-tocotrienol.

Vitamin A also increases postirradiation survival when fed to mice as a dietary supplement.[85] In these experiments, mice were maintained on a diet containing various levels of vitamin A or β-carotene, and the mice fed on supplemented diets displayed better survival after irradiation than those fed the basal diet. Vitamin A fed to mice for 3 days before partial-body irradiation can substantially reduce the effects of localized (hind limb) X-irradiation.[89] In addition to its radioprotective ability, vitamin A or β-carotene may also be able to promote recovery from burn injury by reversing postburn immunosuppression.[90] This point is significant because burns are expected to be one of the collateral injuries on the nuclear battlefield.

Selenium is protective when administered either orally or parenterally. When given orally as sodium selenite in drinking water (4 ppm) or injected (1.6 mg/kg) 24 hours before exposure to 9 Gy of cobalt-60 radiation,[91] selenium provided slight but significant increases in survival. The real potential for using selenium as a radioprotective agent lies in its ability to act synergistically with other agents. Selenium was shown to decrease the toxicity of amifostine and

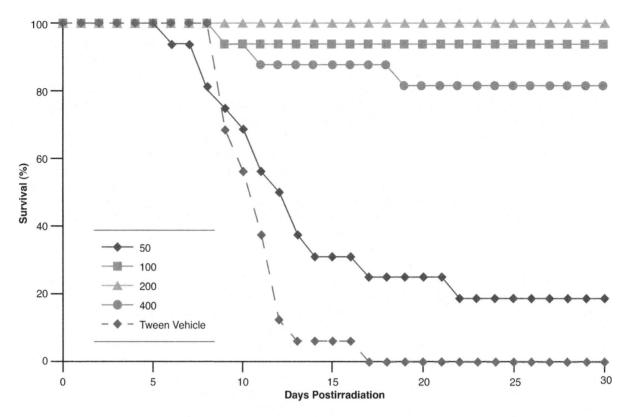

Figure 11-4. Gamma-tocotrienol as a radiation countermeasure at 11 Gy. Thirty-day survival of mice (n = 16 per group) treated 24 hours before receiving 11 Gy of cobalt-60 gamma radiation, with a single subcutaneous injection of a vehicle (5% polysorbate 80) or γ-tocotrienol at doses of 50 to 400 mg/kg body weight. Mice that received a γ-tocotrienol dose of 100, 200, or 400 mg/kg exhibited a significant increase from the vehicle control group.

increase radioprotection when combined with it.[91] Selenium, copper, and zinc were shown to be marginally radioprotective, but they enhance the radioprotection by amifostine.[92]

The parenteral administration of superoxide dismutase increased survival in mice exposed to ionizing radiation.[93] Intravenous injection of this enzyme in mice at a dose of 200 mg/kg given 1 hour before irradiation with X-rays resulted in a DRF of 1.38. A single injection of only 35 mg/kg given 1 hour before irradiation with X-rays also increased survival (DRF: 1.12). The highest DRF reported for this enzyme is 1.56, achieved in mice given two intravenous injections: once at a dose of 200 mg/kg given 1 hour before irradiation with X-rays, and the other at a dose of 35 mg/kg given 1 hour after irradiation.[93] Although further studies on protection by parenteral superoxide dismutase (SOD) were reported, mimetics of SOD showed promise of radioprotection. Eukarion-189, a salen-manganese complex, and superoxide dismutase/catalase mimetic enhanced 30-day survival, with a DRF of 1.15.[94]

Recently, flavonoids were found to be potential nontoxic radioprotectants. Genistein, a nontoxic iso-flavone from soybeans, protected mice when given as a single subcutaneous injection at a dose of 200 mg/kg 24 hours before lethal irradiation.[95] The 30-day survival in the genistein-treated group was 97%, as compared to 31% of the vehicle-treated mice and 0% of untreated mice. One of the reasons for the protection by genistein may be due to the extended quiescence followed by reduced senescence of bone-marrow repopulating LSK⁺ (Lin⁺Sca1⁺Kit⁺) cells.[96]

The ocimum flavonoids orientin and vicenin protected mice from radiation-induced intestinal and bone-marrow syndromes with DRFs of 1.30 and 1.37, respectively.[97] Both of these flavonoids protected mice from prenatal radiation-induced genomic instability and reduced delayed chromosomal aberrations and tumorigenesis in adult mice.[98]

Eicosanoids

The eicosanoids are a large group of potent inflammatory mediators derived from the 20-carbon fatty-acid precursor, arachidonic acid. The compounds in this family that were examined for their abilities to increase the survival of irradiated animals include 16,16-dimethyl prostaglandin E, (DiPGE$_2$, a synthetic analogue of the naturally occurring prostaglandin GE$_2$), leukotriene C (LTC), and platelet-activating factor (PAF). DiPGE$_2$, at a toxic dose that induced diarrhea 5 to 15 minutes before irradiation, elicited a DRF of 1.72, but some protection could still be achieved when the compound was given 1 hour before irradiation.[99] Misoprostol, a stable analogue of prostaglandins, increased the survival of intestinal clonogenic cells by 600%. Diarrhea and other side effects of misoprostol were significantly decreased by mixing misoprostol with iloprost (a prostanoid), which simultaneously decreased the radiation protection efficacy.[100] LTC$_4$ was shown to be effective in increasing the survival of hematopoietic stem cells in mice exposed to cobalt-60 gamma radiation.[101] Despite the high DRFs obtained with these compounds, serious irreversible toxicity associated with prostanoids prevented further exploration for human use.

Biological Response Modifiers, Immunomodulators, and Cytokines

The original immunomodulators were generally crude, whole-cell, microbial preparations (such as Bacillus Calmette-Guérin [BCG] and *Corynebacterium parvum*) used because they could nonspecifically stimulate host immune responses. Later, the active components of these cells (such as endotoxin and zymosan) were identified and isolated from their cell walls. Further work led to the purification, identification, and synthesis of the specific portions of the cell fragments that were responsible for stimulating immune responses (such as endotoxin and glucan from zymosan). Stimulation of cells by immunomodulators results in the release of cytokines, which act as specific stimulators of host immune responses. Recent advances include the development of biologically defined molecules and recombinantly produced cytokines (such as interleukin 1 [IL 1] and granulocyte-macrophage colony-stimulating factor [GM-CSF]), which are relatively nontoxic but allow specific manipulation of various components of the immune and hematological systems.

Bacterial endotoxin was probably the first biological response modifier shown to be a radioprotectant.[102] The window of protection for endotoxin is very narrow due to its high toxicity. A less toxic product from endotoxin obtained by acid hydrolysis was found to have almost the same radioprotective efficacy. This product, 3D-monophosphoryl lipid A (3D-MPL), at a dose of 0.2 to 0.5 mg/kg body weight, given intraperitoneally 16 to 20 hours before radiation, protects mice from radiation-induced lethality, with a DRF of 1.2.

Glucans, which are β-1,3-linked polysaccharides, in soluble and particulate forms showed differential radioprotective efficacy, with the particulate form being more radioprotective. Particulate glucan showed a DRF of 1.22 at a dose of 75 mg/kg, while soluble glucan provided a DRF of only 1.02 at a dose of 250 mg/kg. There are several other biological response modifiers that showed varying degrees of radioprotection.[103] Polysaccharides MNZ, GLP/Bo4, GLP/Bo5 (from *Saccharomyces cerevisiae*) and MNR (from *Rhodotorula rubra*) also provided high DRFs, but these high values may be due to impurities.

Trehalose dimycolate, also known as cord factor, is a glycolipid consisting of 6,6′-diesters of the sugar D-trehalose. It is isolated from the cell walls of *Mycobacteria*, *Nocardia*, and *Corynebacteria*, and is an active component of Freund's complete adjuvant. Like glucan, trehalose dimycolate is a potent immunostimulant that is capable of increasing host defense mechanisms against a variety of organisms and of increasing survival after irradiation.[104,105]

Cytokines are another class of immunomodulators with radioprotective efficacy. Neta et al[106,107] showed IL 1 protected irradiated mice when given either 20 hours before or 2 hours after irradiation. Radioprotection with a DRF in the range of 1.15 to 1.25 was maximized when IL 1 was given 20 hours before radiation at doses of 4 or 8 µg/kg body weight. Acidic fibroblast growth factor (FGF) 1 was radioprotective, with a DRF of 1.16 when given before irradiation.[108] FGF1 and FGF2 induced radiation resistance of crypt cells.[109] A chimeric form of FGF1 and FGF2 augmented activity useful for epithelial proliferation and radioprotection.[110] Tumor necrosis factor α (TNF-α) was also shown to be radioprotective in mice. It has been suggested that TNF-α does not protect tumor cells from radiation, but protects only normal cells. On the other hand, it is also reported that specific inhibition of TNF-α receptors by genetic knock-out protected lungs from radiation.[111] Ammonium trichloro (dioxyethylene-0-0′) tellurate (AS101), a synthetic immunomodulator, was shown to protect mice from hematopoietic injury.[112]

Whitnall et al investigated the mechanisms of action of androst-5-ene-3beta,17beta-diol (5-androstenediol [5-AED]) because of its ability to reduce mortality (Figure 11-5), thrombocytopenia, and neutropenia in irradiated mice and nonhuman primates. 5-AED displays extremely low toxicity and androgenicity.[113–115]

In-vitro studies of human hematopoietic progenitor cells showed they are a direct target of 5-AED.[115] Incubation with 5-AED reduced apoptosis and promoted survival of these cells when exposed to gamma radiation, and this effect was dependent on activation of NFκB and resultant induction of G-CSF, consistent with the demonstration of G-CSF induction in mice treated with 5-AED.[116,117]

Two other cytokines may be potentially useful agents: GM-CSF and interleukin 3 (IL 3). Several growth factors that are specific for different hematological cell populations have been discovered and can be produced by recombinant DNA methods. One of these, a specific human recombinant GM-CSF (rhGM-CSF), accelerates marrow repair or engraftment and may contribute to increased nonspecific resistance. It functions by increasing the number of circulating granulocytes and platelets in normal animals and accelerating the recovery of these cells after irradiation. This factor was used in treating some victims of the radiation exposure accident in Goiânia, Brazil. The effectiveness of GM-CSF in ameliorating radiation-induced cytopenia can be seen from data obtained

in the minimal-shielding experiment.[62] In that experiment, the survival of partially shielded monkeys that were given supportive therapy was enhanced. Unshielded animals rapidly became neutropenic and died within 15 days. In the shielded animals that survived beyond 30 days, peripheral granulocytes began to recover slowly between days 20 and 40. In contrast, shielded animals treated with GM-CSF showed evidence of granulocyte recovery well before day 20, and granulocyte levels quickly reached supranormal levels. Therefore, it appears this factor is a useful adjunct to radiation-injury therapy. However, its effectiveness as a regeneration agent in radioprotective regimens is much lower than that for IL I and TNF. Other evidence suggests that GM-CSF may act synergistically when combined with other cytokines.[118]

IL 3 has not yet been evaluated for its ability to in-

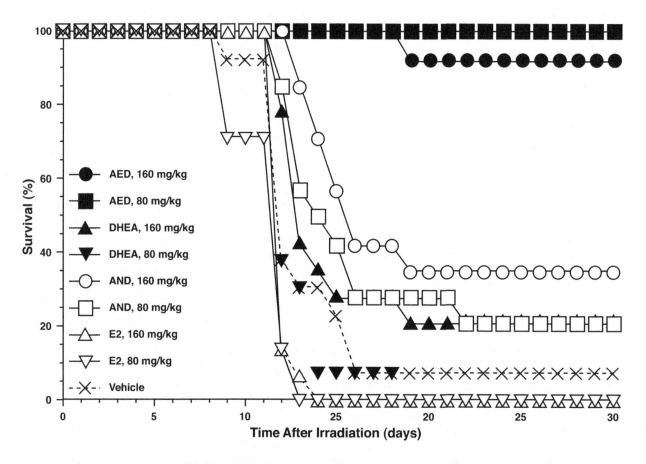

Figure 11-5. Survival time courses of female B6D2F1 mice after subcutaneous injection with 5-androstenediol, dehydroepiandrosterone, 4-androstenedione, or estradiol 24 hours before whole-body gamma-irradiation (11 Gy, 0.6 Gy/min). Survival after 5-androstenediol ($P < 0.001$) or 4-androstenedione (80 mg/kg: $P < 0.05$; 160 mg/kg: $P < 0.01$) was significantly greater than with the vehicle.
AED: 5-androstenediol
AND: 4-androstenedione
DHEA: dehydroepiandrosterone
E2: estradiol

crease survival after irradiation. Unlike the described action of the cytokines (whose major target cells are primarily the more mature functional cells in the system), IL 3 is reported to act specifically in stimulating the growth of pluripotent progenitor cells.[119]

Kiang et al found that the geldanamycin derivative 17-(dimethylaminoethylamino)-17-demethoxygel-danamycin (17-DMAG) improved mouse survival from cobalt-60 gamma irradiation at a lethal dose.[120] 17-DMAG inhibited the radiation-induced activation of the inducible nitric oxide synthase pathway, thereby blocking apoptosis[121] and autophagy.[122] This drug also inhibited the radiation-induced activation of p53–Bax signal transduction[121] and the radiation-induced increases in cytokines (Kiang, unpublished data, 2010).

Combination Agents

Rationale

Agents that act as protectors, mitigators, or therapies contribute in different ways to counter radiation injury by protection, repair, and regeneration. Each of them also has its limitations. Neither chemical nor enzymatic means of protection minimize direct damage. In addition, it is almost impossible for any protective or repair agent to either completely eliminate all of the reactive intermediates formed or repair all of the damaged molecules. Regardless of the efficiency of scavengers and repair agents and their concentration within the cell at the time of irradiation, some molecular damage and cell death still occurs. The effectiveness of agents that function in the regeneration strategy is limited because the agents require a pool of surviving functional cells on which to work. That pool of hematopoietic stem cells and highly radiosensitive progenitor cells becomes depleted even at sublethal radiation doses.

It is reasonable to expect that optional survival would be provided by an agent or combination of agents that would operate using two or more of these strategies. Such a formulation would maximize the effectiveness and minimize its limitations. Protective agents prevent the production of reactive species resulting from the radiolysis of water. Mitigators attenuate the injury. Therapeutic agents repair the damage to critical target molecules and allow regeneration of critical cells. A combination of these agents increases the surviving fraction of stem cells, progenitor cells, and mature cells of the hematopoietic system after irradiation. By allowing stem cells to survive at higher radiation doses, the net effect is to increase the threshold radiation dose that limits the effectiveness of regenerative agents. Taken together or at intervals with protective agents and mitigators, these agents further enhance

the organism's survival by maximizing the proliferation and function of the extra stem cells provided.

It would be difficult to produce one drug that would be able to ameliorate radiation injury by performing protection, repair, and regeneration. Two or more agents might be used either together or at intervals, but this is not ideal; a single dose is the simplest dosing regimen that is desirable for military personnel under battle conditions or for first responders in emergency situations. Therefore, the goal is a single treatment consisting of a combination of two or more agents with the capabilities of protection, repair, and regeneration.

Combination Agents

The concept of using a combination of agents that function by different mechanisms to achieve protection was developed and studied in the 1950s and 1960s.[7,92] In many of the combinations examined, synergistic effects were seen. These results are particularly significant because increased protection with the combinations was often achieved using substantially lower doses of individual drugs than those required for protection when each agent was given separately. For example, one study examined various combinations of five different radioprotective agents: cysteine, β-mercaptoethylamine (MEA), aminoethylisothiouronium bromide-hydrobromide (AET), glutathione, and serotonin.[123] MEA, AET, or serotonin used alone provided similar protection, with a DRF of 1.7; cysteine was less effective, with a DRF of 1.12; and glutathione was marginally protective, with a DRF of 1.05. The most effective regimen was a combination of all five agents, which produced a DRF of 2.8. In this combination, the MEA dose was one half, and the AET dose was two thirds that used when the drugs were given individually.

Additive and synergistic effects were demonstrated with various combinations of aminothiols, antioxidant vitamins and minerals, immunomodulators, prostanoids, and cytokines. It is likely that a first-generation agent will be a combination of subtoxic doses of two or more of these agents (Table 11-3).

Mitigation of Performance Decrement

Because a single, self-administrable agent is sought as a radiation countermeasure, it might also be necessary to include moderators of performance decrements such as nausea, vomiting, diarrhea, or hypotension in any regimen that is developed. While measures to enhance resistance to the lethal effects of radiation have been extensively studied, the application of pharmacological interventions to mitigate performance and behavioral deficiencies has not been addressed sufficiently, even though

TABLE 11-3

RADIOPROTECTIVE EFFICACY OF SELECTED COMBINED AGENTS

Agents		Dose (mg/kg)		Dose Reduction Factor[*]		
A	*B*	*A*	*B*	*A*	*B*	*A+B*
IL 1[1]	TNF	150[†]	5[‡]	1.19	1.12	1.38
Glucan-P[2]	Amifostine	75	200	1.22	1.33	1.51
Selenium[3]	Amifostine	1.6	400	1.1	2.2	2.5
DiPGE₂[§]	Amifostine	0.4	200	1.4	1.9	2.2

[*]Dose reduction factor = radiation $LD_{50/30}$ dose for drug / radiation $LD_{50/30}$ dose for excipient
[†]µg/mouse
[‡]ng/mouse
[§]Unpublished data
$DiPGE_2$: 16,16-dimethyl prostaglandin E_2
IL 1: interleukin 1
$LD_{50/30}$: the dose of radiation expected to cause death to 50% of an exposed population within 30 days
TNF: tumor necrosis factor
Data sources: (1) Neta R, Oppenheim JJ, Douches SD. Interdependence of IL-I, TNF, and CSFs in radioprotection. *J Immunol.* 1988;140:108–111. (2) Patchen ML, MacVittie TJ, Weiss JF. Combined modality radioprotection: the use of glucan and selenium with WR-2721. *Int J Radiat Oncol Biol Phys.* 1990;18:1069–75. (3) Weiss JF, Hoover RL, Kumar KS. Selenium pretreatment enhances the radioprotective effect and reduces the lethal toxicity of WR-2721. *Free Rad Res Communs.* 1987;3:33–38.

these are immediate military concerns. Although it is possible for radioprotective agents to prevent some performance decrements, drugs that increase survival generally have not enhanced performance. In fact, except for a few notable exceptions, they usually exacerbate radiation-induced performance decrements.[73,74] Groups of drugs are being developed that will, perhaps, stabilize performance by modulating cellular permeability, altering regional blood flow, and interrupting the release or action of various mediators. Drugs are being identified that can modulate postirradiation nausea, vomiting, diarrhea, and other performance decrements.

Radiation Countermeasures and Supportive Therapy

Radiation countermeasures will be most effective in personnel exposed to radiation doses within the ranges required to produce the hematopoietic subsyndrome (approximately 2.0–8.0 Gy) and mild gastrointestinal subsyndrome (approximately 8.0–10.0 Gy), and in whom no associated injuries are present. In the event of more severe radiation injury, or if radiation injury is combined with traumatic or burn injuries (a likely occurrence on the battlefield or after a radiation leak or explosion accident), radioprotective measures alone will be insufficient and additional supportive therapy will be required. Although the effectiveness of radiation countermeasures may be reduced in the face of

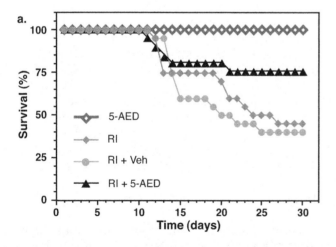 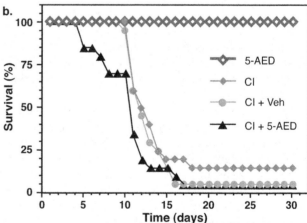

Figure 11-6. Comparative effects of 5-androstenediol on survival in mice receiving either radiation alone (*a*) or radiation followed by wound trauma (*b*). B6F2D1/J female mice received cobalt-60 gamma radiation at 9.75 Gy alone or followed by a 15% body-surface-area wound. Then the mice were subcutaneously injected with a vehicle (polyethylene glycol 400) or 30 mg/kg 5-androstenediol at 2 hours, 24 hours, and 48 hours after radiation alone or combined injury.
5-AED: 5-androstenediol
CI: combined injury
RI: radiation injury
Veh: vehicle

more severe radiation injury or combined injury, it should be noted that their use at the time of irradiation will likely increase the effectiveness of supportive therapies provided days later.

Traumatic injury can reduce the ability of pharmacological agents to increase survival from a lethal radiation dose (Figure 11-6). Ledney et al[124] reported that mice treated with 5-AED dissolved in PEG-400 (polyethylene glycol 400) within 2 hours after exposure to 9.75 Gy of cobalt-60 gamma radiation showed 76% survival, whereas mice treated with just PEG-400 showed 40% survival. However, this protection was not seen in mice receiving 9.75 Gy followed by a 15% total-surface-area wound. In the irradiated and wounded mice, death began to occur about 1 week earlier than in the irradiated-only mice, and all mice died at the same rate regardless of treatment with 5-AED.[124] A similar observation was also found with trehalose dimycolate treatment.[104]

This difference in protective response between irradiated-only and combined-injury mice may be due to a more profound activation of the inducible nitric oxide synthase pathway, increases in serum cytokine concentrations and bacterial infection, reduction of cell adhesion and extracellular matrix, and increases in toll-like receptor signaling, resulting in physiological perturbations[125] so as to induce apoptosis[121] and autophagy.[122] Finally, multiple organ dysfunction and failure occur and mortality is manifested. Various interventions to enhance resistance to radiation and wounds may be used in combination to prevent infection in severely injured subjects. To avoid infection, the natural and artificial defenses must be in balance so that the host resistance is sufficient to control the number of microorganisms. Therefore, as normal defenses are compromised due to suppression by radiation, artificial interventions are required to maintain resistance above the threshold for infection (Figure 11-7).

The potential synergy between therapeutic agents, such as antibiotics, and substances that may be used as radioprotectants is indicated by data on the use of glucan and the antibiotic pefloxacin in the management of postirradiation mortality. In that experiment, only 25% of mice given 7.9 Gy of whole-body cobalt-60 gamma radiation survived. Treatment with either glucan alone at 1 hour or with pefloxacin alone for 24 days after irradiation resulted in 48% and 7% survival,

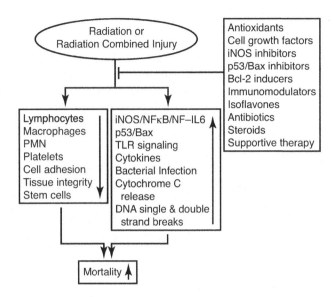

Figure 11-7. Radiation or radiation combined with wound attenuate the normal defenses. Various interventions against radiation injury or radiation injury combined with wound injury may be used in combination to improve the chance of survival in severely injured subjects.
Bax: B-cell-lymphoma-2–associated X protein
Bcl-2: B-cell lymphoma 2
DNA: deoxyribonucleic acid
iNOS: inducible nitric oxide synthase
NFκB: nuclear factor κ-light-chain-enhancer of activated B
NF–IL6: nuclear factor–interleukin-6
p53: protein 53
PMN: polymorphonuclear leukocytes
TLR: toll-like receptor

respectively. However, if the two treatments were combined, survival was 85%.[126] An increase in DRF was demonstrated when glucan was combined with selenium and amifostine.[127] Combining α-tocopherol with WR-3689 (a methylated form of amifostine) reduced the toxic dose of WR-3689 without compromising the DRF.[128] Other combination modality strategies were reviewed by Weiss et al.[92] Recently, a mixture of dietary antioxidants was shown to protect hematopoietic cells and improve survival after total-body irradiation.[129] Curcumin, when combined with copper (II) in a ratio of 1:1, showed higher radioprotection as compared to curcumin alone.[130] Combining salts of copper, selenium, and zinc increased radioprotection by amifostine or 5-aminosalicylic acid.[92,131]

DEVELOPMENT OF A RADIOPROTECTIVE REGIMEN

A variety of factors must be considered when evaluating and developing candidate radiation countermeasure drugs for military use, and a compromise must be reached between the ideal and the achievable. To screen radiation countermeasure agents in animals at the Armed Forces Radiobiology

Research Institute (AFRRI), an optimal drug dose for screening is determined. Drug doses are selected in a stepwise, up-or-down fashion to assess toxicity over 14 days. A drug dose that does not result in any adverse effects is established and known as the "no-observed-adverse-effect" level. The drug dose to be used for initial radioprotection experiments is one fourth the no-observed-adverse-effect level. Then the optimal timing of drug administration, the optimal drug dose, and the optimal administration route can be determined. It should be noted that ease of administration, simplicity of dose schedule, minimal side effects, and a wide safety margin are particularly important because it may be necessary to administer a radioprotective drug repeatedly for several days.

Pharmacological Side Effects

Side effects (ie, toxicity) are a major obstacle in fielding agents to prevent, mitigate, or treat radiation injury. No chronic toxicity is acceptable. Acute toxicity (such as nausea, vomiting, and hypotension) are common, especially with the sulfur compounds. For a fieldable drug, any acute side effects will have to be reduced in severity so that military performance is not impaired. If that is not possible, these effects should at least be controllable by other conveniently applied therapies.

Additionally, these agents must not significantly increase the user's vulnerability to chemical or biological agents or antidotes, exacerbate other battlefield injuries, negatively affect behavior, or interfere significantly with wound healing. The agent should have a wide safety margin (ie, therapeutic index) to compensate for the "if one is good, then two must be better" philosophy.

New Directions

Past nuclear accidents at Chernobyl, Three Mile Island, Goiânia, and Tokaimura, and recent global developments in the possession of weapons-grade nuclear fissionable materials by several nations are indications that a radiological/nuclear incident is only a matter of time. Therefore, there is an urgent need to develop a safe and effective radiation countermeasure. Such a need prompted intense efforts by the National Institute for Allergy and Infectious Diseases and the Department of Defense Threat Reduction Agency to devote considerable resources to developing radiation mitigators and prophylactic agents. These efforts are already yielding sporadic successes. Among the drugs that were screened and exploited under the direction of these two agencies or AFRRI, a few are showing

moderate successes. 5-AED,[111] a toll-like receptor 5 agonist,[132] genistein,[133] SOM230,[134] and Ex-RAD[52] have been observed in completed small-animal studies. Some have already been afforded investigational new drug status by the US Food and Drug Administration and are in phase I clinical trials with humans.

Simultaneously, newer approaches are being explored. One approach being developed involves incorporating the human MnSOD gene into a minicircle plasmid and testing its radioprotective potential.[135] The MnSOD-containing plasmid was radioprotective in vitro and in vivo. One problem encountered in the current radiation countermeasure discovery programs is a lack of efficacy of oral drugs. Application of nanotechnology may make drugs that are currently delivered by injection available orally. In this technology, the drug is encapsulated in a nanoparticle, allowing it to pass through the stomach and be delivered into the bloodstream. Nanoencapsulation has been shown to increase the cellular delivery of drugs as much as 3- to 10-fold.[136]

At AFRRI, a permanent intramural screening program has been instituted to test potential radiation countermeasures that may be developed independently at the institute or referred from various sources. At this writing, four radiation countermeasure candidates have been granted investigational new drug status by the US Food and Drug Administration. All four are AFRRI products: two initiated independently at AFRRI, and two the results of collaborations with biotechnology firms.

Systems Biology Approach

Applying bioinformatics tools, it should be possible to search the database of chemicals maintained by the National Center for Biotechnology Information and identify chemicals that may have chemical structures similar to well-established radiation countermeasures. The compounds can be screened for their abilities to protect cell lines from radiation as measured by clonogenic survival. Selected drugs from this initial screening would be subjected to mechanistic studies in these cells by high-content screening to establish if the clonogenic survival is accompanied by the restoration of pathway-specific genes affected by radiation. Those chemicals surviving these rigorous initial tests will be subjected to in-vivo screening in rodents and further development. Since this approach would miss effective countermeasures that depend on cell interactions or mechanisms not present in the cultures, a parallel program of initial screening in vivo should be maintained.

SUMMARY

The development of radioprotective agents has been dominated by the study of sulphydryl compounds, particularly the aminothiols. These compounds function by a variety of mechanisms, almost all of which increase survival in the irradiated organism by minimizing the radiation-induced damage to critical biological molecules. These compounds suffer from one major drawback: high levels of protection are accompanied by unacceptable side effects. Therefore, it has been necessary to search for less toxic compounds for radiation injury alone and for combined injury.

Among the candidates being evaluated are naturally occurring dietary components such as selenium, vitamin A, vitamin E, genistein, and drugs of low toxicity that are being used clinically, such as MPG. The drawback to these agents is that the protection achieved is relatively low. However, some vitamin E isoforms and genistein display more protection than reported previously for dietary components. These compounds merit further exploration.

The net effect of protective compounds is an increase in the number of stem and progenitor cells that survive the initial radiation insult. To exploit this early benefit, agents that stimulate the proliferation and differentiation of those cells would help optimize cell repopulation of organ systems that were depleted by radiation-induced cell death. The use of regeneration agents, such as immunomodulators and cytokines, alone has been shown to enhance survival after irradiation. When these agents are administered along with a protective agent, additive or synergistic effects are seen. Most importantly, these effects are often achieved using subtoxic doses of the individual agents.

Combining those agents that use a protection or repair strategy with those that promote regeneration offers the advantages of circumventing side effects, enhancing the effectiveness of relatively nontoxic agents that provide only mild protection when given alone, and maximizing the therapeutic benefit provided by each agent. The use of pharmacological agents to increase survival after irradiation will be most effective for personnel exposed to low or intermediate doses of radiation who have minimal associated traumatic or burn injuries. Indeed, in a mass casualty situation, those agents may be the only type of medical intervention available. On the other hand, with smaller numbers of casualties, especially those with combined injuries, it is likely that additional supportive therapies will be available. The early application of radiation countermeasures will minimize the need for subsequent interventions and will enhance the effectiveness of the interventions that are provided.

Many factors must be considered in defining the desired properties of a potentially fieldable first-generation agent. Since the development of WR-2721 (amifostine), emphasis has been placed on studying agents that produce DRFs greater than 2. This emphasis may actually have hampered efforts to field a suitable agent. Some agents with lower DRFs can provide significant protection and may be more appropriate for field use. The agent should also have a high therapeutic index because it will most likely be self-administered. Whether or not the agent can be taken orally is ultimately an important consideration.

Based on candidate agents now available, it may soon be possible to recommend a countermeasure regimen that meets the requirements. The recommendation will probably include a combination of at least two of the candidate agents described above. Fielding a first-generation agent that satisfies most of the requirements discussed above is an achievable goal that will satisfy, at least in part, a critical immediate need of the armed forces.

Fielding the first-generation agent is only an initial step. Much work needs to be done to develop an agent that is effective against high-LET radiation. This need will become increasingly urgent as nuclear terrorism threats inrease. Second- and third-generation agents will be developed only through intense studies that are aimed at defining the mechanisms of radiation injury on the molecular and cellular levels and determining how organisms can be stimulated to protect themselves against this injury. The search for more efficacious radiation countermeasures must continue using newer bioinformatics and systems biology approaches.

REFERENCES

1. Coleman CN, Hrdina C, Bader JL, et al. Medical response to a radiologic/nuclear event: integrated plan from the Office of the Assistant Secretary for Preparedness and Response, Department of Health and Human Services. *Ann Emerg Med.* 2009;53:213–222.

2. Stone HB, Moulder JE, Coleman CN, et al. Models for evaluating agents intended for the prophylaxis, mitigation and treatment of radiation injuries: report of an NCI workshop, December 3–4, 2003. *Radiat Res.* 2004;162:711–728.

3. Pellmar TC, Rockwell S; Radiological/Nuclear Threat Countermeasures Working Group. Priority list of research areas for radiological nuclear threat countermeasures [review]. *Radiat Res*. 2005;163:115–123.

4. Patt HM, Tyree E, Straube RL, Smith DE. Cysteine protection against X irradiation. *Science*. 1949;110:213–214.

5. Mettler FA Jr, Voelz GL. Major radiation exposure—what to expect and how to respond. *N Engl J Med*. 2002;346:1554–1561.

6. Glover D, Riley L, Carmichael K, et al. Hypocalcemia and inhibition of parathyroid hormone secretion after administration of WR2721 (a radioprotective and chemoprotective agent). *N Engl J Med*. 1983;309:1137–1141.

7. Giambarresi L. Prospects for radioprotection. In: Walker RI, Cerveny TJ, eds. *Medical Consequences of Nuclear Warfare*. In: Zajtchuk R, Jenkins DP, Bellamy RF, Ingram VM, eds. *Textbook of Military Medicine*. Washington, DC: Department of the Army, Office of The Surgeon General, Borden Institute; 1989: 245–273.

8. Alper T. *Cellular Radiobiology*. London, England: Cambridge University Press; 1979.

9. Weiss JF, Kumar KS. Antioxidant mechanisms in radiation injury and radioprotection. In: Chow CK, ed. *Cellular Antioxidant Defense Mechanisms*. Vol II. Boca Raton, FL: CRC Press; 1988: 163–189.

10. Singh A, Singh H. Time-scale and nature of radiation-biological damage: approaches to radiation protection and post-irradiation therapy. *Prog Biophys Mol Bio*. 1982;39:69–107.

11. Hagan MP, Holahan EV, Ainsworth EJ. Effects of heavy ions on cycling stem cells. *Adv Space Res*. 1986;6:201–211.

12. United Nations Scientific Committee on the Effects of Atomic Radiation. *Sources, Effects and Risks of Ionizing Radiation: 1988 Report to the General Assembly, with Annexes*. New York, NY: United Nations; 1988.

13. Anno GH, Young RW, Bloom RM, Mercier JR. Dose response relationships for acute ionizing-radiation lethality. *Health Phys*. 2003;84:565–575.

14. Waselenko JK, MacVittie TJ, Blakeley WF, et al. Medical management of the acute radiation syndrome: recommendations of the Strategic National Stockpile Radiation Working Group. *Ann Intern Med*. 2004;140:1037–1051.

15. Kuniak M, Azizova T, Day R, et al. The radiation injury severity classification system: an early injury assessment tool for the frontline health-care provider. *Br J Radiol*. 2008;81:232–243.

16. International Atomic Energy Agency. *Diagnosis and Treatment of Radiation Injuries*. Vienna, Austria: IAEA; 1998. Safety report series 2.

17. Fuchs E, Tumbar T, Guasch G. Socializing with the neighbors: stem cells and their niche. *Cell*. 2004;116:769–778.

18. Scadden DT. The stem-cell niche as an entity of action. *Nature*. 2006;441:1075–1079.

19. Fliedner TM, Nothdurft W, Steinbach KH. Blood cell changes after radiation exposure as an indicator for hematopoietic stem cell function. *Bone Marrow Transplantation*. 1988;3:77–84.

20. Kellett M, Potten CS, Rew DA. A comparison of in vivo cell proliferation measurements in the intestine of mouse and man. *Epith Cell Biol*. 1992;1:147–155.

21. Paris F, Fuks Z, Kang A, et al. Endothelial apoptosis as the primary lesion initiating intestinal radiation damage in mice. *Science*. 2001;293:293–297.

22. Rotolo JA, Maj JG, Feldman R, et al. Bax and bak do not exhibit functional redundancy in mediating radiation-induced endothelial apoptosis in the intestinal mucosa. *Int J Radiat Oncol Biol Phys*. 2008;70:804–815.

23. Demidenko E, Williams BB, Swartz HM. Radiation dose prediction using data on time to emesis in the case of nuclear terrorism. *Radiat Res*. 2009;171:310–319.

24. Quastler H. The nature of intestinal radiation death. *Radiat Res*. 1956;4:303–320.

25. Schultze B, Korr H. Cell kinetic studies of different cell types in the developing and adult brain of the rat and the mouse: a review. *Cell Tissue Kinet*. 1981;14:309–325.

26. Mettler FA, Upton AC. *Medical Effects of Ionizing Radiation*. 3rd ed. Philadelphia, PA: Saunders; 2008.

27. Hawkins RN, Cockerham LG. Postirradiation cardiovascular dysfunction. In: Conklin JJ, Walker RI, eds. *Military Radiobiology*. Orlando, FL: Academic Press; 1987: 153–163.

28. Monti P, Wysocki J, van der Meeren A, Griffiths NM. The contribution of radiation-induced injury to the gastrointestinal tract in the development of multi-organ dysfunction syndrome or failure. *Br J Radiol*. 2005;27(suppl):89–94.

29. Osborne JW. Prevention of intestinal radiation death by removal of the irradiated intestine. *Radiat Res*. 1956;4:541–546.

30. Terry NHA, Travis EL. The influence of bone marrow depletion on intestinal radiation damage. *Int J Radiat Oncol Biol Phys*. 1989;17:569–573.

31. Greenstock CL. Redox processes in radiation biology and cancer. *Radiat Res*. 1981;86:196–211.

32. Chapman WH, Cipte CR, Elizholtz DC, Cronkite EP, Chambers FW Jr. *Sulfhydryl-Containing Agents and the Effects of Ionizing Radiations. Beneficial Effect of Glutathione Injection on X-Ray Induced Mortality Rate and Weight Loss in Mice*. Bethesda, MD: Naval Medical Research Institute; 1949. Naval Medical Research Institute Project NM006012,08.25.

33. Copeland ES. Mechanisms of radioprotection—a review. *Photochem Photobiol*. 1978;28:839–844.

34. Serianni RW, Bruce AK. Role of sulphur in radioprotective extracts of *Micrococcus radiodurans*. *Nature*. 1968;218:485–487.

35. Ijiri K, Potten CS. Response of intestinal cells of differing topographical and hierarchical status to ten cytotoxic drugs and five sources of radiation. *Br J Cancer*. 1983;47:175–185.

36. Uckun FM, Tuel-Ahlgren L, Song CW, et al. Ionizing radiation stimulates unidentified tyrosine-specific protein kinases in human B-lymphocyte precursors, triggering apoptosis and clonogenic cell death. *Proc Natl Acad Sci U S A*. 1992;89:9005–9009.

37. Lotem J, Sachs L. Hematopoietic cells from mice deficient in wild-type p53 are more resistant to induction of apoptosis by some agents. *Blood*. 1993;82:1092–1096.

38. Whitnall MH, Pellmar TC. New directions in development of pharmacological countermeasures for the acute radiation syndrome. In: Kasid UN, Notario V, Haimovitz-Friedman A, Bar-Eli M. eds. *Reviews in Cancer Biology and Therapeutics*. Kerala, India: Transworld Research Network; 2007: 193–209.

39. Potten CS, Grant HK. The relationship between ionizing radiation-induced apoptosis and stem cells in the small and large intestine. *Br J Cancer*. 1998;78:993–1003.

40. Herodin F, Grenier N, Drouet M. Revisiting therapeutic strategies in radiation casualties. *Exp Hematol*. 2007;35:28–33.

41. Radford IR, Murphy TK. Radiation response of mouse lymphoid and myeloid cell lines. Part III. Different signals can lead to apoptosis and may influence sensitivity to killing by DNA double-strand breakage. *Int J Radiat Biol*. 1994;65:229–239.

42. Tanikawa S, Nose M, Aoki Y, Tsuneoka K, Shikita M, Nara N. Effects of recombinant human granulocyte colony-stimulating factor on the hematologic recovery and survival of irradiated mice. *Blood*. 1990;76:445–449.

43. Neelis KJ, Visser TP, Dimjati W, et al. A single dose of thrombopoietin shortly after myelosuppressive total body irradiation prevents pancytopenia in mice by promoting short-term multilineage spleen-repopulating cells at the transient expense of bone marrow-repopulating cells. *Blood*. 1998;92:1586–1597.

44. Xiao M, Whitnall MH. Pharmacological countermeasures for the acute radiation syndrome. *Curr Mol Pharmacol.* 2009;2:122–133.

45. Komarova EA, Christov K, Faerman AI, Gudkov AV. Different impact of p53 and p21 on the radiation response of mouse tissues. *Oncogene.* 2000;19:3791–3798.

46. Valerie K, Yacoub A, Hagan MP, et al. Radiation-induced cell signaling: inside-out and outside-in. *Mol Cancer Ther.* 2007;6:789–801.

47. Moretti L, Cha YI, Niermann K J, Lu B. Switch between apoptosis and autophagy: radiation-induced endoplasmic reticulum stress? *Cell Cycle.* 2007;6:793–798.

48. Sohn D, Graupner V, Neise D, Essmann F, Schulze-Osthoff K, Janicke RU. Pifithrin-alpha protects against DNA damage-induced apoptosis downstream of mitochondria independent of p53. *Cell Death Differ.* 2009;16:869–878.

49. Ahmed KM, Li JJ. NF-kappa B-mediated adaptive resistance to ionizing radiation. *Free Radic Biol Med.* 2008;44:1–13.

50. Pyatt DW, Stillman WS, Yang Y, Gross S, Zheng JH, Irons RD. An essential role for NF-kappaB in human CD34(+) bone marrow cell survival. *Blood.* 1999;93:3302–3308.

51. Burdelya LG, Krivokrysenko VI, Tallant TC, et al. An agonist of toll-like receptor 5 has radioprotective activity in mouse and primate models. *Science.* 2008;320:226–230.

52. Ghosh SP, Perkins MW, Hieber K, et al. Radiation protection by a new chemical entity, Ex-Rad: efficacy and mechanisms. *Radiat Res.* 2009;171:173–179.

53. Thotala DK, Hallahan DE, Yazlovitskaya EM. Inhibition of glycogen synthase kinase 3 beta attenuates neurocognitive dysfunction resulting from cranial irradiation. *Cancer Res.* 2008;68:5859–5868.

54. Deng W, Shuyu E, Tsukahara R, et al. The lysophosphatidic acid type 2 receptor is required for protection against radiation-induced intestinal injury. *Gastroenterology.* 2007;132:1834–1851.

55. Mikkelsen RB, Wardman P. Biological chemistry of reactive oxygen and nitrogen and radiation-induced signal transduction mechanisms. *Oncogene.* 2003;22:5734–5754.

56. Galabova-Kovacs G, Kolbus A, Matzen D, et al. ERK and beyond: insights from B-Raf and Raf-1 conditional knockouts. *Cell Cycle.* 2006;5:1514–1518.

57. Daly MJ. A new perspective on radiation resistance based on *Deinococcus radiodurans. Nat Rev Microbiol.* 2009;7:237–245.

58. He L, Kim SO, Kwon O, et al. ATM blocks tunicamycin-induced endoplasmic reticulum stress. *FEBS Lett.* 2009;583:903–908.

59. Thedieck K, Polak P, Kim ML, et al. PRAS40 and PRR5-like protein are new mTOR interactors that regulate apoptosis. *PLoS ONE.* 2007;2:e1217.

60. Cao C, Subhawong T, Albert JM, et al. Inhibition of mammalian target of rapamycin or apoptotic pathway induces autophagy and radiosensitizes PTEN null prostate cancer cells. *Cancer Res.* 2006;66:10040–10047.

61. Cohen S, Pick E, Oppenheim JJ, eds. *Biology of the Lymphokines.* New York, NY: Academic Press; 1979.

62. Monroy RL, Skelley RR, Taylor P, Dubois A, Donahue RE, MacVittie TJ. Recovery from severe hematopoietic suppression using recombinant human granulocyte macrophage colony stimulating factor. *Exp Hematol.* 1988;16:344–348.

63. Davidson DE, Grenan MM, Sweeney TR. Biological characteristics of some improved radioprotectors. In: Brady LW, ed. *Radiation Sensitizers: Their Use in the Clinical Management of Cancer.* New York , NY: Masson Publishers; 1980: 309–320.

64. Carr CJ, Huff JE, Fisher KD, Huber TE. Protective agents modifying biological effects of radiation. *Arch Environ Health.* 1970;21:88–98.

65. Pizzarello DJ, Colombetti LG, eds. *Radiation Biology.* Boca Raton, FL: CRC Press; 1982.

66. Piper JR, Stringfellow CR Jr, Elliot RD, Johnston TP. S-2-(omega-aminoalkylamino)ethyl dihydrogen phosphorothioates and related compounds as potential antiradiation agents. *J Med Chem.* 1969;12:236–243.

67. Yuhas JM. Biological factors affecting the radioprotective efficiency of S-2-(3-aminopropylamino)ethylphosphorothioic acid (WR-2721): $LD_{50(30)}$ doses. *Radiat Res.* 1970;44:621–628.

68. Yuhas JM, Storer JB. Differential chemoprotection of normal and malignant tissues. *J National Cancer Inst.* 1969;42:331–335.

69. Glover DJ, Glick JH, Weiler C, Hurowitz S, Kligerman M. WR-2721 protects against the hematologic toxicity of cyclophosphamide: a controlled phase II trial. *J Clin Oncol.* 1986;4:584–588.

70. Glover DJ, Glick JH, Weiler C, Fox K, DuPont G. WR-2721 and high dose cisplatin: an active combination in the treatment of metastatic melanoma. *J Clin Oncol.* 1987;5:574–578.

71. Phillips TL. Rationale for initial clinical trials and future development of radioprotectors. *Cancer Clin Trials.* 1980;3:165–173.

72. Turrisi AT, Glover DJ, Hurwitz S, et al. Final report of the Phase I trial of single-dose WR-2721 [5-S-(3-aminopropylamino) ethylphosphorothioic acid]. *Cancer Treat Rep.* 1986;70:1389–1393.

73. Bogo V, Jacobs AJ, Weiss JF. Behavioral toxicity and efficacy of WR-2721 as a radioprotectant. *Radiat Res.* 1985;104:182–190.

74. Landauer MR, Hirsch DD, Dominitz JA, Weiss JF. Dose and time relationships of the radioprotector WR-2721 on locomotor activity in mice. *Pharmacol Biochem Behav.* 1987;27:573–576.

75. Fleckenstein L, Swynnerton N, Ludden TM, Mangold D. Bioavailability and newer methods of delivery of phosphorothioate radioprotectors. *Pharmacol Therap.* 1988;39:203–212.

76. Dubois A, Jacobus JP, Grissom MP, Eng RR, Conklin JJ. Altered gastric emptying and prevention of radiation-induced vomiting in dogs. *Gastroenterology.* 1984;86:444–448.

77. Rasey JS, Magee S, Nelson N, Chin L, Krohn KA. Response of mouse tissues to neutron and gamma radiation: protection by WR-3689 and WR-77913. *Radiother Oncol.* 1990:17:167–173.

78. Rasey JS, Nelson NJ, Mahler P, Anderson K, Krohn KA, Menard T. Radioprotection of normal tissues against gamma rays and cyclotron neutrons with WR-2721: LD_{50} studies and ^{35}S-WR-2721 biodistribution. *Radiat Res.* 1984;97:598–607.

79. Ledney GD, Elliott TE, Harding RA, Jackson WE III, Inal CE, Landauer MR. WR-151327 increases resistance to *Klebsiella pneumoniae* infection in mixed-field- and gamma-photon-irradiated mice. *Int J Radiat Biol.* 2000;76:261–271.

80. Landauer MR, Davis HD, Dominitz JA, Weiss JF. Comparative behavioral toxicity of four sulfhydryl radioprotective compounds in mice: WR-2721, cysteamine, diethyldithiocarbamate, and N-acetylcysteine. *Pharmacol Ther.* 1988;39:97–100.

81. Freeman BA, Crapo JD. Biology of disease: free radicals and tissue injury. *Lab Invest.* 1982;47:412–426.

82. Srinivasan V, Jacobs AJ, Simpson SA, Weiss JF. Radioprotection by vitamin E: effects on hepatic enzymes, delayed type hypersensitivity, and postirradiation survival of mice. In: Prasad KN, ed. *Modulation and Mediation of Cancer by Vitamins.* Basel, Switzerland: Karger; 1983: 119–131.

83. Kumar KS, Srinivasan V, Toles R, Jobe L, Seed TM. Nutritional approaches to radioprotection: vitamin E. *Mil Med.* 2002;167:57–59.

84. Felemovicius I, Bonsack ME, Baptista ML, Delaney JP. Intestinal radioprotection by vitamin E (alpha-tocopherol). *Ann Surg*. 1995;222:504–510.

85. Seifter E, Rettura G, Padawar J, et al. Morbidity and mortality reduction by supplemental vitamin A or beta-carotene in CBA mice given total-body-radiation. *J Natl Cancer Inst*. 1984;73:1167–1177.

86. Kumar KS, Ghosh SP, Hauer-Jensen M. Gamma-tocotrienol: potential as a countermeasure against radiological threat. In: Watson RR and Preedy VR, eds. *Tocotrienols: Vitamin E Beyond Tocopherols*. Boca Raton, FL: CRC Press; 2009: 379–398.

87. Ghosh SP, Kulkarni S, Hieber K, et al. Gamma-tocotrienol, a tocol antioxidant as a potent radioprotector. *Int J Radiat Biol*. 2009;85:598–606.

88. Berbée M, Fu Q, Boerma M, Wang J, Kumar KS, Hauer-Jensen M. Gamma-tocotrienol ameliorates intestinal radiation injury and reduces vascular oxidative stress after total-body irradiation by an HMG-CoA reductase-dependent mechanism. *Radiat Res*. 2009;171:596–605.

89. Seifter E, Mendecki J, Holtzman S, et al. Role of vitamin A and beta-carotene in radiation protection: relation to antioxidant properties. *Pharmacol Ther*. 1988;39:357–365.

90. Fusi S, Kupper TS, Green DG, Ariyan S. Reversal of postburn immunosuppression by the administration of vitamin A. *Surgery*. 1984;96:330–335.

91. Weiss JF, Hoover RL, Kumar KS. Selenium pretreatment enhances the radioprotective effect and reduces the lethal toxicity of WR-2721. *Free Radic Res Commun*. 1987;3:33–38.

92. Weiss JF, Kumar KS, Walden TL, Neta R, Landauer MR, Clark EP. Advances in radioprotection through the use of combined agent regimens. *Int J Radiat Biol*. 1990;57:709–722.

93. Petkau A. Radiation protection by superoxide dismutase. *Photochem Photobiol*. 1978;28:765–774.

94. Srinivasan V, Doctrow S, Singh VK, Whitnall MH. Evaluation of EUK-189, a synthetic superoxide dismutase/catalase mimetic as a radiation countermeasure. *Immunopharmacol Immunotoxicol*. 2008;30:271–290.

95. Davis TA, Clarke TK, Mog SR, Landauer MR. Subcutaneous administration of genistein prior to lethal irradiation supports multilineage, hematopoietic progenitor cell recovery and survival. *Int J Radiat Biol*. 2007;83:141–151.

96. Davis TA, Mungunsukh O, Zins S, Day RM, Landauer MR. Genistein induces radioprotection by hematopoietic stem cell quiescence. *Int J Radiat Biol*. 2008;84:713–726.

97. Uma Devi P, Ganasoundari A, Rao BS, Srinivasan KK. In vivo radioprotection by ocimum flavonoids: survival of mice. *Radiat Res*. 1999;151:74–78.

98. Uma Devi P, Satyamitra M. Protection against prenatal irradiation-induced genomic instability and its consequences in adult mice by Ocimum flavonoids, orientin and vicenin. *Int J Radiat Biol*. 2004;80:653–662.

99. Walden TL Jr, Patchen M, Snyder SL. 16,16-Dimethyl prostaglandin E, increases survival in mice following irradiation. *Radiat Res*. 1987;109:440–448.

100. Kumar KS, Srinivasan V, Palazzolo D, Kendrick JM, Clark EP. Synergistic protection of irradiated mice by a combination of iloprost and misoprostol. *Adv Exp Med Biol*. 1997;400B:831–839.

101. Walden TL Jr, Patchen ML, MacVittie TJ. Leukotriene-induced radioprotection of hematopoietic stem cells in mice. *Radiat Res*. 1988;113:388–395.

102. Ainsworth EJ. From endotoxins to newer immunomodulators: survival-promoting effects of microbial polysaccharide complexes in irradiated animals. *Pharmacol Ther*. 1988;39:223–241.

103. Chirigos MA, Patchen ML. Survey of newer biological response modifiers for possible use in radioprotection. *Pharmacol Ther.* 1988;39:243–246.

104. Madonna GS, Ledney GD, Elliott TB, et al. Trehalose dimycolate enhances resistance to infection in neutropenic animals. *Infect Immun.* 1989;57:2495–2501.

105. Madonna GS, Ledney GD, Funckes DC, Ribi EE. Monophosphoryl lipid A and trehalose dimycolate therapy enhances survival in sublethally irradiated mice challenged with *Klebsiella pneumonia.* In: Masihi KN, Lange W. eds. *Immunomodulators and Non-Specific Host Defense Mechanisms Against Microbial Infections.* Oxford, UK: Pergamon Press; 1988: 351–356.

106. Neta R. Role of cytokines in radioprotection. *Pharmacol Ther.* 1988;39:261–266.

107. Neta R, Monroy R, MacVittie TJ. Utility of interleukin-1 in therapy of radiation injury as studied in small and large animal models. *Biotherapy.* 1989;1:301–311.

108. Okunieff P, Wu T, Huang K, Ding I. Differential radioprotection of three mouse strains by basic or acidic fibroblast growth factor. *Br J Cancer Suppl.* 1996;27:S105–S108.

109. Okunieff P, Mester M, Wang J, et al. In vivo radioprotective effects of angiogenic growth factors on the small bowel of C3H mice. *Radiat Res.* 1998;150:204–211.

110. Motomura K, Hagiwara A, Komi-Kuramochi A, et al. An FGF1:FGF2 chimeric growth factor exhibits universal FGF receptor specificity, enhanced stability and augmented activity useful for epithelial proliferation and radioprotection. *Biochim Biophys Acta.* 2008;1780:1432–1440.

111. Zhang M, Qian J, Xing X, et al. Inhibition of the tumor necrosis factor-alpha pathway is radioprotective for the lung. *Clin Cancer Res.* 2008;14:1868–1876.

112. Kalechman Y, Gafter U, Barkai IS, Albeck M, Sredni B. Mechanism of radioprotection conferred by the immunomodulator AS101. *Exp Hematol.* 1993;21:150–155.

113. Whitnall MH, Villa V, Seed TM, et al. Molecular specificity of 5-androstenediol as a systemic radioprotectant in mice. *Immunopharmacol Immunotoxicol.* 2005;27:15–32.

114. Stickney DR, Dowding C, Authier S, et al. 5-androstenediol improves survival in clinically unsupported rhesus monkeys with radiation-induced myelosuppression. *Int Immunopharmacol.* 2007;7:500–505.

115. Whitnall MH, Wilhelmsen CL, McKinney L, Miner V, Seed TM, Jackson WE III. Radioprotective efficacy and acute toxicity of 5-androstenediol after subcutaneous or oral administration in mice. *Immunopharmacol Immunotoxicol.* 2002;24:595–626.

116. Xiao M, Inal CE, Parekh V, Chang CM, Whitnall MH. 5-Androstenediol promotes survival of gamma-irradiated human hematopoietic progenitors through induction of nuclear factor-kappaB activation and granulocyte colony-stimulating factor expression. *Mol Pharmacol.* 2007;72:370–379.

117. Singh VK, Grace MB, Jacobsen KO, et al. Administration of 5-androstenediol to mice: pharmacokinetics and cytokine gene expression. *Exp Mol Pathol.* 2008;84:178–188.

118. Neta R, Oppenheim JJ, Douches SD. Interdependence of IL-I, TNF, and CSFs in radioprotection. *J Immunol.* 1988;140:108–111.

119. Dinarello CA, Mier JW. Lymphokines. *N Eng J Med.* 1987;317:940–945.

120. Fukumoto R, Kiang JG. Geldanamycin analog 17-DMAG limits apoptosis in human peripheral blood cells by inhibition of p53 activation and its interaction with heat shock protein 90 kDa after ionizing radiation. *Radiat Res.* 176:333-345, 2011.

121. Kiang JG, Smith JT, Agravante NG. Geldanamycin analog 17-DMAG inhibits iNOS and caspases in gamma irradiated human T cells. *Radiat Res*. 2009;172:321–330.

122. Gorbunov NV, Kiang JG. Up-regulation of autophagy in the small intestine Paneth cell in response to total-body gamma-irradiation. *J Pathol*. 2009;217:242–252.

123. Maisin JR, Mattelin G, Fridman-Manduzio A, van der Parren J. Reduction of short-and long-term radiation lethality by mixtures of chemical protectors. *Radiat Res*. 1968;35:26–34.

124. Ledney GD, Jiao W, Elliott TB, Kiang JG. Combined injury: therapeutic studies. In: *55th Radiation Research Society Annual Meeting*. Savannah, GA: Radiation Research Society; 2009. Abstract 112.

125. Kiang JG, Jiao W, Cary L, et al. Wound trauma increases radiation-induced mortality by activation of iNOS pathway and elevation of cytokine concentrations and bacterial infection. *Radiat Res*. 2010;173:319–332.

126. Patchen ML, Brook I, Elliott TB, Jackson WE. Adverse effects of pefloxacin in irradiated C3H/HeN mice: correction with glucan therapy. *Antimicrob Agents Chemother*. 1993;37:1882–1889.

127. Patchen ML, MacVittie TJ, Weiss JF. Combined modality radioprotection: the use of glucan and selenium with WR-2721. *Int J Radiat Oncol Biol Phys*. 1990;18:1069–1075.

128. Srinivasan V, Weiss JF. Radioprotection by vitamin E: injectable vitamin E administered alone or with WR-3689 enhances survival of irradiated mice. *Int J Radiat Oncol Biol Phys*. 1992;23:841–845.

129. Wambi C, Sanzari J, Wan XS, et al. Protective effects of dietary antioxidants on proton total-body irradiation-mediated hematopoietic cell and animal survival. *Radiat Res*. 2009;172:175–186.

130. Kunwar A, Narang H, Priyadarsini KI, Krishna M, Pandey R, Sainis KB. Effect of curcumin and curcumin copper complex (1:1) on radiation-induced changes of anti-oxidant enzymes levels in the livers of Swiss albino mice. *J Cell Biochem*. 2007;102:1214–1224.

131. Mantena SK, Unnikrishnan MK, Chandrasekharan K. Radioprotection by copper and zinc complexes of 5-aminosalicylic acid: a preliminary study. *J Environ Pathol Toxicol Oncol*. 2008;27:123–134.

132. Burdelya LG, Krivokrysenko VI, Tallant TC, et al. An agonist of toll-like receptor 5 has radioprotective activity in mouse and primate models. *Science*. 2008;320:226–230.

133. Davis TA, Mungunsukh O, Zins S, Day RM, Landauer MR. Genistein induces radioprotection by hematopoietic stem cell quiescence. *Int J Radiat Biol*. 2008;84:713–726.

134. Fu Q, Berbée M, Boerma M, Wang J, Schmid HA, Hauer-Jensen M. The somatostatin analog SOM230 (pasireotide) ameliorates injury of the intestinal mucosa and increases survival after total-body irradiation by inhibiting exocrine pancreatic secretion. *Radiat Res*. 2009;171:698–707.

135. Zhang X, Epperly MW, Kay MA, et al. Radioprotection in vitro and in vivo by minicircle plasmid carrying the human manganese superoxide dismutase transgene. *Hum Gene Ther*. 2008;19:820–826.

136. Trickler WJ, Nagvekar AA, Dash AK. The in vitro sub-cellular localization and in vivo efficacy of novel chitosan/GMO nanostructures containing paclitaxel. *Pharm Res*. 2009;26:1963–1973.

CHAPTER 12

CYTOGENETIC BIODOSIMETRY

PATAJE G.S. PRASANNA, PhD,* AND C. NORMAN COLEMAN, MD, FACP, FACR, FASTRO†

INTRODUCTION

BIODOSIMETRY PRINCIPLES
Lymphocyte Cell Cycle
Human Karyotype
Chromosome Structure
Radiation-Induced Chromosome Aberrations

BIODOSIMETRY BY DICENTRIC ASSAY
Blood Sampling, Culturing, and Analysis
Influencing Factors for Dose Assessment
Assay Harmonization, Quality Control, and Assurance
Laboratory Automation and Information Management
Triage Dose Prediction

SUMMARY: TREATMENT IMPLICATIONS

*Program Director, Radiation Research Program, National Cancer Institute, National Institutes of Health, Executive Plaza North, 6015A, Room 6020, 6130 Executive Boulevard, MSC 7440, Bethesda, Maryland 20889; formerly, Principal Investigator, Armed Forces Radiobiology Research Institute, Bethesda, Maryland
†Senior Medical Advisor and Team Leader, Office of the Assistant Secretary for Preparedness and Response, US Department of Health and Human Services, 200 Independence Avenue, Room 638G, Washington, DC 20201; and Associate Director, Radiation Research Program, Division of Cancer Therapeutics and Diagnosis, National Cancer Institute, National Institutes of Health, Executive Plaza North, Room 6014, 6130 Executive Boulevard, MSC 7440, Bethesda, Maryland 20892; formerly, Professor and Chairman, Harvard Joint Center for Radiation Therapy, Boston, Massachusetts

INTRODUCTION

Biological dosimetry is the measurement of radiation-induced changes in the human body to assess acute- and long-term health risks. Biological dose estimation provides an independent means of obtaining dose information otherwise exclusively based on computer modeling, dose reconstruction, and physical dosimetry. Various biodosimetry tools are available and certain characteristics make some more valuable than others (Exhibit 12-1).

Cytogenetic methods now occupy a unique and valuable niche in biological dosimetry.[1] When available, cytogenetic analysis can complement physical dosimetry by confirming or ruling out a radiological exposure. When physical dosimetry is unavailable, cytogenetic analysis is often the only available dose estimation method. Cytogenetic biodosimetry using human peripheral blood lymphocytes (HPBLs) following an accidental overexposure was first used in the 1962 Recuplex criticality accident in Hanford, Washington.[2] Since then it has been used in response to several radiation accidents, such as that at Chernobyl (Ukraine), Goiânia (Brazil), and Tokaimura (Japan), for dose assessment, as well to resolve suspected occupational overexposures.

Estimated doses using cytogenetic methods correlate well with the severity of acute radiation syndrome (ARS).[3] In the Chernobyl accident, dosimetry was approximated by rapid preliminary examination of 50 lymphocyte metaphases per person for several individuals,[4] although accurate dose assessment involves analysis of 500 to 1,000 metaphase spreads taken from the peripheral blood lymphocyte (PBL) cultures obtained from a radiation-exposed individual. The radiation accidents above emphasized the importance of cytogenetic methods in early dose assessment after a radiological event in influencing treatment decisions; as a result, many countries have set up laboratories for

***

EXHIBIT 12-1

CHARACTERISTICS OF AN IDEAL BIODOSIMETER

***

- Shows dose-effect relationship
- Demonstrates radiation specificity
- Persists after exposure
- Shows low interindividual variation
- Provides results within a clinically relevant time
- Estimates fraction of the body irradiated and dose to that fraction in partial-body exposures
- Can assess in fractionated and chronic exposures
- Has known radiation quality effects
- Uses sampling that is noninvasive or semi-invasive
- Is amenable to automation

***

biological dosimetry. Cytogenetic methods, which are standardized and routinely used, are also employed to assess the late effects of irradiation. A technical manual and standards for laboratory accreditations are also available.[5–7]

Small volumes (less than 10 mL) of peripheral blood are obtained by phlebotomy from exposed subjects as soon as practical (generally 1 day after exposure) and sent to a cytogenetic biodosimetry laboratory for dose assessment. The laboratory processes samples according to its established protocols. Cytogenetic damage is then assessed by experts and dose assessment is made by comparison with an appropriate calibration curve, taking into consideration radiation type, dose rate, whole- or partial-body exposures, delay between samplings, and specific cytogenetic assessment.[5]

BIODOSIMETRY PRINCIPLES

Lymphocyte Cell Cycle

PBLs are routinely used for cytogenetic biodosimetry. They have diploid deoxyribonucleic acid (DNA) content (2n) and are predominantly in a "quiescent" state; therefore, they do not normally undergo cell division. There are two types of circulating PBLs: T and B lymphocytes. T lymphocytes (specifically the CD4+ and CD8+ subtypes) can be stimulated by mitogen (eg, phytohemagglutinin) to grow in culture. First-division cycle metaphases are harvested from lymphocyte cultures for assessing radiation dose. Upon stimulation, T lymphocytes undergo a

cell-division cycle, which is divided into two brief periods: interphase (gap 1 [G_1], synthesis [S], and gap 2 [G_2] phases) and mitosis (M phase). In interphase, the cell grows and replicates its DNA; in mitosis, it divides into two distinct daughter cells. In general, regulatory molecules, cyclins, and cyclin-dependent kinases (CDKs) regulate eukaryotic cell cycles.[8] Cyclin D is the first cyclin produced in response to extracellular growth signals. When activated by a bound cyclin, CDKs perform phosphorylation, which in turn activates or inactivates target proteins to a synchronized entry into the next phase of the cell cycle.

Cell-cycle regulation is mediated via cell-cycle

checkpoints[9] such that entry and exit of cells from each phase depends on the proper progression and completion of the previous phase. Cell-cycle checkpoints prevent cycle progression at specific points, allowing completion verification of the necessary phase and DNA damage repair. The cell does not proceed to the next phase until all checkpoint requirements are met. The presence of several checkpoints ensures that damaged or incomplete DNA is not passed on to daughter cells. Two main checkpoints are the G_1/S checkpoint and the G_2/M checkpoint. Genes such as protein 53 play important roles in triggering the control mechanisms at both the G_1/S and G_2/M checkpoints.

G_1 Phase

Within interphase, the stage from the end of the previous M phase until the beginning of DNA synthesis is called the G_1 phase. This phase is marked by the synthesis of enzymes that are required for DNA replication in the S phase. Upon receiving a promitotic extracellular signal, G_1 cyclin-CDK complexes activate to prepare the cell for the S phase, promoting the expression of transcription factors that in turn promote the expression of S cyclins and enzymes required for DNA replication. The G_1 cyclin-CDK complexes also promote the degradation of molecules that function as S-phase inhibitors.

S Phase

The S phase follows the G_1 phase, commencing with DNA synthesis. Upon completion of the S phase, all chromosomes are replicated, quadruplicating the DNA content. Each chromosome now consists of two (sister) chromatids. Ribonucleic acid transcription and protein synthesis rates are very low, barring histone production, which is crucial for chromatin packaging. Active S cyclin-CDK complexes phosphorylate proteins in the prereplication complexes, which are assembled during the G_1 phase. The phosphorylation serves two purposes: (1) to activate the already-assembled prereplication complex, and (2) to prevent new complexes from forming. This ensures that every portion of the cell's genome is replicated only once.

G_2 Phase

The G_2 phase follows the S phase, which lasts until the cell enters mitosis. Again, significant protein synthesis occurs during this phase, mainly involving the production of microtubules that are required for transporting sister chromatids to opposite poles to divide the nucleus. Inhibition of protein synthesis during the G_2 phase prevents the cell from undergoing mitosis.

M Phase

The M phase follows the G_2 phase and sequentially consists of prophase, metaphase, anaphase, and telophase. In mitosis, karyokinesis (division of chromosomes between the two daughter cells), and cytokinesis (division of cytoplasm) occur. Mitotic cyclin-CDK complexes promote the initiation of mitosis by stimulating the synthesis of downstream proteins involved in chromosome condensation and mitotic spindle assembly, preparing for chromosome segregation. Anaphase-promoting complex, a critical protein complex, is activated during this phase, promoting degradation of structural proteins associated with the chromosomal kinetochore. Anaphase-promoting complex also targets the mitotic cyclins for degradation, ensuring the progression of telophase culminates in cytokinesis.

HPBLs are highly differentiated and are in a synchronized quiescent state, called "G_0." Following stimulation in culture, this synchrony is maintained; at least until the first-division cycle is complete. Although the lymphocyte cell-cycle time depends on culture conditions, DNA synthesis starts around 26 hours after culture initiation, and first-division mitoses start to appear around 36 hours after stimulation. DNA synthesis peaks at 34 and 40 hours, resulting in two peaks of respective mitotic activity around 44 and 49 hours of culture initiation.[5] Irradiation of lymphocytes as well as the presence of chromosomal aberrations induce a delay in cell-cycle progression as well as asynchrony, to some extent.

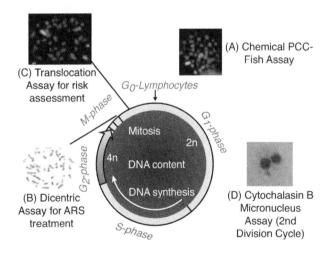

Figure 12-1. Various cytogenetic assays performed using human peripheral blood lymphocytes in different cell cycle phases. (*a*) Chemical premature chromosome condensation assay. (*b*) Dicentric assay. (*c*) Translocation assay. (*d*) Cytochalasin B micronucleus assay.
ARS: acute radiation syndrome
DNA: deoxyribonucleic acid

Various cytogenetic assays (Figure 12-1) can be performed using HPBLs. Premature chromosome condensation (PCC) assay is performed in the G_0/G_1 phase, where chromatin material is condensed prematurely by means of mitotic cell fusion,[10] phosphatase inhibitors,[11] or mitotisis-promoting factors in conjunction with phosphatase inhibitors[12] to study radiation-induced chromosome damage. Dicentric and chromosome translocation assays are performed after DNA replication, using metaphase spreads specifically for analyzing structural chromosomal aberrations (see Figure 12-1, b and c). In the second-division cycle, cytome assay[13] (including micronucleus and nucleoplasmic bridges) is performed (see Figure 12-1, d).

Human Karyotype

Based on the relative size of chromosomes and the position of the centromere (the point of spindle attachment during mitosis or the primary region of constriction) along the longitudinal axis, chromosomes are arranged in the form of a karyotype. The human karyotype consists of 46 chromosomes (44 autosomes and 2 sex chromosomes) and are classified into 7 groups: A, B, C, D, E, F, and G (Figure 12-2).

Group A consists of three pairs of large, metacentric (centromere position is in the middle of the longitudinal axis) chromosomes, 1, 2, and 3. Chromosome 1 is the largest pair of metacentric chromosomes in the human karyotype. Group B consists of chromosomes 4 and 5, which are large, submetacentric chromosomes (the centromere is located off center, dividing the chromosome's arms into "short" and "long" arms). Chromosomes are arranged in the karyotype with the short arm on the top and long arm on the bottom. Group C consists of chromosomes 6 through

12. These are all mid-sized, submetacentric chromosomes relative to group B chromosomes. The D group consists of chromosomes 13 through 15. All three pairs are large acrocentrics, where the centromere is positioned toward the terminal end of the chromosomes. Often these chromosomes display a "satellite," small chromatin material in the form of a dot. A smaller metacentric chromosome (16) and two smaller submetacentric chromosomes (17 and 18) constitute group E. Group F consists of chromosome pairs 19 and 20; the smallest metacentrics. Chromosome pairs 21 and 22, the smallest acrocentics, form group G. The G group chromosomes frequently display satellites. Sex chromosomes in a male karyotype consist of an X chromosome, which is medium sized (similar to C group chromosomes) and a Y chromosome, which is a small, acrocentric chromosome similar to G group chromosomes. Sex chromosomes in a female karyotype consist of two X chromosomes.

Simultaneous visualization of all pairs of chromosomes in different colors is now possible with the use of molecular cytogenetic techniques, using combinatorial labeling to generate many different colors unique to specific chromosomes with limited, spectrally distinct fluorophores. Spectral differences among chromosomes are captured using a fluorescent microscope to analyze structural aberrations.

Chromosome Structure

The DNA backbone is made up of sugar, phosphates, and holding bases, as well as adenine, thymine, guanine, and cytosine, which carry genetic information. The basic premise of cell biology is that the chromosomes are dynamically modified in interphase and condense during mitosis. Cytogenetic examination of radiation-induced damage is mostly analyzed using condensed chromosomes, such as metaphase chromosomes. Historically, three different conceptual classes of models for metaphase chromosome architecture have evolved. They are the chromatin network, hierarchical folding, and radial loop ("scaffold") models, which are quite different in terms of structural motifs, giving rise to chromosome condensation. In the chromatin network model, chromosomes are stabilized by protein cross-links between adjacent chromatin fibers every 15 kilobases, on average.[14] In the hierarchical models of chromosome folding, 10- and 30-nm chromatin fibers fold progressively in larger fibers (chromonema) that coil and form the metaphase chromosomes.[15]

The scaffold model assumes loops of chromatin are attached to an axial chromosome structure, or "scaffold," formed by nonhistone proteins, topoisomerase IIα, and structural maintenance of chro-

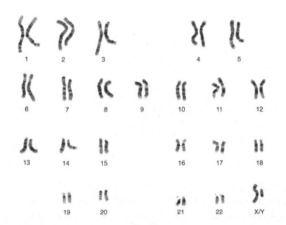

Figure 12-2. The human karyotype.
Courtesy of the National Library of Medicine.

mosomes (SMCs).[16] This model is consistent with the relationships of observed structural dimensions and the "central dogma of molecular biology" related to transcription, replication, and matrix attachment domains.[17] The DNA double helix is folded in alternating coiling-and-loop formation, induced by the packaging of histones and nonhistone proteins spooled in a tight helix. Histones H2A, H2B, H3, and H4 form "core" histones, and H1 and H5 form "linker" histones. Two of each core histones form a nucleosome core by wrapping the DNA double helix. The DNA is locked into place by binding the nucleosome, and entry and exit sites of the DNA double helix by the linker histone, H1.

Condensins and topoisomerase II appear to play an important role in the dynamics of chromosome condensation. The axial distribution of topoisomerase IIα and the condensing subunit, SMC 2, in unextracted metaphase chromosomes, with SMC 2 localizing to 150 to 200 nm diameter central core, is now confirmed by examination of interphase chromosomes.[16] Early prophase condensation occurs through the folding of large-scale chromatin fibers into condensed masses. These resolve into linear, middle prophase chromatids measuring 200 to 300 nm in diameter that double in diameter by late prophase. Hierarchical levels of chromatin folding are stabilized late in mitosis by this axial "glue" of topoisomerase IIα and SMC 2.[17]

Gene analyses are often based on short stretches of only a few kilobases of DNA; however, an orderly transcription and replication can also involve highly folded chromosomal domains containing hundreds of kilobases of DNA. Three-dimensional chromosomal domains within the nucleus may also contribute to phenotypic expression of genes and induced aberrations.

Radiation-Induced Chromosome Aberrations

For cytogenetic biological dosimetry using HPBLs, it is important to quantify aberrations in first-division cycle metaphase spreads, where structural changes are observed in their entirety without the confounding effects of elimination and dilution of aberrations associated with cell division. Classification and relationships of induced chromosomal structural changes are discussed in great detail by Savage.[18] Generally, there are two broad categories of structural chromosomal aberrations induced by irradiation: chromosome type and chromatid type. In the former, the induced changes are always visualized in both the sister chromatids of a chromosome, whereas in the latter only one of the sister chromatids is affected. Chromosome-type aberrations arise from damage of the chromatid thread in its pre-DNA synthesis stage (unreplicated), and this damage

is duplicated along with the chromosome during cell-cycle progression through the S phase. Since HPBLs are largely in a presynthetic phase of the cell cycle, irradiation produces only chromosome-type aberrations (ie, damage affecting both the chromatids); therefore, the description below focuses only on chromosome-type structural aberrations. Chromatid-types of structural aberrations are produced only when the cells are irradiated during or after chromosome duplication. Chromosome-type structural aberrations are rarely found after chemical or drug exposure, when cells are examined in their first-division cycle.

Exchanges

Interchanges. Asymmetrical interchanges (dicentrics) result in a chromosome with two centromeres along with a single acentric fragment. In order to produce a dicentric aberration, DNA lesions are necessary in two unreplicated chromosomes (circulating lymphocytes are in their pre-DNA synthetic stage) in close proximity with respect to time and space so that the damaged chromosomes can undergo an exchange. The exchange is radiation specific and can occur either as a result of a misrepair of DNA strand breaks induced directly by radiation, or as a result of misrepair during excision repair of base damage. The distance between centromeres can vary from being indistinguishable to spanning almost the total length of the arms involved. Dicentrics are the most easily recognizable and unambiguous aberrations to score in the spectrum of radiation-induced chromosomal aberrations. The cells containing dicentrics are rapidly lost from the cell population because of mechanical difficulties during cell division. The associated acentric fragment is usually excluded from the daughter nuclei, often forming a micronucleus resulting in a genetically deficient daughter nucleus.

Symmetrical interchange (reciprocal translocation), the symmetrical counterpart of the dicentric, is a reciprocal transfer of terminal portions of two separate chromosomes. These are often undetected with conventional staining methods. Reciprocal translocations can be transmitted to subsequent cell generations; therefore, they are often referred to as "stable" translocations.

Intrachanges. Interarm intrachanges, when asymmetric and complete, form centric rings and are often scored along with dicentrics for dose estimation. They are analogous to asymmetrical interchanges, where two lesions in different arms of the same chromosomes form a loop around the centromere. An acentric fragment is also formed. At anaphase, because of failure to freely separate, these may form interlocking rings, leading to the formation of bridges.

Symmetrical interarm intrachanges (pericentric inversion), when complete, lead to a pericentric inversion involving inversion of the arms by 180°. Unless this results in a very obvious change in centromere index or the arm ratio, such aberration is undetectable.

In intraarm intrachange (interstitial deletions), the interaction of two lesions within an unduplicated chromosome arm can result in deletion of a region interstitial to the centromere and the telomere. Ends of the deleted portion may rejoin, forming an acentric ring, whereas the chromosome arm may be shortened. At anaphase, interstitial deletions, which lack a centromere or point of spindle attachment like other acentric fragments or terminal deletions (see Breaks, below), lag and form a micronucleus. Occasionally, the interstitial segment between two segments may be reversed or inverted. Since there is no change in the arm ratio, such aberrations are also undetectable.

Breaks (terminal deletions, chromosome breaks). Breaks arise because of a complete severance of a terminal region of a chromosome arm. The size of the deletion may vary. Small deletions are difficult to identify; therefore, often in cytogenetic biodosimetry, these are categorized together with interstitial deletions and called "fragments" or "deletions." However, when scoring, acentric fragments arising from dicentrics or centric rings are invariably excluded from the category of fragments or deletions.

BIODOSIMETRY BY DICENTRIC ASSAY

Because of their radiation specificity, dicentrics, a common structural aberration, in an individual's PBLs indicate radiation exposure. They show a very good dose-effect relationship for different radiation types. For low-LET (linear energy transfer) radiation, the dose-effect relationship is linear–quadratic; for high-LET radiation, the relationship is linear (Figure 12-3). Lymphocyte exposure in vitro or in vivo produces similar levels of dicentrics per gray.[5] Therefore, observed dicentric yield in an exposed person's PBLs can be converted to absorbed dose by comparison with an appropriate calibration curve. Because of low background levels (about 1 dicentric chromosome in 1,000 cells), high sensitivity (a threshold dose of 0.05 Gy), very low interindividual variation, and ability to assess partial-body exposure, dicentric assay (DCA) is considered the "gold standard" biodosimetry method. Estimated doses using DCA correlate well with the severity of ARS.

Blood Sampling, Culturing, and Analysis

Small volumes (less than 10 mL) of peripheral blood are collected from exposed subjects in vacutainers containing a suitable anticoagulant as soon as practical, generally 1 day after exposure, and sent to a cytogenetic biodosimetry laboratory for blood culturing, metaphase spread harvesting, and DCA for dose estimation. The laboratory processes samples in accordance with internationally accepted protocols and guidelines. Briefly, either whole blood, lymphocyte-enriched buffy coat, or isolated PBLs are stimulated by a mitogen (eg, phytohemagglutinin) to grow in culture and cells in first-division cycle metaphases are collected on glass slides. Specimen collection procedures for cytogenetic biodosimetry are described elsewhere in the literature.[19] Metaphase spreads are then stained and dicentric chromosomes are counted by microscopy to estimate dose by comparison with an appropriate calibration.

Influencing Factors for Dose Assessment

Radiation Type and Dose Rate

Most accidental radiation exposures involve gamma or X-rays. Since there is a difference in the yield of dicentrics with energy between gamma and X-rays, it is imperative to equate the dicentric yield with an appropriate calibration curve for dose assessment. Occasionally radiation accidents may also involve degraded neutrons. Since the energy spectrum for degraded neutrons is similar to that for fission spectrum neutrons, the linear dose-effect calibration curve for fission neutrons is normally used for dose estimation. For low-LET radiations, dose rate is an important determinant of dicentric yield, particu-

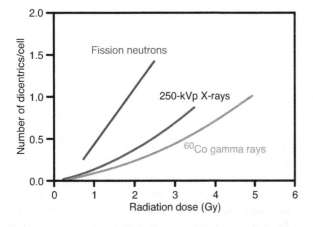

Figure 12-3. Dose-response relationship for dicentrics in human lymphocytes for three radiation qualities.

larly in the quadratic component of a dose-response curve. The dicentric yield reduces with dose rate. For biodosimetry triage during a nuclear detonation, most radiation-only injuries will be caused by fallout. While there may be some neutron component, the dose estimation is done assuming only gamma-ray exposure.

Sampling Delay

The persistence of dicentrics in HPBLs is closely related to the life span of the blood lymphocytes. Renewal of circulating lymphocytes from bone marrow stem cells will result in dilution of dicentric frequency with time following exposure, and hence, dose underestimation. Lymphocyte half-life can vary among individuals; however, no correction for the assessed dose is necessary when sampling is done before 4 to 6 weeks after exposure. Dose assessment is still possible by DCA up to 3 years after exposure, with the appropriate correction based on lymphocyte half-life in circulating pool.

Heterogeneity of Irradiation

Accidental irradiations often result in inhomogeneous dose distribution and irradiated and unirradiated lymphocytes are mixed. In such cases, the overall dicentric frequency following a high-dose exposure of a small part of the body can be equal to the overall frequency after exposure of a large portion of the body to a lower dose. With uniform whole-body exposures to low-LET radiations, the dicentrics follow a Poisson distribution; with significant partial-body exposures, the distribution is non-Poisson. Two statistical methods are generally used to assess partial-body exposures: Dolphin's contaminated Poisson method and Sasaki's QDR (Quantity of Dicentrics and Rings) method.[5] The frequency of metaphase spreads without dicentric aberrations can be used to identify patients with partial-body exposure and cohorts suitable for cytokine therapy after radiation accidents.[20] Dose estimations following internal radionuclide contamination are difficult and estimated doses are less certain. However, since incidence of dicentrics in circulating lymphocytes is radiation-specific, the presence of dicentrics may be used in identifying internal contamination of radionuclides.

Statistical Considerations

Dose estimation requires constructing a calibration curve by the maximum likelihood method and deriving dose and confidence intervals by comparing observed dicentric yield with a chosen calibration curve. Deriving a dose from the measured yield of dicentrics is relatively easy, but the degree of accuracy and precision on the assessed dose depends on the confidence limits of the calibration curve used, number of metaphase spreads analyzed, or number of dicentrics observed in a given number of metaphase spreads. Generally, a 95% confidence limit is chosen to express uncertainty on the assessed dose, and at lower doses, dose estimate is based on the analysis of at least 500 metaphases.

However, for risk-based stratification in radiation mass casualty and emergency situations, scoring 20 to 50 metaphase spreads is adequate to provide information on dose and the nature of dose distribution (ie, whether the irradiation is partial- or whole-body based on the distribution of dicentrics among the analyzed cell population).[20] Statistical methods for constructing calibration curves and assessing dose are not available in routine statistical software. Several laboratories have generic programs, which are not especially user-friendly, quality controlled, or widely available. Two cytogenetic dose assessment software tools, Chromosomal Aberration Calculation Software (CABAS; this free program can be downloaded at http://www.ujk.edu.pl/ibiol/cabas/index.htm)[21] and Dose Estimate (Health Protection Agency Centre for Radiation, Chemical and Environmental Hazards, Didcot, England)[22] are now available.

Other factors that influence dose assessment (to a lesser degree) in DCA include age, whether or not the individual smokes, and genetic predisposition.

Assay Harmonization, Quality Control, and Assurance

The DCA's variability and accuracy among different cytogenetic laboratories was determined in an interlaboratory comparison study. Minimum variability was found in calibration curves among established laboratories, and biologically predicted dose was accurate against physical doses (Figure 12-4).[1] However, it is important to determine dose based on each laboratory's own calibration. For a given number of dicentrics, comparison with another laboratory's calibration curve may lead to erroneous dose assessment if the calibration curves are inherently different.

Laboratory protocols and quality-control standards are available. The International Atomic Energy Agency revised technical details of laboratory protocols, standardizing methodologies,[19,23] and the International Organization for Standardization developed compliance standards for laboratory accreditation.[6] Performance criteria for cytogenetic triage in a radiation mass casualty situation are also available.[7]

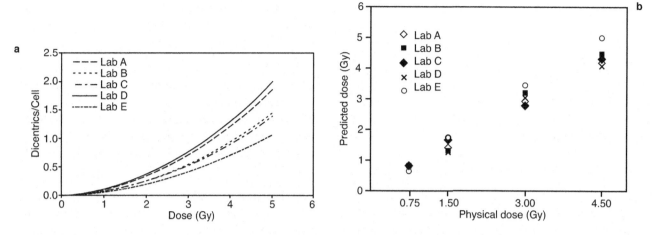

Figure 12-4. Comparison of radiation dose-effect calibration curves for (*a*) cobalt-60 gamma radiation for dicentric yield among established cytogenetic laboratories and (*b*) distribution of predicted biological doses to dose-blinded samples for actual physical doses in all laboratories. Reproduced with permission from: Wilkins RC, Romm H, Kao TC, et al. Interlaboratory comparison of the dicentric assay for radiation biodosimetry in mass casualty events. *Radiat Res.* 2008;169:551–560.

Laboratory Automation and Information Management

Laboratory automation and information management is essential for practical applications of cytogenetic assays in radiation mass casualties. Cytogenetic sample preparation, DCAs for dose assessments, and cytogenic data management are time-consuming and laborious in a large-scale disaster. For dose-based stratification of exposed subjects to estimate risk for developing ARS in mass casualties, whole blood is processed through a cytogenetic laboratory's various automated equipment stations. A laboratory information management system (LIMS) will allow sample tracking and prioritization as well as data and resource management. LIMS should be flexible, scalable, and upgradable for automated cytogenetic sample processing of metaphase spreads from whole blood. Automation by customization and integration of commercial, off-the-shelf technologies can support quality control and assurance, as well as increase throughput and the occupational safety of laboratory personnel in a biologically hazardous, high-throughput laboratory environment.[24] In the Armed Forces Radiobiology Research Institute's automated cytogenetic laboratory, a customized, automated, liquid-handling robot enclosed in an engineered Biosafety Level 2 environment and integrated with an automated cell viability analyzer and automated centrifuge performs high-throughput blood-sample processing, eliminating an important rate-limiting bottleneck in sample processing for cytogenetic dose assessment and maintaining sample chain-of-custody via barcoding and sample

tracking in LIMS. Because there is no difference in radiation-induced dicentric yield between whole blood and isolated lymphocyte cultures,[25] a whole-blood culture method may be preferred in mass casualty situations to enhance throughput. Metaphase harvesters are used to eliminate the labor-intensive and repetitive tasks involved in metaphase harvesting from blood cultures (ie, centrifugation, aspiration and disposal of supernatant, treatment with hypotonic and fixative solutions) under controlled environmental conditions in a one-step protocol, thus enhancing quality and reproducibility. Similarly, a metaphase spreader provides optimal environmental conditions of temperature and humidity for spreading cell suspension on glass slides. An autostainer provides a rapid and consistent method of staining slides with Giemsa and requires minimal human involvement. Intelligent, flexible, and tandem sample scheduling can allow up to 1,000 samples per week in such an automated cytogenetic laboratory. A sample priority assignment feature in LIMS can allow specific sample batches to be queued and processed ahead of others with no user involvement.

Automated metaphase spread analysis is currently limited to differentially locating metaphase spreads on microscope slides and computer-assisted manual scoring, at best.[26] Nevertheless, automated metaphase finders further enhance a laboratory's sample analysis throughput.[27] A metaphase finder generally consists of a high-end computer, a digital camera, a high-quality microscope, an automated stage with autofocus, and a robotic slide delivery system. The computer is loaded with automated metaphase-finding software and interactive automated scoring and annotation software for chromosome aberration analysis. Such metaphase finders can scan up to 250 slides per run, locating metaphase spreads on slides. As it scans, the data (pictures and locations of metaphase spreads on slides) are stored on the hard disk or a centralized server for subsequent relocation and analysis of metaphases either at the metaphase finder station itself or at multiple remote satellite scoring stations.[28] While automated sample processing for cytogenetic analysis increases throughput, downstream DCA for dose estimation may rely on one or all of the following:

- A physical transfer of slides to various satellite laboratories or laboratories in a network for manual analysis.
- Digital encryption and transfer via a virtual private network for downstream analysis and assessment (for virtual high-resolution images of metaphase spreads acquired by metaphase finders). The technological advances in terms of required bandwidth and capability to stream data and images are already available. Virtual digitization can be coupled with real-time data and image monitoring, further enhancing the speed and accuracy at which samples from irradiated personnel can be treated in a mass casualty event.
- Development of an automatic, ultrafast, high-

capacity digital-pathology scanning platform to build and validate a reliable and walk-away analysis system based on artificial intelligence for rapid downstream DCA.

Triage Dose Prediction

A triage dose prediction model (Figure 12-5) uses the dose-response calibration curve data from the interlaboratory comparison study[1] for rapid, risk-based stratification of a radiation-exposed population. It applies DCA after whole-body and partial-body exposures following a radiation mass casualty event.[29] A single HPBL count (after 12 hours) or serial counts are used to estimate dose, as is the individual's medical history. DCA would be used selectively after a radiation mass casualty event. DCA is proposed following receipt of blood samples from a radiation event to confirm irradiation by an initial screening involving analysis of only 20 metaphase spreads. Accordingly, radiation doses greater than 2 Gy are confirmed by the presence of four dicentrics in 20 metaphases. For cases with confirmed doses of 2 Gy or more, analysis is then increased to 50 metaphases to evaluate homogeneity of the dicentric distribution. Partial-body exposures are indicated by variation from the expected dose-dependent distribution of the number of dicentrics per cell. In cases of uniform whole-body exposures, samples

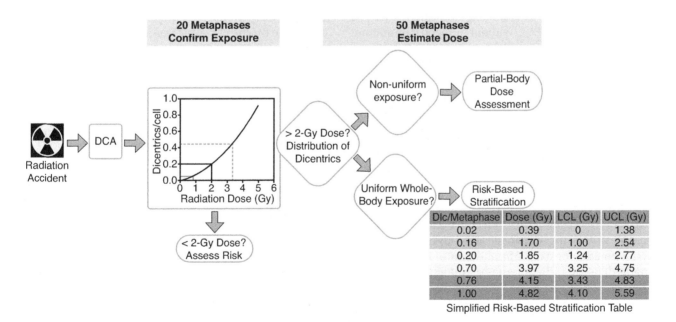

Dic/Metaphase	Dose (Gy)	LCL (Gy)	UCL (Gy)
0.02	0.39	0	1.38
0.16	1.70	1.00	2.54
0.20	1.85	1.24	2.77
0.70	3.97	3.25	4.75
0.76	4.15	3.43	4.83
1.00	4.82	4.10	5.59

Simplified Risk-Based Stratification Table

Figure 12-5. Rapid risk-based stratification by cytogenetic dose assessment in radiation mass casualties. Reproduced with permission from: Prasanna PG, Moroni M, Pellmar TC. Triage dose assessment for partial-body exposure: dicentric analysis. *Health Phys.* 2009;98:244–251.

DCA: dicentric assay; Dic: dicentric; LCL: lower confidence limit; UCL: upper confidence limit

are categorized based on a risk-based stratification table into the following categories: not life threatening, potentially life threatening, and significantly life threatening (see Figure 12-5). For acute moderate exposure, DCA is more suitable.

Acute High-Dose Exposures

HPBLs and complete blood counts (white count, differential, and platelets) will be used in triage decision-making. In cases of acute, high-dose, life-threatening exposures, the PCC assay is useful for estimating dose because radiation-induced cell death and cell-cycle progression delay will not interfere. Traditionally, PCC is induced in HPBLs by fusing Chinese hamster ovary mitotic cells, obtained from cell cultures, using polyethylene glycol as a fusogen to allow radiation-induced chromosome damage in an extended dose range to be measured.[30] Specific inhibitors of protein phosphatases (eg, calyculin A or okadaic acid) are also used to induce PCC in various cell-cycle stages in proliferating cells, such as mitogen-stimulated HPBLs.[11,31] Further, chromosome damage in chemically induced PCC can also be studied using whole-chromosome–specific hybridization probes.[32] Differentiated and nonproliferating cells, such as resting HPBLs, do not normally respond to phosphatase inhibitor treatment and do not induce PCC. However, incubating resting HPBLs in a cell culture medium containing a phosphatase inhibitor, such as calyculin A, along with a mitosis-promoting factor, p34cd2/cyclin B kinase, and adenosine triphosphate, induces PCC without mitogen stimulation. This method results in a high yield of PCC suitable for fluorescence in situ hybridization (FISH) and biological dosimetry.[12,33] Chromosome-specific aberrations are detected using a single whole chromosome probe[12] or a set of whole chromosome probes.[33] Upon FISH, undamaged (normal) cells display two fluorescent spots representing specific chromosomes, and cells with an aberrant specific chromosome show more than two spots per chromosome. Irradiation increases the frequency of damaged cells. The PCC-FISH method was useful in estimating dose in cases of localized high-dose irradiation to skin.[34] Nevertheless, because of limited sample processing and analysis throughput, as well as requirements for expert application of the PCC-FISH method, use in radiation mass casualties is limited.

Acute Low-Dose Exposures

Managing radiation mass casualties will require early dose estimation, both for treatment and assessment of long-term health risks. The cytochalasin-B blocked micronucleus assay[35] may be suitable for early dose estimation. In this assay, radiation-induced chromosome damage is measured as micronuclei in cytokinesis-blocked HPBL. It has undergone extensive development and evolved as a "cytome" assay.[13] The cytome assay is a "catch all" method for measuring induced genetic insult and includes a radiation-specific biomarker: nucleoplasmic bridges. A strong correlation was observed between nucleoplasmic bridges and dicentric chromosmes and centric rings.[36] Therefore, nucleoplasmic bridges can be considered "surrogate" radiation exposure markers for early dose assessment, particularly at doses below 2 Gy in radiological mass casualties. In addition, micronuclei in interphase cells represent chromosome damage transmitted through cell division to daughter cells after radiation exposure; concurrent measurement of micronuclei can also serve as an early biomarker for late effects.

Retrospective Biological Dosimetry

Analysis of persistent chromosomal aberrations, such as stable translocations, is relevant for retrospective biological dosimetry. With advances in molecular cytogenetic techniques, translocations are easily recognizable by chromosome painting. Specific DNA sequences attached to flourochromes are used as probes to either detect a part of a chromosome or paint entire chromosomes, enabling observation of chromosome rearrangements. Translocation analysis is normally used for retrospective estimation of dose rather than for acute exposures in populations without prior personal dosimetry. However, important confounders for using translocation analysis for prospective acute biodosimetry include (*a*) interindividual differences in radiosensitivity, (*b*) inability to distinguish between chronic and acute exposures, (*c*) whole- and partial-body exposures, (*d*) reproducibility of data among laboratories, (*e*) want of standardized scoring criteria, and (*f*) possible radiation-quality–dependent variation in persistency.[5]

SUMMARY: TREATMENT IMPLICATIONS

Medical management of radiation exposure depends on the dose received, organs exposed, and individual susceptibility. The scenario of exposure is critical, ranging from a potential overdose from a diagnostic procedure or radiation therapy, to an industrial accident, to a mass casualty event as large as a nuclear detonation. The extent of diagnostic and therapeutic resources and personnel available will be determined by the event. For medical or industrial incidents, there will likely be sufficient resources so that healthcare workers can conduct a medical history, physical examination, and laboratory studies on each person involved. For a mass casualty event, priorities will be established based on the resources available.

Details on medical evaluation are available from the Radiation Event Medical Management Web site (www. remm.nlm.gov).[37] In general, medical management is based on both dose and organ dysfunction score.[38] Radiation syndromes (eg, ARS) are organ based, with the hematological system predominating at the lower doses, gastrointestinal and cutaneous syndrome next, and central nervous system syndrome at doses of about 10 Gy. It is now recognized that all organs are affected by irradiation to some extent, so radiation sickness really is a multiorgan injury.[39] Radiation doses greater than 2 Gy to a substantial part of the body would raise the issue of prompt initiation of mitigating agents; doses in excess of 4 Gy would require immediate medical attention. For mitigation to be effective, it must be administered in a timely manner, probably within the first 24 hours. For people with lower exposure not at risk for ARS, the concern is for radiation-induced cancers, the discussion of which is beyond the scope of this chapter.

If time of an exposure is known, the initial dose assessment will be made on symptoms and possible physical dosimetry. The initial laboratory assessment will include a complete blood count, and the decline in lymphocytes and possibly the ratio of neutrophils to lymphocytes will be used to estimate dose. Should these data indicate the need for immediate treatment, a blood sample would be stored, if possible, for eventual cytogenetic assay. For those who have received a dose that does not require medical intervention, at least in a mass casualty setting, no further evaluation would be done at this time, although later a blood sample may be taken to estimate long-term risk. There may be a group of victims with doses between 2 and 4 Gy for whom the need for ARS treatment is uncertain. Since the hematological syndrome has an onset of 2 to 4 weeks, it is logical that further blood analysis, including blood count and cytogenetic biodosimetry, be done as rapidly as possible, and those at risk for developing bone marrow dysfunction be sent to the appropriate experts for management (for example, to the Radiation Injury Treatment Network).[40]

Potentially exposed victims concerned about radiation-induced cancer could undergo cytogenetic biodosimetry. For a mass casualty event, the cutoff may be estimated exposure of 0.75 Gy, but that decision would be made based on the size of the event and the laboratory capacity. Individuals deemed at increased risk of radiation-induced cancer could undergo counseling to improve their general health (eg, eliminate smoking) and to understand their increase in lifetime cancer risk in terms they could understand. The latter may help reduce anxiety and stress-related illnesses.

REFERENCES

1. Wilkins RC, Romm H, Kao TC, et al. Interlaboratory comparison of the dicentric assay for radiation biodosimetry in mass casualty events. *Radiat Res.* 2008;169:551–560.

2. Bender MA, Gooch PC. Somatic chromosome aberrations induced by human whole-body irradiation: the "Recuplex" criticality accident. *Radiat Res.* 1966;29:568–582.

3. Sevan'kaev A. Results of cytogenetic studies of the consequences of the Chernobyl accident [in Russian]. *Radiats Biol Radioecol.* 2000;40:589–595.

4. Pyatkin EK, Nugis VY, Chrikov AA. Absorbed dose estimation according to the results of cytogenetic investigations of lymphocyte cultures of persons who suffered in the accident at Chernobyl atomic power station. *Radiat Med.* 1989;4:52.

5. International Atomic Energy Agency. *Cytogenetic Analysis for Radiation Dose Assessment: A Manual.* Vienna, Austria: IAEA; 2001.

6. International Organization for Standardization. *Radiation Protection-Performance Criteria for Service Laboratories Performing Biological Dosimetry by Cytogenetics.* Geneva, Switzerland: ISO: 2004.

7. International Organization for Standardization. *Performance Criteria for Service Laboratories Performing Cytogenetic Triage for Assessment of Mass Casualties in Radiological or Nuclear Emergencies.* Geneva, Switzerland: ISO; 2008.

8. Nurse P. Regulation of eukaryotic cell cycle. *Eur J Cancer.* 1997;33:1002–1004.

9. Elledge SJ. Cell cycle checkpoints: preventing an identity crisis. *Science*. 1996;274:1664–1672.

10. Pantelias GE, Mallie HD. Direct analysis of radiation-induced fragments and rings in unstimulated human peripheral blood lymphocytes by means of the premature chromosome condensation technique. *Mutat Res*. 1985;149:67–72.

11. Gotoh E, Asakawa Y. Detection and evaluation of chromosomal aberrations induced by high doses of gamma-irradiation using immunogold-silver painting of prematurely condensed chromosomes. *Int J Radiat Biol*. 1996;70:517–520.

12. Prasanna PG, Escalada ND, Blakely WF. Induction of premature chromosome condensation by a phosphatase inhibitor and a protein kinase in unstimulated human peripheral blood lymphocytes: a simple and rapid technique to study chromosome aberrations using specific whole-chromosome DNA hybridization probes for biological dosimetry. *Mutat Res*. 2000;466:131–141.

13. Fenech M. Cytokinesis-block micronucleus cytome assay. *Nature Protoc*. 2007;2:1084–1104.

14. Poirier MG, Marko JF. Mitotic chromosomes are chromatin networks without a mechanically contiguous protein scaffold. *Proc Natl Acad Sci U S A*. 2002;99:15393–15397.

15. Belmont AS, Bruce K. Visualization of G1 chromosomes: a folded, twisted, supercoiled chromonema model of interphase chromatid structure. *J Cell Biol*. 1994;127:287–302.

16. Kireeva N, Lakonishok M, Kireev I, Hirano T, Belmont AS. Visualization of early chromosome condensation: a hierarchical folding, axial glue model of chromosome structure. *J Cell Biol*. 2004;166:775–785.

17. Manuelidis L, Chen TL. A unified model of eukaryotic chromosomes. *Cytometry*. 1990;11:8–25.

18. Savage JR. Classification and relationships of induced chromosomal structural changes. *J Med Genet*. 1976;13:103–122.

19. Armed Forces Radiobiology Research Institute. *Medical Management of Radiological Casualties Handbook*. Bethesda, MD: AFRRI; 2003.

20. Lloyd DC. Chromosomal analysis to assess radiation dose. *Stem Cells*. 1997;15(Suppl 2):195–201.

21. Deperas J, Szluinska M, Deperas-Kaminska M, et al. CABAS: a freely available PC program for fitting calibration curves in chromosome aberration dosimetry. *Radiat Prot Dosimetry*. 2007;124:115–123.

22. Ainsbury EA, Lloyd DC. Dose estimation software for radiation biodosimetry. *Health Phys*. 2010;98:290–295.

23. International Atomic Energy Agency. *Cytogenetic Dosimetry: Applications in Preparedness for and Response to Radiation Emergencies: A Manual*. Vienna, Austria: IAEA; 2011.

24. Martin PR, Berdychevski RE, Subramanian U, Blakely WF, Prasanna PG. Sample tracking in an automated cytogenetic biodosimetry laboratory for radiation mass casualties. *Radiat Meas*. 2007;42:1119–1124.

25. Moroni M, Krasnopolsky K, Subramanian U, Martin PR, Doherty KM, Prasanna PG. Does cell culture type and blood transport temperature affect dicentric yield and radiation dose assessment? *J Med Chem Biol Radiol Def*. 2008;6. http://www.jmedcbr.org/issue_0601/Prasanna/Prasanna_10_08.html. Accessed January 12, 2011.

26. Schunck C, Johannes T, Varga D, Lörch T, Plesch A. New developments in automated cytogenetic imaging: unattended scoring of dicentric chromosomes, micronuclei, single cell gel electrophoresis, and fluorescence signals. *Cytogenet Genome Res*. 2004;104:383–389.

27. Weber J, Scheid W, Traut H. Time-saving in biological dosimetry by using the automatic metaphase finder Metafer2. *Mutat Res*. 1992;272:31–34.

28. Blakely WF, Prasanna PG, Kolanko CJ, et al. Application of the premature chromosome condensation assay in simulated partial-body radiation exposures: evaluation of the use of an automated metaphase-finder. *Stem Cells*. 1995;13(Suppl 1):223–230.

29. Prasanna PG, Moroni M, Pellmar TC. Triage dose assessment for partial-body exposure: dicentric analysis. *Health Phys.* 2009;98:244–251.

30. Pantelias GE, Maillie HD. Direct analysis of radiation-induced chromosome fragments and rings in unstimulated human peripheral blood lymphocytes by means of the premature chromosome condensation technique. *Mutat Res.* 1985;149:67–72.

31. Durante M, Furusawa Y, Gotoh E. A simple method for simultaneous interphase-metaphase chromosome analysis in biodosimetry. *Int J Radiat Biol.* 1998;74:457–462.

32. Coco-Martin JM, Begg AC. Detection of radiation-induced chromosome aberrations using fluorescence in situ hybridization in drug-induced premature chromosome condensations of tumor cell lines with different radiosensitivities. *Int J Radiat Biol.* 1997;71:265–273.

33. Pathak R, Ramakumar A, Subramanian U, Prasanna PG. Differential radio-sensitivities of human chromosomes 1 and 2 in one donor in interphase- and metaphase-spreads after 60Co gamma-irradiation. *BMC Med Phys.* 2009;9:6.

34. Pouget JP, Laurent C, Delbos M, et al. PCC-FISH in skin fibroblasts for local dose assessment: biodosimetric analysis of a victim of the Georgian radiological accident. *Radiat Res.* 2004;162:365–376.

35. Fenech M, Morley AA. Measurement of micronucleus in lymphocytes. *Mutat Res.* 1985;147:29–36.

36. Fenech M. The lymphocyte cytokinesis-block micronucleus cytome assay and its application in radiation biodosimery. *Health Phys.* 2010;98:234–243.

37. Bader J, Namhauser J, Coleman NC, et al. Radiation event medical management. http://www.remm.nlm.gov. Accessed June 20, 2009.

38. Berger ME, Christensen DM, Lowry PC, Jones OW, Wiley AL. Medical management of radiation injuries: current approaches. *Occup Med (Lond).* 2006;56:162–172.

39. Fliedner TM, Chao NJ, Bader JL, et al. Stem cells, multiorgan failure in radiation emergency medical preparedness: a U.S./European Consultation Workshop. *Stem Cells.* 2009;27:1205–1211.

40. Weinstock DM, Case CJ Jr, Bader JL, et al. Radiologic and nuclear events: contingency planning for hematologists/oncologists. *Blood.* 2008;111:5440–5445.

ABBREVIATIONS and ACRONYMS

A

ACH: acetylcholine
5-AED: androst-5-ene-3beta,17beta-diol; 5-androstenediol
AET: aminoethyl thiouronium bromide
AFRRI: Armed Forces Radiobiology Research Institute
ALARA: as low as reasonably achievable
AND: 4-androstenedione
ARS: acute radiation syndrome (sickness)
AS101: ammonium trichloro (dioxyethylene-0-0') tellurate
ASMase: acid sphingomyelinase
ATF6: activating transcription factor 6
ATM: ataxia telangiectasia mutated protein

B

BAT: Biodosimetry Assessment Tool
BAX: Bcl-2–associated X protein
BCG: Bacillus Calmette-Guérin
Bcl-2: B-cell lymphoma 2
Bcl-XL: B-cell lymphoma-extra large

C

cAMP: cyclic adenosine monophosphate
c-FLIP: caspase 8 and fas-associated protein with death domain-like apoptosis regulator
Ca-DTPA: calcium diethylenetriamine pentaacetic acid
Ca: calcium
CBRN: chemical, biological, radiological, and nuclear
CDK: cyclin-dependent kinases
CFU: colony-forming unit
CHOP: controlled amino acid therapy/enhancer binding protein homologous protein
CI: combined injury
CNS: central nervous systems
Co: cobalt
CRP: C-reactive protein
CSF: colony-stimulating factor

D

17-DMAG: 17-(dimethylaminoethylamino)-17-demethoxygeldan-amycin
D: dose
DCA: dicentric assay
DHEA: dehydroepiandrosterone
DIME: delayed, immediate, minimal, expectant
DiPGE$_2$: 16,16-dimethyl prostaglandin E
DNA: deoxyribonucleic acid
DoD: Department of Defense
DRF: dose reduction factor
DTPA: diethylenetriamine pentaacetic acid
e-CFU: endogenous colony forming units
DTRA: Defense Threat Reduction Agency

E

E2: estradiol
ECM: extracellular matrix
ED$_{50}$: effective dose; the amount of drug that produces a therapeutic response in 50% of the subjects taking it
EDTA: ethylenediaminetetraacetic acid
EMP: electromagnetic pulse
EMT: emergency medical technician
EPD: early performance decrement

EPD: electronic personal dosimeter
EPR: electron paramagnetic resonance
ER: endoplasmic reticulum
ERW: enhanced radiation weapon
ETI: early transient incapacitation

F

FDA: Food and Drug Administration
FGF: fibroblast growth factor
FISH: fluorescence in situ hybridization
Flt-3: FMS-like tyrosine kinase 3
Flt-3L: FMS-like tyrosine kinase 3 ligand
FQ: fluoroquinolone
FRAT: First-Responders Radiological Assessment Triage

G

G-CSF: granulocyte colony-stimulating factor
G$_1$: gap 1 (phase of interphase)
G$_2$: gap 2 (phase of interphase)
GADD45β: growth arrest- and DNA-damage–inducible, beta
GI: gastrointestinal
GM-CSF: granulocyte-macrophage colony-stimulating factor
GSK: glycogen synthase kinase

H

H$_2$O: water
HEPA: high-efficiency particulate air
HER-2: human epidermal growth factor receptor 2
HIAP-1: human inhibitor of apoptosis protein-1
HPBL: human peripheral blood lymphocyte
HSC: hematopoietic stem cell
5HT: 5 hydroxytrytapine

I

ICRP: International Commission on Radiological Protection
IL: interleukin
IM: intramuscular
iNOS: inducible nitric oxide synthase
IRE1: inositol-requiring 1
IV: intravenous

J

JNK: c-Jun N-terminal kinases

K

KGF: keratinocyte growth factor

L

LCL: lower confidence limit
LD$_{50/30}$: the dose required to kill 50% of the test population within 30 days
LD$_{50}$: the amount necessary to kill 50% of the subject population
LD$_{50/60}$: the dose at which 50% of the exposed population will die within 60 days
LET: linear energy transfer
LIMS: laboratory information management system
LPA: proapoptotic signal lysophosphatidic acid
LSK$^+$: Lin$^+$ Sca 1$^+$ Kit$^+$
LTC: leukotriene C

M

3D-MPL: 3D-monophosphoryl lipid A
M phase: mitotic phase
MAPK: mitogen-activated protein kinase
MEA: β-mercaptoethylamine
MEV: mega electron volts
MMP: matrix metalloproteinases
MnSOD: manganese superoxide dismutase
MOD: multiorgan dysfunction
MOF: multiorgan failure
MOPP: mission-oriented protective posture
MPG: mercaptopropionyl glycine
MRI: magnetic resonance imaging
MTF: medical treatment facility
mTOR: mammalian target of rapamycin

N

n: neutrons
N: nitrogen
NATO: North Atlantic Treaty Organization
NCRP: National Council on Radiation Protection
NF-IL6: nuclear factor interleukin 6
NFκB: nuclear factor k-light-chain-enhancer of activated B
NO: nitric oxide

O

O, O_2: oxygen
OEG: operatonal exposure guidance
OTP: octadecenyl thiophosphate

P13K: phosphatidylinositol 3-kinases
p53: protein 53
PAF: platelet-activating factor
PBL: peripheral blood lymphocyte
PCC: premature chromosome condensation
PDF: portable document format
PEG-400: polyethylene glycol 400
pegG-CSF: pegfilgrastim
PERK: protein kinase RNA-like endoplasmic reticulum kinase
PMN: polymorphonuclear leukocytes
PPE: personal protective equipment
PPF: paired-pulse facilitation
PTSD: posttraumatic stress disorder

R

RBE: relative biologic effectiveness
RDD: radiological dispersal device
RED: radiological exposure device
rem: roentgen equivalents mamal
rhGM-CSF: human recombinant GM-CSF
RI: radiation injury
RIF: radiation-induced fibrosis
ROS: reactive oxygen species

S

S: synthesis (phase of interphase)
SAA: serum amyloid A
SALT: sort, assess, life-saving interventions, treatment and/or transport
SCBA: self-contained breathing apparatus
SED: skin erythema disease
SMC: structural maintenance of chromosomes
SOD: superoxide dismutase
START: simple triage and rapid treatment

T

TE: time to emesis
TGF-β: transforming growth factor β
TLD: thermoluminescent dosimeter
TLR: toll-like receptor
TNF-α: tumor necrosis factor alpha
TNT: trinitrotoluene

U

UCL: upper confidence interval

X

XIAP: X-linked inhibitor of apoptosis protein

Z

Zn: zinc
Zn-DTPA: zinc diethylentriamene pentaacetate

INDEX

Made in the USA
Monee, IL
01 October 2020